MEDSURG-BC Study Guide

MedSurg BC Review Book + 500 Practice Questions for the ANCC Medical-Surgical Nursing Certification Exam | Med Surg Nursing Book (Includes 4 Full-Length Tests)

Audrey Windrow
Miraiam Web N.

Printed in USA.

Disclaimer:

Printed in the United States of America.

CONTENTS

1 Assessment And Diagnosis:
2 Planning, Implementation, And Evaluation:
3 Professional Role:

MEDSURG-BC Practice Test 1
Answers with Explanation for Practice Test 1
MEDSURG-BC Practice Test 2
Answers with Explanation for Practice Test 2
MEDSURG-BC Practice Test 3
Answers with Explanation for Practice Test 3
MEDSURG-BC Practice Test 4
Answers with Explanation for Practice Test 4

Key to Success: Do's to pass the exam with ease:

1. Study Smart:

To easily pass the MEDSURG-BC exam, it is important to study smart. Instead of trying to memorize every single detail, focus on understanding the key concepts and information that are most likely to be tested on the exam. This will help you retain the information better and be more prepared for the questions that you will encounter. We give you the key concepts that is covered in the exam.

2. Set a Study Schedule:

Create a study schedule that works for you and allows you to dedicate enough time to each section of the exam. Consistency is key in retaining information and mastering the material.

3. Review Content Outline:

Familiarize yourself with the content outline provided by the organization to understand what topics will be covered on the exam. Focus on areas where you may need extra study time.

4. Practice, Practice, Practice: Take Practice Tests

One of the best ways to prepare for the MEDSURG-BC exam is to take practice tests. This will not only familiarize you with the format of the exam but also help you gauge your level of readiness. Make sure to take multiple practice tests and review the questions you missed to further strengthen your knowledge.

5. Seek Support:

Reach out to peers, mentors, or online communities for support and guidance throughout your study process. Surround yourself with people who understand the challenges of preparing for the MEDSURG-BC exam and can offer advice or encouragement.

6. Stay Positive:

Believe in yourself and your ability to pass the MEDSURG-BC exam. Stay positive, focused, and determined to achieve your certification. Visualize success and keep your goals in mind. Success is definitely yours.

Why this book is your key to success in the MEDSURG-BC Exam:

Stay Ahead with Updated Content:

This study guide is your go-to resource for the most current information and practice questions tailored for the MEDSURG-BC Exam. With regular updates to match exam standards, you can be confident that you are well-prepared to excel.

Learn from the Best with Expert Guidance:

Written by experts who have conquered the MEDSURG-BC Exam, this book offers priceless guidance and strategies for achieving success. Benefit from their experience and expertise to approach the exam with assurance.

Understand Deeper with Insightful Explanations:

Enhance your understanding of the material with detailed explanations accompanying each question. By exploring the reasoning behind the answers, you will improve your comprehension and be better equipped to handle challenging questions on exam day.

Get Familiar with Exam Format:

Practice with questions mirroring the actual MEDSURG-BC Exam structure to build confidence and readiness for test day. Familiarize yourself with the exam format to set yourself up for success.

Sharpen Your Critical Thinking:

Engage with the questions, answers, and explanations in this book to boost your critical thinking skills and ability to analyze and respond effectively. Strengthen your cognitive skills and problem-solving abilities as you prepare for the MEDSURG-BC Exam.

Study with Confidence in a Clear and Concise Manner:

This MEDSURG-BC Prep simplifies complex concepts in a straightforward and easy-to-understand style, ensuring clarity without overwhelming you with technical jargon. Dive into the material knowing that this resource will help you grasp key concepts and excel on exam day.

MEDSURG-BC Certification Review

1 Assessment And Diagnosis:

Assessment and diagnosis are fundamental components of the nursing process, particularly within the realm of medical-surgical nursing. These stages are critical for developing effective care plans and ensuring optimal patient outcomes.

Assessment is the systematic collection, verification, and organization of relevant patient data. It involves gathering comprehensive information about the patient's physiological, psychological, sociocultural, spiritual, economic, and lifestyle factors. The goal is to establish a thorough understanding of the patient's health status and needs. This process begins with a health history interview, which includes questions about the patient's current condition, medical history, family history, lifestyle habits, and any symptoms they may be experiencing.

Physical examination is another crucial aspect of assessment. It involves inspecting, palpating, percussing, and auscultating the body to gather objective data. Nurses must be skilled in recognizing normal versus abnormal findings and understanding their implications for the patient's health. Vital signs, such as temperature, pulse, respiration rate, and blood pressure, are routinely measured to establish baseline data and monitor changes over time.

In addition to direct patient interaction, nurses also review diagnostic test results, such as laboratory findings and imaging studies. This data is integrated with subjective information from the patient to form a complete picture of their health status.

Once assessment data is collected and analyzed, the next step is diagnosis. Nursing diagnosis involves interpreting assessment data to identify patient problems that nurses can address independently or collaboratively with other healthcare professionals. The North American Nursing Diagnosis Association International (NANDA-I) provides a standardized classification system for nursing diagnoses that helps ensure consistency in identifying patient problems.

Nursing diagnoses are distinct from medical diagnoses; they focus on the patient's response to health conditions rather than the conditions themselves. For example, while a medical diagnosis might identify pneumonia as a disease process, a nursing diagnosis would address issues such as impaired gas exchange or ineffective airway clearance resulting from pneumonia.

Formulating accurate nursing diagnoses requires critical thinking skills. Nurses must synthesize assessment data to identify patterns or clusters of related information that suggest specific health issues. They must also prioritize these diagnoses based on factors such as severity, urgency, and potential impact on the patient's overall health.

Each nursing diagnosis consists of three components: the problem statement (what's wrong), the etiology (the cause or contributing factors), and defining characteristics (signs and symptoms). This structure helps guide nurses in planning appropriate interventions tailored to each patient's unique needs.

The accuracy of both assessment and diagnosis directly influences subsequent steps in the nursing process: planning, implementation, and evaluation. A thorough assessment ensures that all relevant information is considered when identifying patient problems. Accurate diagnoses enable nurses to develop targeted care plans that effectively address those problems.

In summary, assessment and diagnosis are integral parts of medical-surgical nursing practice. They require a combination of technical skills for data collection and critical thinking abilities for data interpretation. By mastering these processes, nurses can deliver high-quality care that meets patients' individual needs and promotes positive health outcomes. Understanding these concepts is essential for success on the Medical-Surgical Nursing (MEDSURG-BC) certification exam and in clinical practice.

1.1.1 Health History Collection:

Health history collection is a critical skill for medical-surgical nurses, serving as the foundation for patient assessment and diagnosis. It involves systematically gathering comprehensive information about the patient's past and present health status, which aids in identifying health problems and planning effective care. This process encompasses various components, including biographical data, chief complaint, history of present illness, past medical history, family history, social history, and review of systems.

Biographical data includes basic information such as the patient's name, age, gender, ethnicity, and contact details. This data helps identify any cultural or demographic factors that may influence the patient's health.

The chief complaint is a concise statement describing the primary reason for the patient's visit. It is usually expressed in the patient's own words and provides direction for further inquiry.

The history of present illness (HPI) expands on the chief complaint by detailing the onset, duration, location, intensity, and progression of symptoms. It also includes any associated factors or alleviating/aggravating circumstances. This section is crucial for understanding the context of the current health issue and guides diagnostic reasoning.

Past medical history (PMH) involves documenting previous illnesses, surgeries, hospitalizations, allergies, immunizations, and ongoing treatments. This information helps identify patterns or recurrent issues that may affect the current health status.

Family history provides insight into genetic predispositions or familial diseases that could impact the patient's health. Understanding hereditary conditions enables proactive management and preventive strategies.

Social history assesses lifestyle factors such as occupation, education level, living conditions, marital status, dietary habits, exercise routines, substance use (tobacco, alcohol, drugs), and sexual practices. These elements are significant, as they can directly or indirectly influence health outcomes.

The review of systems (ROS) is a systematic approach to evaluating each body system through a series of questions aimed at uncovering symptoms not previously discussed. This thorough review ensures that no potential health concerns are overlooked.

Effective health history collection requires strong communication skills to build rapport with patients and encourage open dialogue. Nurses must be adept at using both open-ended questions to elicit detailed responses and closed-ended questions to clarify specific points. Active listening is vital for fully understanding patient narratives and for picking up on non-verbal cues that may indicate distress or discomfort.

Cultural competence is also essential during this process. Nurses must be sensitive to cultural differences that may influence how patients perceive their health and healthcare interactions. Understanding these nuances helps tailor questions appropriately and ensures respectful communication.

Documentation of the collected health history should be accurate and thorough. It forms part of the legal medical record and serves as a reference for all healthcare providers involved in the patient's care. Accurate documentation ensures continuity of care and facilitates effective communication among multidisciplinary teams.

In summary, health history collection is an indispensable component of patient assessment in medical-surgical nursing. It provides a holistic view of the patient's health status by integrating diverse aspects of their medical background and current condition. Mastery of this skill enables nurses to identify potential health issues early, formulate accurate diagnoses, and develop personalized care plans that address the unique needs of each patient. For those preparing for the MEDSURG-BC exam, understanding the intricacies of this process is crucial for demonstrating competency in assessment and diagnosis within clinical practice.

1.1.2 Physical Assessment:

Physical assessment is a systematic process used by medical-surgical nurses to collect, analyze, and interpret data about a patient's physiological status. It forms the cornerstone of clinical decision-making and patient care planning. This process involves a comprehensive evaluation of the body systems to determine health status, identify any deviations from normal, and establish a baseline for future comparisons.

The physical assessment begins with obtaining a thorough patient history, which includes collecting subjective data such as symptoms described by the patient. This history provides context and guides the nurse in focusing on specific areas during the physical examination.

The physical examination itself is typically organized into four primary techniques: inspection, palpation, percussion, and auscultation. These methods are applied systematically to assess each body system.

1. Inspection involves visually examining the patient for any abnormalities or changes in appearance. This includes observing skin color, posture, gait, and overall demeanor. Nurses should also note any signs of distress or discomfort.

2. Palpation requires using the hands to feel body parts for size, shape, firmness, or the location of certain structures. It helps in assessing temperature, texture, moisture, organ location and size, swelling, vibration or pulsation, rigidity or spasticity, crepitation, presence of lumps or masses, and tenderness or pain.

3. Percussion involves tapping on specific areas of the body to produce sounds that help determine the underlying structure's density. Different sounds can indicate whether an area is filled with air (as in the lungs), fluid (as in ascites), or solid tissue (as in the liver).

4. Auscultation is listening to sounds produced within the body using a stethoscope. This technique is crucial for evaluating heart sounds (rate, rhythm), lung sounds (breath sounds), and bowel sounds (presence and frequency).

Each body system is assessed methodically:

- Neurological System: Assess mental status, cranial nerve function, motor function (strength and coordination), sensory function (pain, temperature), reflexes, and balance.

- Cardiovascular System: Evaluate heart rate and rhythm through auscultation; inspect for jugular vein distention; palpate peripheral pulses for strength and equality; assess for edema; measure blood pressure.

- Respiratory System: Inspect chest symmetry and effort; auscultate lung fields for breath sounds; note any abnormal breathing patterns or adventitious sounds such as wheezes or crackles.

- Gastrointestinal System: Inspect the abdomen for distention; auscultate bowel sounds in all quadrants; palpate for tenderness or masses; percuss to assess liver span and fluid presence.

- Musculoskeletal System: Observe posture and gait; inspect joints for swelling or deformity; assess range of motion and muscle strength; palpate bones and muscles for tenderness.

- Integumentary System: Inspect the skin for color changes, lesions, and moisture level; palpate for temperature and texture differences.

- Genitourinary System: Evaluate bladder distention through palpation; inquire about urinary patterns and symptoms.

Documentation of findings is critical for continuity of care. Accurate recording ensures effective communication among healthcare providers and supports clinical reasoning processes.

In conclusion, physical assessment is an essential skill that enables medical-surgical nurses to provide high-quality care by identifying potential health issues early on. Mastery of this skill requires practice and a keen understanding of normal versus abnormal findings across different body systems.

1.1.2.1 Vital Signs:

Vital signs are fundamental physiological measurements that provide critical information about a patient's health status. They are essential components of a physical assessment and serve as indicators of the body's basic functions. The primary vital signs include temperature, pulse, respiration rate, and blood pressure. Each of these parameters offers insights into the functioning of various body systems and can indicate the presence of medical conditions or the need for further investigation.

Temperature is a measure of the body's ability to generate and dissipate heat. It reflects the balance between heat produced by metabolic processes and heat lost to the environment. Normal body temperature can vary depending on the individual, the time of day, and the method of measurement (oral, rectal, axillary, tympanic). Fever may indicate infection or inflammation, whereas hypothermia may suggest exposure to cold environments or metabolic disorders.

Pulse, or heart rate, is the number of heartbeats per minute. It provides insight into cardiac function and circulatory status. A normal resting heart rate for adults ranges from 60 to 100 beats per minute. Tachycardia (elevated heart rate) can occur due to stress, fever, anemia, or cardiac conditions, while bradycardia (reduced heart rate) might be seen in athletes or as a result of medication effects or cardiac disease. The rhythm and strength of the pulse also offer valuable clinical information.

Respiration rate is the number of breaths taken per minute and is an indicator of respiratory function. The normal range for adults is typically 12 to 20 breaths per minute. Tachypnea (increased respiratory rate) may be associated with conditions such as anxiety, lung disease, or metabolic acidosis. Bradypnea (decreased respiratory rate) might occur with opioid use or neurological impairment. Observing the depth and effort involved in breathing can provide additional insights into respiratory health.

Blood pressure measures the force exerted by circulating blood on the walls of blood vessels. It consists of two readings: systolic pressure (pressure during heartbeats) and diastolic pressure (pressure between beats). Normal blood pressure is usually around 120/80 mmHg. Hypertension (high blood pressure) increases the risk for cardiovascular diseases such as stroke and myocardial infarction. Hypotension (low blood pressure) might result in dizziness or fainting and could indicate dehydration or endocrine disorders.

In addition to these primary vital signs, some healthcare settings may also monitor oxygen saturation using pulse oximetry and pain level as an additional fifth vital sign due to its impact on patient well-being and recovery.

Accurate measurement and interpretation of vital signs are crucial in identifying changes in a patient's condition early on. Medical-surgical nurses must be proficient in obtaining these measurements using appropriate techniques and equipment while considering factors that might affect readings, such as patient activity level, emotional state, or environmental influences.

Documentation of vital signs should be precise and consistent to facilitate effective communication among healthcare providers and enable comparison over time. Prompt recognition of abnormal vital signs allows for timely intervention, which can significantly impact patient outcomes.

In summary, vital signs are key indicators that reflect a patient's physiological status and are integral to comprehensive patient assessment in medical-surgical nursing practice. Understanding how to accurately measure, interpret, and respond to changes in these parameters is essential for providing high-quality care and ensuring patient safety.

1.1.2.2 Disease Process:

The disease process refers to the sequence of events that occur in the body as a result of a pathological condition. It encompasses the onset, progression, and resolution of a disease, providing a framework for understanding how diseases develop and affect the body. For medical-surgical nurses, comprehending the disease process is crucial for effective patient assessment and management.

The disease process begins with etiology, which is the cause or origin of the disease. Etiologies can be infectious (caused by pathogens like bacteria or viruses), genetic (resulting from inherited genetic mutations), environmental (due to exposure to harmful substances), or multifactorial (involving multiple contributing factors). Understanding the etiology helps in identifying risk factors and implementing preventive measures.

Following etiology, pathogenesis describes the mechanism by which the disease develops. This involves understanding how etiological factors lead to cellular and tissue changes, ultimately causing clinical manifestations. For instance, in infectious diseases, pathogenesis may involve pathogen invasion, replication, and immune response activation. In chronic diseases like diabetes, it includes insulin resistance and subsequent metabolic disturbances.

Once pathogenesis is established, the disease progresses through various stages. The initial stage is often asymptomatic or presents with mild symptoms, known as the incubation or latent period. As the disease advances, symptoms become more pronounced, marking the acute phase. During this phase, patients may experience significant discomfort and require immediate medical attention.

The body's response to disease involves both local and systemic reactions. Locally, inflammation is a common response characterized by redness, heat, swelling, pain, and loss of function. Systemically, the body may exhibit fever, fatigue, or malaise as it attempts to combat the disease. These responses are mediated by complex interactions between immune cells and chemical mediators.

As the disease progresses, complications may arise due to direct damage caused by the pathogen or secondary effects on other organ systems. For example, in pneumonia, respiratory failure can occur due to impaired gas exchange in the lungs. Recognizing potential complications is vital for timely intervention and prevention of further morbidity.

Eventually, the disease reaches a resolution phase where recovery occurs either spontaneously or with medical intervention. Resolution can be complete, with full restoration of health, or partial, with lingering deficits or chronic conditions. In some cases, diseases may become chronic, with periods of remission and exacerbation.

Throughout this process, diagnostic tools such as laboratory tests and imaging studies play a crucial role in identifying specific abnormalities associated with different stages of the disease. These tools aid in confirming diagnoses and monitoring progression or response to treatment.

Management of the disease process involves a multidisciplinary approach tailored to each patient's needs. Treatment strategies may include pharmacological interventions to target specific pathways involved in pathogenesis or supportive care to alleviate symptoms and improve quality of life.

In summary, understanding the disease process is fundamental for medical-surgical nurses, as it informs patient assessment and guides clinical decision-making. By recognizing etiological factors, pathogenesis mechanisms, progression stages, and potential complications, nurses can provide comprehensive care that addresses both immediate needs and long-term outcomes for their patients. This knowledge not only enhances clinical practice but also contributes to improved patient education and empowerment in managing their health conditions effectively.

1.1.2.3 Review Of Systems:

The Review of Systems (ROS) is a systematic approach used by healthcare professionals, including medical-surgical nurses, to gather comprehensive information about a patient's overall health status. It involves a series of questions organized by body systems, aimed at identifying any symptoms the patient may be experiencing. This method is crucial for detecting underlying conditions that may not be immediately apparent during the physical examination or initial patient history.

The ROS is typically divided into various categories corresponding to different bodily systems. These include the integumentary, respiratory, cardiovascular, gastrointestinal, musculoskeletal, neurological, endocrine, hematologic, and genitourinary systems, among others. Each category involves specific questions designed to elicit information about symptoms or issues related to that system.

For the integumentary system, questions might focus on changes in skin color, texture, or the presence of rashes or lesions. In the respiratory system review, inquiries may cover symptoms such as coughing, wheezing, or shortness of breath. Cardiovascular assessment questions often include chest pain, palpitations, or edema. The gastrointestinal system review might involve asking about nausea, vomiting, diarrhea, or constipation.

The purpose of conducting a ROS is multifaceted. Firstly, it helps in identifying symptoms that may not have been mentioned during the initial history-taking process. Patients might not consider certain symptoms relevant or may forget to mention them unless specifically asked. Secondly, it aids in correlating symptoms with potential diagnoses. By systematically reviewing each body system, nurses can piece together information that might point toward a specific condition or disease process.

Furthermore, the ROS serves as a tool for risk assessment and preventive care planning. For instance, discovering symptoms suggestive of cardiovascular issues could prompt further investigation and early intervention to prevent complications such as heart disease.

In practice, the ROS should be tailored to each patient based on their presenting complaints and medical history. While a comprehensive ROS is ideal for new patients or those with complex medical histories, a focused ROS may be more appropriate for follow-up visits where specific issues are being monitored.

Medical-surgical nurses must possess strong communication skills to effectively conduct a ROS. This involves not only asking the right questions but also listening attentively to the patient's responses and observing non-verbal cues that might indicate discomfort or distress. Additionally, cultural competence is essential in understanding how different patients might perceive and report their symptoms.

Documentation of the ROS findings is crucial for continuity of care. Accurate and thorough documentation ensures that all healthcare team members are aware of any potential issues and can collaborate effectively in managing the patient's care.

In summary, the Review of Systems is an integral component of patient assessment in medical-surgical nursing. It provides valuable insights into a patient's health status by systematically exploring each body system for potential symptoms or concerns. By conducting a thorough ROS, nurses can enhance diagnostic accuracy, improve patient outcomes through early detection and intervention, and contribute to comprehensive care planning. Mastery of this skill is essential for success in the Medical-Surgical Nursing (MEDSURG-BC) certification exam and in professional practice as a competent and effective medical-surgical nurse.

1.1.2.4 Understanding Activities of Daily Living (ADLs):

Activities of Daily Living (ADLs) are fundamental tasks that individuals perform daily to maintain personal health and well-being. These activities are essential for independent living and serve as a measure to assess an individual's functional status, particularly in healthcare settings. ADLs are typically categorized into basic and instrumental activities.

Basic ADLs include self-care tasks that are necessary for fundamental functioning. These consist of:

1. Bathing: The ability to wash oneself and maintain personal hygiene.
2. Dressing: The capacity to select appropriate clothing and dress oneself.
3. Eating: The ability to feed oneself, which may also involve preparing food.
4. Toileting: The capability to use the restroom independently, including maintaining continence.
5. Transferring: The ability to move from one position to another, such as from a bed to a chair.

Instrumental Activities of Daily Living (IADLs) are more complex skills that enable an individual to live independently within a community. These include:

1. Managing Finances: The ability to handle money, pay bills, and budget expenses.
2. Handling Transportation: The capability to drive or use public transportation.
3. Shopping and Meal Preparation: The skills needed to purchase groceries and prepare meals.
4. Housekeeping and Home Maintenance: The ability to clean and maintain the home environment.
5. Managing Medications: The capacity to obtain and take medications correctly.

In the context of medical-surgical nursing, assessing ADLs is crucial for developing care plans tailored to the individual needs of patients. A thorough evaluation of ADLs helps identify patients who may require assistance or adaptive devices to enhance their independence.

The assessment of ADLs involves direct observation, patient interviews, and sometimes input from family members or caregivers. Standardized tools such as the Katz Index of Independence in Activities of Daily Living or the Barthel Index are often employed to quantify an individual's level of independence.

Understanding a patient's ability to perform ADLs is important not only for evaluating their current health status but also for predicting outcomes such as recovery time, discharge planning, and the need for rehabilitation services or long-term care placement.

Nurses play a pivotal role in promoting the independence of patients by encouraging them to perform ADLs as much as possible within their capabilities. This includes providing education on adaptive techniques or equipment that can assist in performing these tasks more effectively.

Furthermore, nurses must be vigilant in identifying changes in a patient's ability to perform ADLs, which could indicate deterioration in health status or the need for further medical intervention. For instance, a sudden decline in an elderly patient's ability to manage finances or medications might signal cognitive impairment that requires further evaluation.

In summary, Activities of Daily Living are a critical component of patient assessment in medical-surgical nursing. They provide valuable insights into a patient's functional abilities and guide healthcare professionals in delivering personalized care aimed at maximizing independence and quality of life. By comprehensively understanding and assessing ADLs, nurses can significantly impact patient outcomes and contribute positively to their overall well-being.

1.1.3 Psychosocial Assessment:

Psychosocial assessment is a critical component of nursing practice, particularly in the field of medical-surgical nursing, where understanding the psychological and social dimensions of a patient's life can significantly influence their health outcomes. This assessment involves a comprehensive evaluation of a patient's mental health, emotional well-being, social context, and coping mechanisms. It is an integral part of holistic patient care, enabling nurses to identify potential psychosocial stressors that may impact a patient's recovery and overall health.

The primary goal of a psychosocial assessment is to gather detailed information about the patient's psychological state and social environment to develop an individualized care plan that addresses these factors alongside their physical health needs. This process typically includes several key components:

1. Patient History: The assessment begins with collecting a thorough patient history. This includes demographic information, cultural background, educational level, occupation, and living situation. Understanding these elements helps nurses identify any social determinants of health that may affect the patient's medical condition or treatment adherence.

2. Mental Health Evaluation: Nurses assess the patient's mental health status by exploring their mood, behavior, thought processes, and cognitive function. This involves asking questions about any history of mental illness, current psychiatric symptoms (such as depression or anxiety), and any past or present treatments for mental health issues.

3. Emotional Well-being: Evaluating emotional well-being is crucial, as it affects how patients cope with illness and stress. Nurses inquire about the patient's feelings regarding their diagnosis, treatment, and prognosis. They also assess for signs of emotional distress or maladaptive coping strategies that could hinder recovery.

4. Social Support Systems: Understanding the patient's social support network is vital. Nurses assess the availability and quality of support from family members, friends, community resources, and healthcare professionals. A strong support system can positively influence a patient's ability to manage their illness and adhere to treatment plans.

5. Coping Mechanisms: Identifying how patients cope with stress and illness is essential for tailoring interventions that promote effective coping strategies. Nurses explore both adaptive (e.g., problem-solving, seeking social support) and maladaptive (e.g., substance abuse, denial) coping mechanisms.

6. Spirituality and Beliefs: Spiritual beliefs can significantly impact how patients perceive their illness and the recovery process. Nurses assess the role of spirituality in the patient's life and how it may influence their healthcare decisions.

7. Economic Factors: Financial stability can affect access to healthcare services, medication adherence, and overall well-being. Nurses evaluate economic factors such as insurance coverage, employment status, and financial concerns that might impact treatment.

8. Cultural Influences: Cultural beliefs and practices can shape health behaviors and attitudes towards medical care. Nurses need to be culturally competent to recognize these influences and incorporate them into the care plan.

Conducting a thorough psychosocial assessment requires effective communication skills, empathy, cultural sensitivity, and clinical judgment. Nurses must create a trusting environment where patients feel comfortable sharing personal information. The data gathered through this assessment informs the development of a comprehensive care plan that addresses not only the physical but also the psychosocial needs of the patient.

In summary, psychosocial assessment is an essential aspect of medical-surgical nursing that facilitates understanding of the complex interplay between psychological factors and physical health. By integrating this knowledge into patient care, nurses can enhance therapeutic outcomes and improve the quality of life for their patients.

1.1.3.1 Developmental Stages:

Developmental stages refer to the distinct phases of growth and development that individuals undergo from birth through adulthood. Each stage is characterized by specific physical, cognitive, emotional, and social changes. Understanding these stages is crucial for medical-surgical nurses, as it aids in assessing patients' psychosocial needs and providing age-appropriate care.

The developmental stages are typically divided into several key periods: infancy, early childhood, middle childhood, adolescence, early adulthood, middle adulthood, and late adulthood. Each stage presents unique challenges and milestones that influence an individual's health and well-being.

Infancy (Birth to 2 years): This stage is marked by rapid physical growth and development. Infants learn to trust their caregivers and the environment through consistent care and nurturing, a concept known as Erikson's Trust vs. Mistrust. Cognitive development during this period involves sensory exploration and the beginnings of language acquisition.

Early Childhood (2 to 6 years): Also known as the preschool years, this stage involves significant language development and the emergence of basic motor skills. Children begin to assert their independence while learning to cooperate with others. Erikson describes this phase as Autonomy vs. Shame and Doubt, where children develop a sense of personal control over physical skills and a sense of independence.

Middle Childhood (6 to 12 years): During this stage, children refine their motor skills and begin formal education. Cognitive development is characterized by logical thinking processes, as described by Piaget's Concrete Operational Stage. Socially, children start forming friendships outside the family unit, which plays a crucial role in their self-esteem and identity formation.

Adolescence (12 to 18 years): Adolescence is a period of rapid physical changes due to puberty. It is also a time of identity exploration as teenagers work through Erikson's Identity vs. Role Confusion. Cognitive abilities advance into Piaget's Formal Operational Stage, allowing for abstract thought processes. Emotional regulation becomes more complex as adolescents seek autonomy from parents while relying on peer relationships for support.

Early Adulthood (18 to 40 years): This stage focuses on building intimate relationships and establishing careers. Erikson's Intimacy vs. Isolation highlights the importance of forming deep connections with others while balancing personal ambitions. Cognitive development continues with the refinement of practical problem-solving skills.

Middle Adulthood (40 to 65 years): Individuals in this stage often experience stability in career and family life but may face challenges such as midlife crises or health issues. Erikson's Generativity vs. Stagnation emphasizes contributing to society through work or family while avoiding feelings of stagnation or unproductiveness.

Late Adulthood (65 years and older): This final stage involves reflection on life achievements and coping with physical decline. Erikson's Integrity vs. Despair centers on finding meaning in life experiences while dealing with loss or regret. Cognitive abilities may decline; however, wisdom and accumulated knowledge often compensate for these changes.

For medical-surgical nurses, understanding developmental stages is vital for providing holistic care that considers patients' emotional and social contexts alongside their physical health needs. By recognizing where a patient falls within these stages, nurses can tailor interventions that support developmental tasks and effectively address potential psychosocial stressors.

In summary, developmental stages provide a framework for understanding human growth across the lifespan. Each stage presents unique challenges that impact an individual's healthcare needs, making it essential for nurses to incorporate this knowledge into their practice for optimal patient outcomes.

1.1.3.2 Suicide Risk:

Suicide risk refers to the likelihood that an individual will attempt or complete suicide. It is a critical component of psychosocial assessment in medical-surgical nursing, as early identification and intervention can prevent tragic outcomes. Understanding suicide risk involves evaluating a range of factors that may contribute to an individual's vulnerability to suicidal thoughts and behaviors.

The assessment of suicide risk begins with recognizing potential warning signs and risk factors. Warning signs are immediate indicators that someone may be contemplating suicide, such as expressing feelings of hopelessness, withdrawing from social interactions, or exhibiting sudden mood changes. Risk factors, on the other hand, are characteristics or conditions that increase the likelihood of suicidal behavior over time. These include mental health disorders like depression and anxiety, a history of previous suicide attempts, substance abuse, chronic medical conditions, and significant life stressors such as loss or trauma.

A thorough suicide risk assessment involves direct communication with the patient. Nurses should approach this conversation with sensitivity and empathy, ensuring a safe and non-judgmental environment. Key questions to explore include whether the patient has had thoughts of self-harm, if they have a specific plan for suicide, and whether they have access to means for carrying out this plan. Understanding the patient's intent and the lethality of their plan is crucial in determining the immediacy of risk.

Protective factors should also be considered during the assessment process. These are elements that can mitigate the risk of suicide, such as strong personal relationships, effective coping strategies, access to mental health care, and a sense of purpose or responsibility towards others. Identifying these factors can help in developing a comprehensive care plan aimed at reducing suicide risk.

In addition to individual assessments, nurses must be aware of environmental factors that could influence suicide risk. Hospital settings may inadvertently increase vulnerability due to stressors like isolation from family or overwhelming medical diagnoses. Ensuring that patients do not have access to means of self-harm within these environments is vital.

Documentation is a critical component of managing suicide risk. Accurate and detailed records of assessments, interventions, and communications with patients are essential for continuity of care and legal protection. Nurses should document any expressed suicidal ideations, plans discussed during assessments, protective factors identified, and actions taken to ensure patient safety.

Interventions for individuals identified as at risk for suicide should be tailored to their specific needs and circumstances. Immediate actions may include ensuring patient safety through supervision or hospitalization if necessary, initiating psychiatric consultations, and developing a safety plan with the patient that outlines steps they can take when experiencing suicidal thoughts.

Education plays a pivotal role in managing suicide risk. Nurses should provide patients and their families with information about warning signs of suicide and available resources for support. Encouraging open communication about mental health can reduce stigma and promote early intervention.

In summary, assessing suicide risk is an integral part of psychosocial evaluation in medical-surgical nursing. It requires a comprehensive approach that considers individual characteristics, environmental influences, and protective factors. Through empathetic communication, thorough documentation, tailored interventions, and education, nurses play a crucial role in identifying individuals at risk for suicide and implementing strategies to safeguard their well-being.

1.1.3.3 Abuse:

Abuse is a critical aspect of psychosocial assessment in medical-surgical nursing, encompassing various forms of maltreatment that can have significant physical and psychological impacts on individuals. It is imperative for medical-surgical nurses to recognize the signs of abuse, understand its implications, and know how to intervene appropriately.

Abuse can be broadly categorized into physical, emotional, sexual, and neglect. Each type has distinct characteristics but may often overlap, complicating the identification and intervention process.

1. Physical Abuse: This involves the intentional use of force against a person that results in bodily injury, pain, or impairment. Signs may include unexplained bruises, fractures, burns, or other injuries that are inconsistent with the explanation provided. Nurses should be vigilant for patterns such as repeated injuries or multiple emergency room visits.

2. Emotional Abuse: Also known as psychological abuse, it includes behaviors that harm an individual's self-worth or emotional well-being. This can manifest as verbal assaults, threats, humiliation, or isolation. Victims may exhibit signs of depression, anxiety, low self-esteem, or withdrawal from social interactions.

3. Sexual Abuse: This refers to any non-consensual sexual contact or behavior. It can occur at any age and often leaves profound psychological scars. Physical signs may include injuries to the genital area or sexually transmitted infections. Psychological indicators might include fearfulness around certain individuals or situations, changes in behavior or mood, and inappropriate sexual knowledge for their age.

4. Neglect: Often considered a form of abuse, neglect involves the failure to provide necessary care, assistance, guidance, or attention to individuals who are unable to care for themselves. This can lead to malnutrition, poor hygiene, untreated medical conditions, and other health issues.

Medical-surgical nurses play a pivotal role in identifying abuse through comprehensive assessments and observations. They should maintain a high index of suspicion when clinical findings do not align with the provided history or when patients exhibit fearfulness around caregivers.

During assessment:

- Interview Techniques: Use open-ended questions in a private setting to encourage disclosure without leading the patient's responses.

- Observation: Note any non-verbal cues, such as flinching at touch or avoidance of eye contact.

- Documentation: Accurately document findings with detailed descriptions of injuries and patient statements, using direct quotes when possible.

Intervention involves:

- Reporting: Nurses are mandated reporters and must report suspected abuse to appropriate authorities following institutional policies.

- Supportive Care: Provide emotional support and ensure the patient's immediate safety.

- Referrals: Facilitate referrals to social services, mental health professionals, or protective services as needed.

Understanding cultural factors is also essential, as perceptions of abuse can vary widely among different cultures. Sensitivity towards these differences while adhering to legal obligations is crucial in providing effective care.

Education is another key component; nurses should educate patients about resources available for those experiencing abuse and empower them with information about their rights and options for seeking help.

In conclusion, recognizing and addressing abuse requires vigilance, sensitivity, and a thorough understanding of its multifaceted nature. Medical-surgical nurses must integrate this knowledge into their practice to effectively support affected individuals and contribute to their safety and well-being. Through continuous education and adherence to ethical standards, nurses can play a transformative role in mitigating the impact of abuse on patients' lives.

1.1.3.4 Substance Use Disorders:

Substance Use Disorders (SUDs) are complex conditions characterized by the uncontrolled use of a substance despite harmful consequences. These disorders are considered brain disorders because they involve changes in the brain's structure and function, which can lead to compulsive behavior related to substance use. SUDs encompass a range of problems associated with the misuse of alcohol, tobacco, and other drugs, including prescription medications.

The diagnosis of SUDs is based on criteria outlined in the Diagnostic and Statistical Manual of Mental Disorders, Fifth Edition (DSM-5). According to the DSM-5, SUDs are classified into mild, moderate, or severe categories based on the number of criteria met. These criteria include a strong desire or craving to use the substance, unsuccessful efforts to cut down or control use, significant time spent obtaining or using the substance, and continued use despite social or interpersonal problems caused by the substance's effects.

The pathophysiology of SUDs involves several neurotransmitter systems in the brain, with dopamine playing a key role. Substances often increase dopamine levels in the brain's reward pathways, reinforcing drug-taking behaviors. Over time, repeated exposure to substances can lead to adaptations in these pathways, resulting in tolerance (requiring more of the substance to achieve the same effect) and withdrawal symptoms when not using the substance.

Risk factors for developing SUDs include genetic predisposition, environmental influences such as exposure to drug-using peers or family members, stress, a history of trauma, and mental health disorders like depression or anxiety. Adolescents and young adults are particularly vulnerable due to ongoing brain development during these stages.

The clinical presentation of SUDs varies depending on the substance involved but commonly includes physical signs such as weight loss or gain, poor hygiene, changes in sleep patterns, and unusual odors on breath or clothing. Behavioral signs may include neglecting responsibilities at work or home, engaging in risky activities while under the influence, legal issues related to substance use, and social withdrawal from family and friends.

Assessment of patients with suspected SUDs involves a comprehensive psychosocial evaluation that includes a detailed history of substance use patterns, previous treatment attempts, psychiatric history, and assessment of social support systems. Screening tools such as the CAGE questionnaire for alcohol use or the Drug Abuse Screening Test (DAST) for drug use can aid in identifying individuals at risk.

Management of SUDs requires a multidisciplinary approach that combines pharmacological and non-pharmacological strategies. Pharmacotherapy may include medications like methadone or buprenorphine for opioid use disorder or naltrexone for alcohol dependence. Behavioral therapies such as cognitive-behavioral therapy (CBT), motivational interviewing (MI), and contingency management are effective components of treatment plans.

Nurses play a crucial role in managing patients with SUDs by providing education about the disorder and its treatment options, supporting patients through withdrawal symptoms during detoxification processes, advocating for their needs within healthcare settings, and facilitating connections with community resources for ongoing support.

In summary, Substance Use Disorders are chronic but treatable conditions that require comprehensive care tailored to individual needs. Medical-surgical nurses must possess a thorough understanding of these disorders to effectively assess and manage affected patients while promoting recovery and reducing the stigma associated with substance misuse.

1.1.4 Cognitive Assessment:

Cognitive assessment is a crucial process in the medical-surgical nursing field, aimed at evaluating an individual's mental functions to identify any impairments or changes in cognitive status. It encompasses a range of tests and observations designed to assess various aspects of cognition, including memory, attention, language, problem-solving skills, and executive functions. This evaluation is essential for diagnosing cognitive disorders, planning appropriate care, and monitoring the progression or improvement of cognitive conditions.

In the context of medical-surgical nursing, cognitive assessment is particularly important because patients may experience cognitive changes due to a variety of factors, such as surgery, medication side effects, metabolic imbalances, or neurological disorders. Nurses play a vital role in the early detection of cognitive impairment, which can significantly impact patient outcomes and quality of life.

The cognitive assessment process typically begins with thorough history-taking to understand the patient's baseline cognitive function and any recent changes. This includes gathering information from the patient, family members, or caregivers about memory lapses, episodes of confusion, difficulty concentrating, or changes in behavior. Understanding the patient's medical history and current medications is also essential, as these can influence cognitive function.

Once the initial information is gathered, nurses may utilize standardized cognitive assessment tools to obtain objective data. Commonly used tools include the Mini-Mental State Examination (MMSE), the Montreal Cognitive Assessment (MoCA), and the Clock Drawing Test. These tools are designed to assess different domains of cognition and provide a quantitative measure of cognitive function.

The MMSE is a widely used tool that evaluates orientation, registration, attention and calculation, recall, language, and visuospatial skills. It provides a score that helps determine the severity of cognitive impairment. The MoCA is another comprehensive screening tool that assesses similar domains but is more sensitive to mild cognitive impairment. The Clock Drawing Test is a simple yet effective tool for assessing executive function and visuospatial abilities.

In addition to these standardized tests, nurses must observe patients' behavior and interactions during their hospital stay. Changes in mood, disorientation to time or place, difficulty following instructions, or an inability to perform activities of daily living may indicate cognitive decline.

Interpreting the results of a cognitive assessment requires careful consideration of various factors, such as age, education level, cultural background, and any sensory impairments that might affect test performance. It is crucial to differentiate between temporary delirium caused by acute illness or medication effects and more permanent conditions like dementia.

Once cognitive impairment is identified, nurses collaborate with the healthcare team to develop an individualized care plan. This may involve addressing reversible causes such as dehydration or infection, adjusting medications that may contribute to cognitive decline, providing orientation aids like clocks or calendars in the patient's room, and involving occupational therapy for cognitive rehabilitation.

Furthermore, educating patients and their families about the nature of cognitive impairment and its management is an essential aspect of nursing care. Providing support resources such as counseling services or support groups can help patients and families cope with the challenges associated with cognitive decline.

In summary, cognitive assessment in medical-surgical nursing involves a comprehensive evaluation of mental functions using standardized tools and clinical observations. It plays a critical role in identifying cognitive impairments early on, enabling timely interventions that improve patient outcomes. Nurses must be adept at conducting these assessments and interpreting their results within the broader context of each patient's unique circumstances.

1.1.4.1 <u>Neuro Status:</u>

Neuro status, or neurological status, refers to the assessment and evaluation of a patient's nervous system function. This assessment is critical for identifying potential neurological disorders, monitoring changes in neurological function, and guiding clinical decisions. For medical-surgical nurses, understanding and accurately assessing neuro status is essential for providing comprehensive patient care.

The evaluation of neuro status involves a systematic approach to assess various components of the nervous system, including mental status, cranial nerves, motor function, sensory function, reflexes, and coordination. Each of these components provides valuable information about the patient's neurological health.

Mental status assessment focuses on evaluating the patient's level of consciousness, orientation, memory, attention, language abilities, and cognitive functions. The Glasgow Coma Scale (GCS) is commonly used to assess the level of consciousness by scoring eye-opening, verbal response, and motor response. Orientation involves checking whether the patient is aware of their person, place, time, and situation. Memory assessment includes evaluating both short-term and long-term recall abilities.

Cranial nerve assessment involves testing the function of the twelve cranial nerves responsible for various sensory and motor functions. This includes evaluating smell (olfactory nerve), vision (optic nerve), eye movements (oculomotor, trochlear, and abducens nerves), facial sensation and movement (trigeminal and facial nerves), hearing and balance (vestibulocochlear nerve), taste (glossopharyngeal and vagus nerves), shoulder shrug and head turn (accessory nerve), and tongue movement (hypoglossal nerve).

Motor function assessment evaluates muscle strength, tone, bulk, and involuntary movements. Nurses assess muscle strength by asking patients to perform specific movements against resistance. Muscle tone is evaluated by passively moving the patient's limbs to detect any rigidity or flaccidity. Observing for involuntary movements such as tremors or fasciculations provides additional information about motor function.

Sensory function assessment includes evaluating the patient's ability to perceive different sensations such as pain, temperature, touch, vibration, and proprioception. This is done using various tools, like a pin for pain sensation or a tuning fork for vibration sense. The nurse compares sensations on both sides of the body to identify any asymmetries or deficits.

Reflex assessment involves testing deep tendon reflexes, such as the patellar or Achilles reflexes, using a reflex hammer. Abnormal reflex responses can indicate neurological issues such as hyperreflexia or hyporeflexia. Additionally, pathological reflexes like Babinski's sign are assessed to detect upper motor neuron lesions.

Coordination assessment evaluates the patient's ability to perform coordinated movements smoothly. Tests like finger-to-nose or heel-to-shin assess cerebellar function, which is responsible for coordination. Observing gait can also provide insights into coordination and balance issues.

Throughout the neuro status assessment process, it is crucial for nurses to document findings accurately and report any significant changes promptly. Changes in neuro status can indicate worsening conditions or complications that require immediate medical intervention.

In conclusion, neuro status assessment is a fundamental component of nursing practice in medical-surgical settings. It provides critical insights into a patient's neurological health and guides clinical decision-making. By systematically assessing mental status, cranial nerves, motor function, sensory function, reflexes, and coordination, medical-surgical nurses play a vital role in ensuring optimal patient outcomes through early detection and intervention in neurological disorders.

1.1.4.2 Developmental Age:

Developmental age refers to the measure of a person's physical, cognitive, emotional, and social development in comparison to typical age norms. Unlike chronological age, which is the actual time elapsed since birth, developmental age considers the maturity and functional capabilities of an individual. This concept is particularly significant in medical-surgical nursing as it helps practitioners tailor care plans that are appropriate for the patient's developmental stage rather than relying solely on their chronological age.

In medical-surgical settings, understanding developmental age is crucial for assessing cognitive abilities, communication skills, and the capacity for self-care. It is essential for nurses to recognize that patients may not always align with their chronological peers in terms of development due to various factors such as congenital conditions, chronic illnesses, or environmental influences. Therefore, comprehensive assessment tools are employed to evaluate developmental milestones across different domains.

Cognitive development encompasses abilities such as memory, problem-solving skills, and comprehension. In adults, cognitive developmental age may be affected by neurological disorders, brain injuries, or psychiatric conditions. For instance, a patient with early-onset Alzheimer's disease may exhibit a developmental age significantly lower than their chronological age. Nurses must adapt communication strategies and interventions to match the patient's cognitive abilities to ensure effective care delivery.

Emotional and social development are also critical components of developmental age. Emotional maturity involves the ability to manage emotions effectively and develop coping mechanisms in response to stressors. Social development pertains to interpersonal skills and the ability to form relationships. Patients with delayed emotional or social development may require additional support in understanding medical procedures or adhering to treatment regimens. Medical-surgical nurses should be adept at identifying these needs and providing appropriate resources or referrals.

Physical development can influence a patient's functional status and ability to participate in self-care activities. Conditions such as muscular dystrophy or cerebral palsy may impact physical developmental age, necessitating modifications in care approaches. Assessing physical capabilities allows nurses to create individualized care plans that accommodate any limitations while promoting independence where possible.

The assessment of developmental age often involves a multidisciplinary approach, utilizing standardized tools such as the Denver Developmental Screening Test or the Bayley Scales of Infant and Toddler Development for pediatric populations. In adult patients, neuropsychological assessments or functional status evaluations may be conducted to determine cognitive and physical developmental levels.

Understanding developmental age is vital for patient-centered care in medical-surgical nursing. It ensures that interventions are appropriate for the patient's true level of functioning rather than solely based on their chronological age. This approach enhances patient engagement, compliance with treatment plans, and overall outcomes.

In summary, developmental age provides a comprehensive framework for evaluating an individual's maturity across various domains relative to typical norms. In medical-surgical nursing practice, recognizing and assessing developmental age enables nurses to deliver personalized care that addresses the unique needs of each patient. By considering cognitive, emotional, social, and physical development, nurses can optimize care strategies and improve patient experiences within healthcare settings.

1.1.4.3 Impairment:

In the context of cognitive assessment, impairment refers to a reduction or loss of cognitive function, which can affect a person's ability to perform everyday activities. Cognitive impairment can vary in severity, ranging from mild deficits that may not significantly impact daily life to severe impairments that can interfere with basic functioning and independence. Understanding cognitive impairment is crucial for medical-surgical nurses, as they play a key role in assessing, identifying, and managing patients with these challenges.

Cognitive impairment encompasses a broad spectrum of conditions characterized by difficulties with memory, attention, language, problem-solving, and other cognitive processes. It is important to recognize that cognitive impairment is not synonymous with dementia; rather, it can be a feature of various medical conditions or an effect of aging. Cognitive impairment can be transient or chronic, reversible or irreversible, depending on its underlying cause.

Medical-surgical nurses must be adept at recognizing signs of cognitive impairment in patients. These signs may include confusion, disorientation, difficulty concentrating, forgetfulness, impaired judgment, and changes in behavior or personality. The onset of these symptoms can be sudden or gradual, and their progression may vary based on the underlying etiology.

Several factors can contribute to cognitive impairment. Acute conditions such as delirium often result from infections, metabolic imbalances, medication side effects, or surgical procedures. Chronic conditions like Alzheimer's disease or vascular dementia are progressive and typically irreversible. Additionally, psychiatric disorders such as depression and anxiety can mimic or exacerbate cognitive impairment.

When assessing a patient for cognitive impairment, medical-surgical nurses should conduct a thorough history and physical examination. This includes evaluating the patient's mental status using standardized tools like the Mini-Mental State Examination (MMSE) or the Montreal Cognitive Assessment (MoCA). These assessments help quantify the level of cognitive function and identify specific areas of deficit.

Nurses should also consider potential reversible causes of cognitive impairment. For instance, addressing nutritional deficiencies (e.g., vitamin B12 deficiency), managing chronic diseases (e.g., diabetes mellitus), optimizing medication regimens to avoid polypharmacy, and ensuring adequate sleep can improve cognitive outcomes. In cases where cognitive impairment is due to neurodegenerative diseases, early identification allows for timely intervention and planning for future care needs.

Interprofessional collaboration is essential in managing patients with cognitive impairment. Medical-surgical nurses work closely with physicians, neurologists, psychiatrists, social workers, and occupational therapists to develop comprehensive care plans tailored to each patient's unique needs. These plans often involve pharmacological interventions to manage symptoms and non-pharmacological strategies, such as cognitive rehabilitation exercises and environmental modifications, to enhance safety and quality of life.

Education and support for patients and their families are vital components of care. Medical-surgical nurses should provide information about the nature of cognitive impairment, potential treatments, and strategies for coping with daily challenges.

Encouraging family involvement in care planning helps ensure continuity of care and emotional support for both patients and caregivers.

In summary, understanding cognitive impairment is critical for medical-surgical nurses involved in patient assessment and management. By recognizing the signs of impairment and identifying its underlying causes, nurses can implement appropriate interventions to enhance patient outcomes. Through interdisciplinary collaboration and patient-centered care approaches, nurses contribute significantly to improving the quality of life for individuals experiencing cognitive challenges.

1.1.5 Diagnostic and Laboratory Testing:

Diagnostic and laboratory testing are critical components in the field of medical-surgical nursing, serving as essential tools for assessing, diagnosing, and managing patient health. These tests provide objective data that guide clinical decision-making and patient care planning. As a medical-surgical nurse, understanding the purpose, process, and interpretation of these tests is vital to ensure optimal patient outcomes.

Diagnostic testing encompasses a wide range of procedures used to identify diseases or conditions. These tests can include imaging studies such as X-rays, CT scans, MRIs, and ultrasounds. Each modality offers unique insights into the body's structure and function. For instance, X-rays are often used to evaluate bone fractures or infections, while CT scans provide detailed cross-sectional images that are useful in diagnosing conditions like tumors or internal bleeding. MRIs offer high-resolution images of soft tissues, making them valuable in assessing neurological disorders or musculoskeletal injuries. Ultrasounds use sound waves to visualize organs and structures and are commonly employed in evaluating abdominal organs or monitoring fetal development.

Laboratory testing involves analyzing samples of blood, urine, stool, or tissue to assess physiological and biochemical states. Common laboratory tests include complete blood counts (CBC), basic metabolic panels (BMP), liver function tests (LFTs), and coagulation profiles. A CBC provides information on red and white blood cell counts and hemoglobin levels, which can indicate anemia or infection. BMPs assess electrolyte balance, kidney function, and glucose levels, which are essential for identifying metabolic imbalances or renal impairment. LFTs evaluate enzymes and proteins produced by the liver, aiding in the diagnosis of liver diseases such as hepatitis or cirrhosis. Coagulation profiles measure clotting factors to monitor the effectiveness of anticoagulation therapy or detect bleeding disorders.

Understanding normal versus abnormal values is crucial for interpreting these tests accurately. Nurses must be familiar with reference ranges for various age groups and recognize factors that can influence test results, such as medications or comorbid conditions. For example, dehydration can elevate blood urea nitrogen (BUN) levels independent of kidney function.

Nurses also play a pivotal role in preparing patients for diagnostic procedures. This includes educating patients about the purpose of the test, any necessary pre-test preparations (such as fasting), potential risks or discomforts, and post-test care instructions. Proper preparation ensures accurate results and minimizes patient anxiety.

Furthermore, nurses must be adept at recognizing critical test results that require immediate intervention. This involves understanding which values indicate life-threatening conditions and necessitate rapid communication with the healthcare team. For instance, a critically low hemoglobin level may require an urgent blood transfusion.

In addition to technical knowledge, nurses must maintain ethical standards when handling diagnostic information. This includes ensuring patient confidentiality and obtaining informed consent when necessary.

In summary, diagnostic and laboratory testing are integral to medical-surgical nursing practice. They provide essential data for diagnosis and treatment planning while requiring nurses to possess a thorough understanding of test purposes, procedures, interpretation of results, and patient care implications. Mastery of these skills is crucial for delivering high-quality care and improving patient outcomes in the dynamic field of medical-surgical nursing.

1.1.5.1 Patient Preparation:

Patient preparation is a critical aspect of diagnostic and laboratory testing in medical-surgical nursing. It involves a systematic approach to readying a patient physically, emotionally, and psychologically for diagnostic procedures or laboratory tests. Proper patient preparation ensures the accuracy of test results, minimizes complications, enhances patient comfort, and promotes positive outcomes.

The process of patient preparation begins with thorough patient education. Nurses must provide clear explanations about the purpose, procedure, and potential risks associated with the test or diagnostic procedure. This includes outlining what the patient should expect before, during, and after the test. Effective communication helps alleviate anxiety and fosters cooperation, ensuring that patients are informed participants in their care.

Physical preparation varies depending on the type of test or procedure. For instance, fasting may be required for certain blood tests to avoid interference from recent food intake. Similarly, bowel preparation might be necessary for procedures like colonoscopy to ensure optimal visualization. Nurses must verify specific instructions from healthcare providers and communicate these to patients well in advance.

Medication management is another crucial component of patient preparation. Nurses need to review the patient's current medications to identify any that should be temporarily discontinued or adjusted prior to testing. For example, anticoagulants might need to be held before invasive procedures to reduce the risk of bleeding. Coordination with prescribing physicians is essential to ensure safe medication practices.

Informed consent is an integral part of patient preparation. Nurses must ensure that patients understand the nature of the procedure and have voluntarily agreed to it. This involves verifying that consent forms are signed and addressing any questions or concerns patients may have about the procedure.

Emotional support is vital in preparing patients for diagnostic tests. Anxiety and fear are common emotions experienced by patients facing medical procedures. Nurses should assess patients' emotional states and provide reassurance as needed. Techniques such as deep breathing exercises or guided imagery can be taught to help manage stress.

For some tests, specific positioning or immobilization may be required during the procedure. Nurses should instruct patients on how they will need to position themselves and offer assistance if necessary. Ensuring comfort with pillows or supports can help maintain required positions without causing undue discomfort.

Patient safety is paramount throughout the preparation process. This includes confirming patient identity using at least two identifiers and verifying allergies to prevent adverse reactions. Additionally, nurses should ensure that any necessary equipment or supplies are available and functioning properly before proceeding with the test.

Documentation plays a crucial role in patient preparation. Nurses must accurately record all relevant information, including patient education provided, consent obtained, medications administered or withheld, and any special instructions given. This documentation serves as a legal record and facilitates continuity of care.

In summary, patient preparation is a comprehensive process that encompasses education, physical readiness, medication management, informed consent, emotional support, positioning guidance, safety checks, and thorough documentation. By meticulously preparing patients for diagnostic and laboratory testing, nurses play a pivotal role in optimizing test accuracy, minimizing risks, and enhancing the overall patient experience in medical-surgical settings.

1.1.5.2 **Response To Abnormal Values:**

In the realm of medical-surgical nursing, responding to abnormal laboratory values is a critical skill that ensures patient safety and optimal outcomes. Abnormal values can indicate underlying health issues, necessitate immediate intervention, or require monitoring and further investigation. Understanding how to effectively respond to these abnormalities involves recognizing the significance of specific lab results, implementing appropriate interventions, and collaborating with the healthcare team.

Abnormal laboratory values refer to test results that fall outside the established normal range for a particular analyte. These deviations can be indicative of physiological dysfunctions, disease processes, or the effects of treatments. The response to these values must be swift, informed, and systematic to prevent adverse outcomes.

The first step in responding to abnormal values is accurate interpretation. Medical-surgical nurses must be proficient in understanding lab results within the context of the patient's clinical presentation. This includes considering factors such as age, gender, medical history, and current medications that might influence lab outcomes. For example, an elevated white blood cell count could suggest infection but may also be a response to stress or medication.

Once an abnormal value is identified, the nurse must determine its clinical significance. This involves assessing whether the value represents a critical change that requires immediate action or if it is a non-critical deviation that warrants monitoring. Critical values often necessitate urgent interventions; for instance, severe hyperkalemia (elevated potassium levels) may require prompt administration of calcium gluconate or insulin and glucose to prevent cardiac complications.

Communication is a pivotal component in managing abnormal lab values. The nurse must promptly report critical findings to the physician or advanced practice provider responsible for the patient's care. Clear and concise communication ensures that appropriate medical decisions are made swiftly. Documentation of both the abnormal value and the subsequent actions taken is essential for maintaining an accurate medical record and facilitating continuity of care.

Interventions following abnormal values may vary depending on the specific test result and its implications. For instance, low hemoglobin levels might necessitate a blood transfusion, whereas high creatinine levels could indicate renal impairment requiring fluid management or a nephrology consultation. Nurses must also educate patients and their families about the implications of abnormal lab results and any necessary lifestyle modifications or treatment plans.

Monitoring is another key aspect of responding to abnormal laboratory values. Continuous assessment allows nurses to evaluate the effectiveness of interventions and detect any further deviations from normal ranges. Regular follow-up testing may be required to ensure stabilization of the patient's condition.

Collaboration with other healthcare professionals enhances patient outcomes when dealing with abnormal lab values. Interdisciplinary teamwork involving physicians, pharmacists, dietitians, and others can provide comprehensive care tailored to address the root cause of the abnormalities.

In summary, responding to abnormal laboratory values involves a multifaceted approach encompassing interpretation, communication, intervention, education, monitoring, and collaboration. Medical-surgical nurses play a vital role in this process by ensuring timely recognition and management of deviations from normal ranges. Mastery of these skills not only contributes to passing the MEDSURG-BC exam but also enhances patient care delivery in clinical practice.

1.1.5.3 **Medication Considerations:**

Medication considerations in the context of medical-surgical nursing involve a comprehensive understanding of pharmacological principles, patient-specific factors, and clinical implications that influence medication administration and management. As a medical-surgical nurse, it is crucial to ensure the safe and effective use of medications in diverse patient populations by considering various factors that can impact drug therapy outcomes.

Firstly, understanding pharmacokinetics and pharmacodynamics is essential. Pharmacokinetics involves the absorption, distribution, metabolism, and excretion of drugs. Nurses must be aware of how these processes can vary among patients due to age, weight, organ function, and concurrent medical conditions. For instance, renal or hepatic impairment can significantly alter drug metabolism and excretion, necessitating dosage adjustments to prevent toxicity.

Pharmacodynamics refers to the effects of drugs on the body and involves understanding the mechanism of action, therapeutic effects, side effects, and potential adverse reactions. Nurses must be vigilant in monitoring for expected therapeutic outcomes as well as any signs of adverse effects or drug interactions. This includes recognizing symptoms that may indicate an allergic reaction or toxicity.

Patient-specific factors play a critical role in medication considerations. These factors include age-related changes in pharmacokinetics and pharmacodynamics. For example, older adults often experience decreased renal function and altered body composition, which can affect drug distribution and elimination. Pediatric patients may require weight-based dosing to ensure efficacy and safety.

Polypharmacy is another important consideration, particularly in patients with multiple chronic conditions. The risk of drug-drug interactions increases with the number of medications a patient takes. Nurses must review all medications, including over-the-counter drugs and supplements, to identify potential interactions that could compromise patient safety or therapeutic efficacy.

Additionally, adherence to prescribed medication regimens is a common challenge. Factors such as complex dosing schedules, side effects, cognitive impairment, or financial constraints can affect adherence. Nurses should assess for barriers to adherence and collaborate with patients to develop strategies that promote consistent medication use.

Cultural and psychosocial factors also influence medication considerations. Cultural beliefs may affect a patient's willingness to take certain medications or adhere to specific treatment plans. Nurses should engage in culturally sensitive communication to ensure patients understand their medication regimens and feel comfortable discussing any concerns.

Informed consent is another critical aspect of medication administration. Patients have the right to understand the purpose of their medications, potential benefits and risks, alternative treatments, and the consequences of refusing treatment. Nurses play a key role in educating patients and advocating for their autonomy in decision-making.

Lastly, legal and ethical considerations must not be overlooked. Nurses are responsible for ensuring that medication orders are complete, accurate, and appropriate for the patient's clinical condition. This includes verifying correct dosages, routes of administration, timing, and ensuring that all orders are signed by authorized prescribers.

In summary, medication considerations in medical-surgical nursing encompass a broad spectrum of knowledge areas, including pharmacological principles, patient-specific variables, polypharmacy management, adherence challenges, cultural competence, informed consent processes, and legal/ethical responsibilities. By integrating these considerations into practice, nurses can optimize medication therapy outcomes while ensuring patient safety and promoting holistic care.

1.1.6 Nursing Diagnosis: Identification & Prioritization

Nursing diagnosis identification and prioritization is a critical component of the nursing process, serving as a foundation for developing effective care plans tailored to individual patient needs. A nursing diagnosis is a clinical judgment concerning a human response to health conditions or life processes, or a vulnerability to that response, by an individual, family, group, or community. It provides the basis for selecting nursing interventions to achieve outcomes for which the nurse is accountable.

The process of identifying nursing diagnoses begins with a comprehensive assessment of the patient. This involves collecting data through observation, interviews, physical examinations, and reviewing medical records. The nurse must gather both subjective data (what the patient says) and objective data (what can be observed or measured) to form a complete picture of the patient's health status.

Once data collection is complete, the nurse analyzes the information to identify patterns or clusters of symptoms that indicate potential health problems. This analysis requires critical thinking skills to differentiate between normal and abnormal findings and to recognize relationships among data points. Nursing diagnoses are then formulated using standardized language provided by systems such as NANDA International (formerly known as the North American Nursing Diagnosis Association), which ensures clarity and consistency in communication among healthcare providers.

After identifying potential nursing diagnoses, prioritization is necessary to determine which issues require immediate attention and which can be addressed later. Prioritization is guided by several factors:

1. Maslow's Hierarchy of Needs: This model prioritizes physiological needs (such as breathing and circulation) over higher-level needs (such as self-esteem). Issues affecting basic survival are addressed first.

2. Patient Safety: Diagnoses that pose immediate threats to patient safety or life are prioritized. For example, the risk of aspiration or impaired gas exchange would take precedence over less critical concerns like a disturbed sleep pattern.

3. Patient Preferences: Whenever possible, patient preferences should be considered in prioritization decisions. Engaging patients in their care plan fosters collaboration and improves adherence to interventions.

4. Potential for Complications: Conditions that could lead to serious complications if untreated should be prioritized. For instance, effectively managing acute pain can prevent complications such as immobility or chronic pain syndromes.

5. Time Sensitivity: Some diagnoses require prompt intervention due to their time-sensitive nature; for example, administering insulin for hyperglycemia or providing anticoagulation therapy for thrombosis prevention.

6. Available Resources: The availability of resources such as staffing levels, equipment, and support services can influence prioritization decisions.

Effective prioritization requires ongoing evaluation and adjustment as patient conditions change. Nurses must remain vigilant in reassessing priorities based on new information or changes in patient status.

In summary, nursing diagnosis identification and prioritization involve systematic assessment and analysis of patient data to formulate accurate nursing diagnoses, followed by strategic decision-making to prioritize care based on urgency, safety, patient preferences, potential complications, time sensitivity, and available resources. Mastery of this process is essential for delivering high-quality care that meets individual patient needs while optimizing outcomes in medical-surgical settings.

1.1.7 Fluids And Electrolytes:

Fluids and electrolytes are essential components of the human body, playing a critical role in maintaining homeostasis, which is the body's ability to maintain a stable internal environment despite changes in external conditions. The balance of fluids and electrolytes is vital for normal cellular function, nerve transmission, muscle contraction, and overall physiological stability.

Fluids refer to the water content within the body, which is distributed between two main compartments: intracellular fluid (ICF) and extracellular fluid (ECF). The ICF, which constitutes about two-thirds of the body's total water content, is found within cells. The ECF, making up the remaining one-third, includes interstitial fluid (the fluid between cells), plasma (the liquid component of blood), and transcellular fluids (e.g., cerebrospinal fluid, synovial fluid).

Electrolytes are minerals that carry an electric charge and are dissolved in body fluids. They include sodium (Na+), potassium (K+), calcium (Ca2+), magnesium (Mg2+), chloride (Cl-), bicarbonate (HCO3-), phosphate (PO4^3-), and sulfate (SO4^2-). Each electrolyte plays a specific role in physiological processes. For instance, sodium is crucial for maintaining fluid balance and nerve function; potassium is essential for muscle contraction and heart function; calcium is vital for bone health and blood clotting; and magnesium aids in enzyme function and neuromuscular activity.

The regulation of fluids and electrolytes involves several mechanisms to ensure equilibrium. The kidneys play a primary role by filtering blood, reabsorbing needed substances, and excreting waste products. Hormones such as antidiuretic hormone (ADH), aldosterone, and atrial natriuretic peptide (ANP) also regulate fluid balance by influencing kidney function. ADH promotes water reabsorption in the kidneys, reducing urine output when the body needs to conserve water. Aldosterone increases sodium reabsorption and potassium excretion, affecting fluid volume and blood pressure. ANP counteracts these effects by promoting sodium excretion.

Disruptions in fluid and electrolyte balance can lead to various clinical conditions. Dehydration occurs when fluid loss exceeds intake, potentially resulting from excessive sweating, vomiting, diarrhea, or insufficient fluid consumption. Symptoms include dry skin, decreased urine output, dizziness, and confusion. Conversely, overhydration or fluid overload may result from excessive fluid intake or impaired excretion due to renal failure or heart failure.

Electrolyte imbalances can have serious consequences. Hyponatremia (low sodium levels) can cause headache, confusion, seizures, and coma. Hypernatremia (high sodium levels) may lead to thirst, agitation, or even neurological impairment. Hypokalemia (low potassium levels) can cause muscle weakness, cramps, and arrhythmias, while hyperkalemia (high potassium levels) poses risks of cardiac arrest. Hypocalcemia (low calcium levels) can result in tetany or convulsions, whereas hypercalcemia may lead to bone pain or kidney stones.

Medical-surgical nurses must be adept at recognizing signs of fluid and electrolyte imbalances through patient assessment and laboratory data interpretation. Interventions may include administering intravenous fluids or electrolytes as needed based on clinical judgment and physician orders. Patient education on maintaining adequate hydration and dietary modifications to manage electrolyte levels is also crucial.

In summary, understanding the intricate roles of fluids and electrolytes is fundamental for medical-surgical nurses to provide effective care. Maintaining this balance is essential for optimal health outcomes across diverse patient populations.

1.1.7.1 Imbalances:

Fluid and electrolyte imbalances are critical concepts in medical-surgical nursing, as they significantly impact patient health and recovery. Imbalances occur when there is a disruption in the normal balance of fluids and electrolytes within the body, which can lead to various clinical manifestations and require prompt intervention.

Electrolytes are minerals in body fluids that carry an electric charge. They are crucial for maintaining numerous physiological functions, including nerve conduction, muscle function, acid-base balance, and fluid balance. The primary electrolytes include sodium, potassium, calcium, magnesium, chloride, bicarbonate, and phosphate. Each of these plays a unique role in maintaining homeostasis.

Fluid imbalances can be categorized into two main types: fluid volume deficit (FVD) and fluid volume excess (FVE). Fluid volume deficit, often referred to as dehydration, occurs when there is a loss of water and electrolytes from the extracellular space. This can result from conditions such as excessive sweating, vomiting, diarrhea, or inadequate fluid intake. Clinically, FVD may present with symptoms such as dry mucous membranes, decreased skin turgor, hypotension, tachycardia, and concentrated urine. Management involves replacing lost fluids orally or intravenously and addressing the underlying cause.

Conversely, fluid volume excess is characterized by an overload of water in the body's extracellular space. This can result from conditions like heart failure, renal failure, or excessive sodium intake leading to water retention. Patients with FVE may exhibit symptoms such as edema, hypertension, jugular venous distention, pulmonary congestion, and weight gain. Treatment focuses on fluid restriction, diuretic administration, and managing the underlying condition.

Electrolyte imbalances involve deviations in the levels of specific electrolytes. Hyponatremia and hypernatremia refer to low and high sodium levels, respectively. Hyponatremia can arise from factors like excessive water intake or SIADH (Syndrome of Inappropriate Antidiuretic Hormone), leading to symptoms such as confusion, seizures, and muscle weakness. Hypernatremia often results from inadequate water intake or excessive water loss and presents with thirst, agitation, or even coma if severe. Management strategies include careful correction of sodium levels with appropriate fluids.

Hypokalemia and hyperkalemia denote low and high potassium levels, respectively. Hypokalemia may result from diuretic use or gastrointestinal losses and presents with muscle cramps, arrhythmias, or fatigue. Hyperkalemia can occur due to renal dysfunction or tissue breakdown (e.g., trauma) and may lead to life-threatening cardiac arrhythmias. Treatment involves addressing the underlying cause while carefully correcting potassium levels using supplements or medications like insulin with glucose for hyperkalemia.

Calcium imbalances include hypocalcemia and hypercalcemia. Hypocalcemia might be caused by vitamin D deficiency or hypoparathyroidism and manifests as tetany or seizures. Hypercalcemia often results from malignancies or hyperparathyroidism, presenting with fatigue or renal stones. Managing calcium imbalances involves dietary adjustments or medications that alter calcium absorption/excretion.

Magnesium imbalances are less common but equally significant. Hypomagnesemia could occur due to chronic alcoholism or malabsorption syndromes, leading to neuromuscular irritability or arrhythmias. Conversely, hypermagnesemia might be seen in renal failure patients receiving magnesium-containing medications, presenting with lethargy or respiratory depression.

In summary, understanding fluid and electrolyte imbalances is vital for medical-surgical nurses, as they play a critical role in accurately assessing patients' conditions and implementing appropriate interventions promptly. Mastery of this knowledge ensures optimal patient outcomes through effective management of these complex physiological processes.

1.1.7.2 Disease-related:

Disease-related fluid and electrolyte imbalances are critical considerations in medical-surgical nursing, as they can significantly impact patient outcomes. These imbalances often arise due to underlying pathophysiological processes associated with various diseases. Understanding these mechanisms is essential for effective assessment, diagnosis, and management.

In the context of disease-related fluid and electrolyte disturbances, several conditions commonly contribute to these imbalances. For instance, heart failure can lead to fluid overload due to impaired cardiac output, resulting in increased venous pressure and subsequent edema formation. The renin-angiotensin-aldosterone system (RAAS) is often activated in heart failure, promoting sodium and water retention, which exacerbates fluid overload.

Renal disorders such as acute kidney injury (AKI) or chronic kidney disease (CKD) are also pivotal in causing electrolyte disturbances. In AKI, there is an abrupt decline in renal function, leading to the accumulation of waste products and electrolytes like potassium and phosphate. Hyperkalemia is a frequent complication, posing risks for cardiac arrhythmias. CKD patients often exhibit chronic imbalances such as hyperphosphatemia and hypocalcemia due to impaired renal excretion and altered vitamin D metabolism.

Liver disease, particularly cirrhosis, is another condition where fluid and electrolyte imbalances are prevalent. Ascites formation in cirrhosis results from portal hypertension and hypoalbuminemia, leading to third-spacing of fluids. Additionally, hyponatremia is common due to the dilutional effect of retained water relative to sodium.

Endocrine disorders such as diabetes insipidus (DI) and the syndrome of inappropriate antidiuretic hormone secretion (SIADH) directly affect fluid balance. DI leads to excessive water loss due to a deficiency of antidiuretic hormone (ADH), resulting in hypernatremia and dehydration. Conversely, SIADH causes water retention and dilutional hyponatremia due to inappropriate ADH secretion.

Gastrointestinal diseases can also precipitate fluid and electrolyte issues. Conditions like vomiting or diarrhea lead to significant losses of electrolytes such as sodium, potassium, and bicarbonate, potentially resulting in metabolic alkalosis or acidosis. Pancreatitis is another example where inflammatory processes can cause third-spacing of fluids into the peritoneal cavity, leading to hypovolemia.

In surgical patients, postoperative complications such as ileus or bowel obstruction may contribute to fluid shifts and electrolyte imbalances. The stress response associated with surgery can activate hormonal pathways that alter sodium and water retention.

Furthermore, malignancies can induce paraneoplastic syndromes affecting fluid and electrolyte balance. For example, certain cancers produce ectopic hormones like parathyroid hormone-related peptide (PTHrP), causing hypercalcemia.

Management of disease-related fluid and electrolyte imbalances involves addressing the underlying condition while correcting specific deficits or excesses. This may include pharmacologic interventions such as diuretics for fluid overload or electrolyte supplements for deficiencies. Monitoring laboratory values closely is crucial for guiding treatment decisions.

In conclusion, disease-related fluid and electrolyte imbalances are multifaceted issues that require a comprehensive understanding of the underlying pathophysiology associated with various conditions. Medical-surgical nurses must be adept at recognizing these imbalances early through vigilant assessment and applying evidence-based interventions tailored to each patient's unique clinical scenario. By mastering these concepts, nurses play a vital role in optimizing patient care outcomes in the medical-surgical setting.

1.1.7.3 Blood Products:

Blood products are biological materials derived from human blood that are used in the treatment and management of various medical conditions. These products play a crucial role in medical-surgical nursing, as they are often necessary for patients undergoing surgery, experiencing trauma, or suffering from conditions that affect blood volume or function. Understanding the different types of blood products, their indications, and the principles of safe administration is essential for medical-surgical nurses.

There are several types of blood products, each with specific components and uses:

1. Whole Blood: This is unmodified human blood that contains red blood cells (RBCs), white blood cells (WBCs), platelets, and plasma. Whole blood is rarely used today due to the availability of component therapy but may be indicated in cases of massive hemorrhage where both volume replacement and oxygen-carrying capacity are needed.

2. Red Blood Cells (RBCs): Also known as packed red blood cells (PRBCs), these are used to increase the oxygen-carrying capacity of the blood in patients with anemia or acute blood loss. RBC transfusions are indicated when hemoglobin levels fall below critical thresholds or when symptoms of anemia become severe.

3. Platelets: Platelet transfusions are indicated for patients with thrombocytopenia (low platelet count) or platelet dysfunction who are at risk for bleeding. They are commonly used in patients undergoing chemotherapy, those with aplastic anemia, or following massive transfusion protocols.

4. Plasma: Plasma is the liquid component of blood that contains clotting factors, electrolytes, and proteins. Fresh frozen plasma (FFP) is used to treat patients with coagulopathy due to liver disease, disseminated intravascular coagulation (DIC), or massive transfusion. It is also used in cases of warfarin overdose when rapid reversal is needed.

5. Cryoprecipitate: This product is rich in clotting factors such as fibrinogen, factor VIII, von Willebrand factor, and factor XIII. It is used primarily to treat conditions like hemophilia A, von Willebrand disease, and hypofibrinogenemia.

6. Albumin: Albumin solutions are used as volume expanders in patients with hypovolemia or hypoalbuminemia. They help maintain oncotic pressure and fluid balance in conditions such as burns, nephrotic syndrome, or liver cirrhosis.

7. Clotting Factor Concentrates: These include specific factor concentrates such as factor VIII or IX for patients with hemophilia or other clotting disorders. They provide targeted therapy for bleeding disorders without the need for large-volume plasma transfusions.

The administration of blood products requires careful consideration of compatibility testing (crossmatching) to prevent transfusion reactions. Medical-surgical nurses must be vigilant in monitoring for adverse reactions such as febrile non-hemolytic reactions, allergic reactions, acute hemolytic reactions, and transfusion-related acute lung injury (TRALI). Vital signs should be closely monitored before, during, and after transfusion.

Informed consent must be obtained prior to transfusion, and patients should be educated about potential risks and benefits. Documentation should include the type and amount of product administered, patient response, and any adverse events observed.

In summary, blood products are essential therapeutic agents in medical-surgical nursing care. Understanding their indications, administration protocols, and potential complications ensures safe and effective patient management. Mastery of this knowledge is crucial for success on the Medical-Surgical Nursing (MEDSURG-BC) certification exam.

2 Planning, Implementation, And Evaluation:

In the realm of medical-surgical nursing, the concepts of planning, implementation, and evaluation form the cornerstone of effective patient care management. These processes are integral to the nursing process, ensuring that patient care is both systematic and individualized.

Planning: Planning in nursing is a critical phase where nurses develop strategies to address the identified health problems of their patients. It involves setting priorities, establishing goals and expected outcomes, and selecting appropriate nursing interventions. The planning phase requires collaboration with patients and other healthcare team members to ensure that the care plan is comprehensive and feasible. Goals should be SMART: Specific, Measurable, Achievable, Relevant, and Time-bound. This means that each goal must be clearly defined, its success measurable by specific criteria, achievable given the patient's current condition and available resources, relevant to the patient's overall health objectives, and time-bound with a clear deadline for reassessment.

Implementation: Implementation is the action phase where the nurse executes the care plan. This involves performing nursing interventions as outlined in the plan of care. These interventions can be direct or indirect actions aimed at improving patient outcomes. Direct care interventions include activities such as administering medications, providing wound care, or educating patients and their families. Indirect care involves actions such as documentation, coordination of care with other healthcare professionals, and advocacy on behalf of the patient. During implementation, it is crucial for nurses to use clinical judgment to adapt interventions as needed based on ongoing assessments of patient responses.

Effective communication skills are vital during this phase to ensure that all team members are informed of any changes in patient status or care requirements. Nurses must also maintain accurate documentation of all interventions performed and the patient responses to these interventions.

Evaluation: Evaluation is an ongoing process that occurs throughout all phases of nursing care but is formally addressed after implementation. It involves assessing whether the goals and expected outcomes have been achieved. This step requires critical thinking and analysis to determine if the interventions were successful or if revisions are necessary.

During evaluation, nurses compare actual patient outcomes with expected outcomes to determine effectiveness. If goals are not met or only partially met, nurses must reassess the situation to identify barriers to success and modify the plan accordingly. This may involve revisiting assessment data to ensure accuracy or adjusting goals or interventions based on new information or changes in the patient's condition.

Evaluation also provides an opportunity for reflection on practice and professional development. By analyzing what worked well and what did not, nurses can improve their clinical skills and knowledge base for future practice.

In conclusion, planning, implementation, and evaluation are dynamic processes that require critical thinking, clinical expertise, and effective communication skills. They ensure that nursing care is tailored to meet individual patient needs while promoting optimal health outcomes. For medical-surgical nurses preparing for the MEDSURG-BC exam, mastering these processes is essential for delivering high-quality, patient-centered care in diverse healthcare settings. Understanding how to effectively plan, implement, and evaluate nursing interventions will not only aid in exam success but also enhance professional practice throughout one's nursing career.

2.1.1 Nursing Care Planning:

Nursing care planning is a critical component of the nursing process, serving as a structured framework for identifying and addressing patient needs through individualized care strategies. It involves the systematic development of a plan that outlines specific nursing interventions tailored to achieve desired health outcomes for patients. The nursing care plan acts as a roadmap that guides nurses in delivering holistic, patient-centered care, ensuring that all aspects of the patient's health are addressed comprehensively.

The process of nursing care planning begins with a thorough assessment of the patient. This initial step involves collecting and analyzing data related to the patient's physical, psychological, social, and spiritual health. Nurses gather information through observation, interviews, physical examinations, and reviewing medical records. This comprehensive assessment forms the foundation for identifying actual or potential health problems that require intervention.

Once the assessment is complete, nurses move on to the diagnosis phase. Here, they use clinical judgment to interpret the data collected and identify nursing diagnoses. These diagnoses are distinct from medical diagnoses and focus on the patient's response to health conditions or life processes. Nursing diagnoses provide a basis for selecting appropriate interventions and setting achievable goals.

The next step in nursing care planning is formulating goals and expected outcomes. Goals are broad statements that reflect what the patient will achieve as a result of nursing interventions. Expected outcomes are specific, measurable criteria used to evaluate whether goals have been met. Goals and outcomes must be realistic, patient-centered, and time-bound to ensure they are attainable within the context of the patient's condition and resources.

Following goal setting, nurses develop individualized nursing interventions designed to address each identified diagnosis. These interventions can include direct care activities such as administering medications or performing wound care, as well as indirect actions like coordinating with other healthcare professionals or providing patient education. The selection of interventions is based on evidence-based practice, clinical expertise, and patient preferences.

Implementation is the phase where nurses put the care plan into action. This involves carrying out the planned interventions while continuously monitoring the patient's response. Effective communication and collaboration with other members of the healthcare team are essential during this phase to ensure coordinated care delivery.

Evaluation is the final step in the nursing care planning process. During evaluation, nurses assess whether the goals and expected outcomes have been achieved. This involves comparing actual patient outcomes with those predicted in the care plan. If goals are not met or if new issues arise, nurses must reassess and modify the care plan accordingly. This iterative process ensures that nursing care remains responsive to changes in the patient's condition.

Nursing care planning is not a static process but rather a dynamic one that requires ongoing assessment and adaptation. It emphasizes critical thinking, clinical reasoning, and decision-making skills to provide safe and effective care. Through careful planning, implementation, and evaluation, nurses play a pivotal role in promoting positive patient outcomes and enhancing the overall quality of care.

In summary, nursing care planning is an essential aspect of professional nursing practice that involves assessing patient needs, diagnosing responses to health conditions, setting goals, implementing interventions, and evaluating outcomes. By following this structured approach, medical-surgical nurses can deliver comprehensive and individualized care that meets the unique needs of each patient while adhering to best practices in nursing standards.

2.1.1.1 Interventions:

In the context of nursing care planning, interventions are specific actions and strategies that nurses implement to address patient needs, achieve desired health outcomes, and promote overall well-being. These interventions are based on the nursing diagnosis and are an integral part of the nursing process, which involves assessment, diagnosis, planning, implementation, and evaluation.

Interventions are categorized into three main types: independent, dependent, and interdependent (or collaborative). Independent nursing interventions are actions that a nurse can perform without a physician's order. These include activities such as educating patients on self-care practices, providing emotional support, and performing basic care procedures like repositioning a patient to prevent pressure ulcers. Independent interventions rely on a nurse's clinical judgment and expertise.

Dependent nursing interventions require an order from a physician or another healthcare provider. These interventions involve tasks such as administering medications, performing wound care as prescribed, or initiating intravenous therapy. Nurses must have a comprehensive understanding of these orders to ensure they are executed safely and effectively.

Interdependent or collaborative interventions involve working alongside other healthcare team members to provide comprehensive care. This could include coordinating with physical therapists for rehabilitation exercises or collaborating with dietitians to create a nutrition plan tailored to the patient's needs. Effective communication and teamwork are essential for successful collaborative interventions.

The selection of appropriate interventions is guided by evidence-based practice. This means that nurses use the best available research findings, clinical expertise, and patient preferences to determine the most effective strategies for care. Evidence-based practice ensures that interventions are not only scientifically sound but also tailored to individual patient circumstances.

Once interventions are selected, they must be clearly documented in the nursing care plan. Documentation should include detailed descriptions of each intervention, including frequency, duration, and any specific instructions necessary for implementation. This ensures continuity of care and allows all members of the healthcare team to understand the planned approach.

During the implementation phase, nurses carry out the planned interventions while continuously assessing the patient's response. This requires critical thinking skills to adapt interventions as needed based on real-time observations and feedback from the patient. For example, if a pain management intervention is not achieving the desired effect, adjustments may be necessary to better address the patient's discomfort.

Evaluation is an ongoing process that involves determining the effectiveness of interventions in achieving desired outcomes. Nurses assess whether goals have been met and make necessary modifications to the care plan based on evaluation findings. If an intervention is not yielding expected results, alternative strategies may be explored.

In summary, interventions are a cornerstone of nursing care planning and play a crucial role in promoting patient health and recovery. They encompass a range of activities, from independent actions performed by nurses to collaborative efforts involving multiple disciplines. The success of these interventions hinges on their alignment with evidence-based practice, thorough documentation, skilled implementation, and rigorous evaluation. By mastering these elements, medical-surgical nurses can ensure high-quality care that meets the complex needs of their patients while effectively preparing for the Medical Surgical Nursing (MEDSURG-BC) certification exam.

2.1.1.2 Modifications:

In the context of nursing care planning, modifications refer to the strategic adjustments made to the initial nursing care plan based on ongoing assessments, patient responses, and evolving clinical conditions. These modifications are crucial for ensuring that the care provided is responsive, individualized, and effective in meeting the dynamic needs of patients.

A comprehensive understanding of modifications involves recognizing their role in the nursing process. Initially, a nursing care plan is developed based on a thorough assessment of the patient's condition, needs, and goals. However, as patients respond to interventions or as their conditions change, nurses must be prepared to modify these plans. This adaptability is essential for delivering high-quality care and optimizing patient outcomes.

The process of making modifications begins with continuous assessment. Nurses gather data through observation, patient interviews, physical examinations, and monitoring vital signs. This information is compared against expected outcomes and baseline data. If discrepancies arise or if new issues are identified, it signals the need for potential modifications.

For example, consider a patient recovering from surgery who was initially expected to ambulate independently within two days. If the patient experiences unexpected pain or complications that impede mobility, the nurse must modify the care plan to include additional pain management strategies or assistive devices to facilitate movement.

Modifications can include changes in interventions, goals, or even priorities within the care plan. Interventions may be adjusted in terms of frequency, intensity, or type. For instance, if a patient's wound is not healing as anticipated with standard dressing changes, a nurse might modify the plan to incorporate advanced wound care techniques or consult with a wound care specialist.

Goals may also need modification if they prove unrealistic or if patient progress exceeds expectations. For instance, if a patient's rehabilitation progresses more rapidly than planned, goals can be adjusted to reflect higher levels of function and independence.

Prioritization within the care plan may shift as well. A patient's condition might evolve such that new issues take precedence over previously identified problems. In such cases, nurses must reprioritize interventions to address the most pressing needs first.

Effective communication and collaboration are essential components of implementing modifications. Nurses must communicate changes in the care plan to all members of the healthcare team to ensure continuity of care. This includes discussing rationales for modifications with patients and their families to maintain transparency and encourage adherence to the revised plan.

Documentation is another critical aspect of making modifications. Detailed records of assessments leading to modifications, the changes made, and patient responses provide a comprehensive account that supports continuity of care and legal accountability.

Furthermore, nurses must evaluate the effectiveness of modifications through ongoing assessments. This iterative process ensures that adjustments lead to desired outcomes and informs further refinements as needed.

In summary, modifications in nursing care planning are essential for providing responsive and individualized patient care. They involve adjusting interventions, goals, and priorities based on continuous assessment and evaluation of patient responses and conditions. By maintaining flexibility and open communication within the healthcare team and with patients, nurses can ensure that care plans remain relevant and effective throughout the patient's healthcare journey. This dynamic approach not only optimizes patient outcomes but also enhances the overall quality of nursing practice in medical-surgical settings.

2.1.1.3 Outcomes:

In the context of nursing care planning, Outcomes refer to the anticipated, measurable changes in a patient's health status or behavior that result from specific nursing interventions. Outcomes serve as benchmarks for evaluating the effectiveness of nursing care and are integral to the nursing process. They are patient-centered goals that guide the planning and implementation phases, ensuring that care is tailored to meet the individual needs of patients.

A comprehensive understanding of outcomes involves recognizing their role in enhancing the quality, safety, and satisfaction of patient care. Outcomes are typically classified into short-term and long-term categories. Short-term outcomes are expected to be achieved in a relatively brief period, often within hours to days, and focus on immediate improvements in patient conditions. Long-term outcomes, on the other hand, are achieved over weeks or months and pertain to sustained changes in health status or behavior.

The formulation of outcomes begins with a thorough assessment of the patient's current condition and needs. This involves collecting data through various methods such as physical examinations, patient interviews, and reviewing medical records. Based on this assessment, nurses identify specific problems or diagnoses that require intervention.

Once problems are identified, outcomes are developed using a SMART framework—Specific, Measurable, Achievable, Relevant, and Time-bound. This framework ensures that each outcome is clearly defined and provides a precise target for evaluation. For instance, instead of stating a vague outcome like improve mobility, a SMART outcome would specify, the patient will ambulate 50 feet with assistance by the end of two days.

Measurability is crucial for determining whether an outcome has been achieved. This involves setting quantifiable criteria that can be objectively assessed. For example, measuring pain reduction using a numerical pain scale allows nurses to evaluate progress accurately.

Achievability considers the patient's condition and the resources available. Outcomes should be realistic given the patient's health status and potential barriers, such as limited mobility or cognitive impairments. Setting achievable outcomes prevents frustration for both patients and healthcare providers.

Relevance ensures that outcomes align with the patient's overall care plan and priorities. They should address significant health issues that impact the patient's quality of life or recovery process. Engaging patients in setting relevant outcomes fosters collaboration and increases their motivation to participate actively in their care.

Time-bound outcomes establish a clear timeline for achievement, promoting timely evaluation and adjustment of care plans if necessary. This aspect is essential for maintaining momentum in patient progress and ensuring that interventions remain effective over time.

Evaluation is an ongoing process where nurses assess whether outcomes have been met based on established criteria. If outcomes are not met, it prompts a re-evaluation of the care plan to identify potential barriers or ineffective interventions. This iterative process allows for continuous improvement in patient care.

In summary, outcomes are critical components of nursing care planning that guide interventions and evaluate effectiveness. By setting SMART outcomes tailored to individual patient needs, nurses can enhance the quality of care provided while ensuring it remains patient-centered and goal-oriented. Understanding how to effectively develop and evaluate outcomes is essential for medical-surgical nurses preparing for the MEDSURG-BC exam, as it underscores their role in delivering high-quality healthcare services that improve patient outcomes across diverse clinical settings.

2.1.2 Postoperative Complication Strategies:

Postoperative complication prevention and management are critical aspects of medical-surgical nursing, focusing on identifying, preventing, and managing complications that may arise following surgical procedures. Effective postoperative care is essential to ensure patient safety, promote recovery, and minimize the risk of complications that can lead to prolonged hospital stays, increased healthcare costs, and adverse patient outcomes.

The prevention of postoperative complications begins with thorough preoperative assessments. This involves evaluating the patient's medical history, current health status, and potential risk factors for complications. Nurses play a vital role in educating patients about the surgical procedure, expected outcomes, and postoperative care instructions. This education helps set realistic expectations and encourages patient compliance with postoperative care plans.

Intraoperative measures also contribute significantly to preventing postoperative complications. Maintaining aseptic techniques, ensuring proper positioning during surgery, and monitoring vital signs are crucial for minimizing the risk of infections, pressure injuries, and other intraoperative complications.

Postoperatively, nurses must conduct comprehensive assessments to detect early signs of complications. Frequent monitoring of vital signs, wound assessments, pain evaluation, and observation for signs of infection are essential components of postoperative care. Early detection allows for timely intervention, reducing the severity of complications.

Pain management is a critical aspect of postoperative care. Effective pain control not only enhances patient comfort but also facilitates early mobilization and respiratory function. Nurses should assess pain regularly using appropriate pain scales and administer analgesics as prescribed while monitoring for adverse effects.

Preventing infections is a primary focus in postoperative care. Nurses must adhere to strict hand hygiene practices and follow protocols for wound care and dressing changes. Educating patients on signs of infection and proper wound care techniques empowers them to participate actively in their recovery process.

Thromboembolism prevention is another key area in postoperative management. Nurses should assess patients for risk factors such as immobility, obesity, or a previous history of thromboembolic events. Implementing interventions like early ambulation, leg exercises, and the use of compression devices or anticoagulant therapy can significantly reduce the risk of deep vein thrombosis (DVT) or pulmonary embolism (PE).

Respiratory complications such as atelectasis or pneumonia are common after surgery. Encouraging deep breathing exercises, using incentive spirometry, and promoting early mobilization are effective strategies to prevent these complications. Positioning patients appropriately and ensuring adequate hydration also support respiratory function.

Gastrointestinal complications like nausea, vomiting, or ileus can hinder recovery. Nurses should monitor bowel sounds, encourage gradual dietary progression as tolerated, and administer antiemetics or prokinetic agents if necessary.

Fluid and electrolyte imbalances can occur postoperatively due to blood loss or fluid shifts during surgery. Close monitoring of intake and output, laboratory values, and signs of dehydration or overload is essential for maintaining homeostasis.

Finally, effective communication among healthcare team members is crucial in managing postoperative complications. Interdisciplinary collaboration ensures comprehensive care planning and timely interventions.

In summary, postoperative complication prevention and management involve a multifaceted approach encompassing preoperative preparation, vigilant intraoperative practices, thorough postoperative assessments, patient education, effective pain management, infection control measures, thromboembolism prevention strategies, respiratory support techniques, gastrointestinal care considerations, fluid balance monitoring, and interdisciplinary communication. By implementing these strategies diligently, medical-surgical nurses play a pivotal role in optimizing patient outcomes following surgical procedures.

2.1.2.1 Bleeding:

Bleeding, also known as hemorrhage, refers to the loss of blood from the circulatory system. It can occur internally, where blood leaks from damaged blood vessels inside the body, or externally, through a natural opening or a break in the skin. In the context of postoperative care, bleeding is a critical complication that requires prompt identification and management to prevent significant morbidity and mortality.

Postoperative bleeding can be classified into primary, reactionary, and secondary bleeding. Primary bleeding occurs during surgery and is typically controlled by the surgeon. Reactionary bleeding happens within 24 hours post-surgery due to factors such as increased blood pressure or dislodgement of clots. Secondary bleeding occurs several days after surgery, often due to infection or the erosion of a blood vessel.

The pathophysiology of postoperative bleeding involves various mechanisms. Surgical trauma can damage blood vessels, leading to immediate bleeding. Coagulation disorders, whether pre-existing or acquired perioperatively, can impair clot formation. Medications such as anticoagulants or antiplatelet agents may exacerbate bleeding tendencies. Additionally, conditions like hypertension or liver dysfunction can contribute to an increased risk of bleeding.

Clinically, signs of postoperative bleeding include visible external bleeding at the surgical site, hematoma formation, ecchymosis, hypotension, tachycardia, and decreased urine output. Internally, patients may present with abdominal distension if intra-abdominal bleeding occurs or respiratory distress if there is thoracic involvement. Hemoglobin and hematocrit levels may drop upon laboratory evaluation.

Management of postoperative bleeding requires a systematic approach. The initial assessment should focus on hemodynamic stability; vital signs must be monitored closely for indications of hypovolemia or shock. Intravenous access should be secured for fluid resuscitation and potential transfusion of blood products if indicated by significant blood loss or symptomatic anemia.

Local measures to control external bleeding include applying direct pressure to the site and elevating the affected area if feasible. For internal bleeding or when conservative measures fail, surgical intervention may be necessary to identify and repair the source of hemorrhage.

Pharmacologic interventions may involve reversing anticoagulation with agents such as vitamin K for warfarin reversal or protamine sulfate for heparin reversal. In cases where coagulopathy is suspected, fresh frozen plasma or platelet transfusions may be required to restore hemostasis.

Preventive strategies are integral in minimizing the risk of postoperative bleeding. Preoperative assessment should identify patients at higher risk due to coagulopathy or medication use. Optimizing medical conditions preoperatively and ensuring appropriate cessation or adjustment of anticoagulant therapy is crucial. Intraoperative techniques that minimize tissue trauma and ensure meticulous hemostasis are essential components of prevention.

Education for healthcare providers regarding early recognition and standardized protocols for management can significantly improve patient outcomes. Nurses play a pivotal role in monitoring for signs of bleeding, administering medications as prescribed, and educating patients about symptoms that warrant immediate attention.

In conclusion, postoperative bleeding is a significant complication that necessitates prompt recognition and intervention by medical-surgical nurses. Understanding its pathophysiology, clinical presentation, and management strategies is vital for ensuring patient safety and optimal recovery outcomes following surgery. Through vigilant monitoring and effective communication within the healthcare team, nurses can contribute significantly to preventing adverse events associated with postoperative hemorrhage.

2.1.2.2 Infection:

Infection is a critical concern in the postoperative setting, representing a significant complication that can impact patient recovery and outcomes. It occurs when pathogenic microorganisms such as bacteria, viruses, fungi, or parasites invade the body, proliferate, and elicit an immune response. In the context of surgery, infections can develop at the site of the incision (surgical site infections or SSIs), within the organ space involved in the procedure, or systemically if pathogens enter the bloodstream.

Surgical site infections are among the most common types of postoperative infections. They are classified into superficial incisional, deep incisional, and organ/space infections. Superficial incisional infections involve only the skin and subcutaneous tissue of the incision, while deep incisional infections extend into the fascial and muscle layers. Organ/space infections occur in any part of the anatomy other than the incision that was opened or manipulated during surgery.

The risk factors for postoperative infections include patient-related factors such as age, nutritional status, diabetes, obesity, smoking, immunosuppression, and colonization with resistant organisms. Procedural factors include the type and duration of surgery, the use of prosthetic implants, and adherence to aseptic techniques during surgery. Environmental factors, such as operating room sterility and postoperative wound care, also play significant roles.

Prevention of infection is paramount in surgical practice. Preoperative measures include optimizing patient health by controlling blood glucose levels in diabetics, encouraging smoking cessation, and possibly using antiseptic showers. Prophylactic antibiotics are often administered within one hour before incision to reduce microbial load at the surgical site. Intraoperative strategies focus on maintaining sterile technique, minimizing operative time, and ensuring proper ventilation in operating rooms to reduce airborne contaminants.

Postoperatively, vigilant monitoring for signs of infection is crucial. These signs include redness, warmth, swelling around the incision site, fever, increased pain at the site of surgery, purulent drainage from the wound, and delayed healing. Laboratory tests such as white blood cell count and cultures may be employed to identify pathogens and guide antibiotic therapy.

Management of postoperative infections involves both pharmacological and non-pharmacological interventions. Antibiotic therapy should be targeted based on culture results to effectively eradicate the causative organism while minimizing the development of resistance. In cases where abscess formation occurs or necrotic tissue is present, surgical intervention may be necessary to drain purulent material or debride infected tissue.

Additionally, supportive care measures such as adequate nutrition to support immune function and wound healing are essential components of infection management. Pain management should be optimized to ensure patient comfort and facilitate mobility and respiratory function.

The role of medical-surgical nurses in preventing and managing postoperative infections is pivotal. Nurses are responsible for implementing evidence-based practices such as hand hygiene protocols, maintaining sterile dressing changes, educating patients about signs of infection to watch for after discharge, and ensuring adherence to prescribed antibiotic regimens.

In conclusion, understanding the dynamics of infection in the postoperative period allows medical-surgical nurses to play a crucial role in prevention and early detection. By employing comprehensive strategies that encompass preoperative optimization, meticulous intraoperative technique, and vigilant postoperative care, nurses can significantly reduce infection rates and improve surgical outcomes for patients.

2.1.2.3 Emboli:

An embolus refers to a substance that travels through the bloodstream and lodges in a blood vessel, causing an obstruction. This obstruction can lead to serious complications, particularly if it occurs in vital organs such as the lungs, brain, or heart. Emboli can be composed of various materials, including blood clots, fat globules, air bubbles, or other foreign substances. Understanding the nature and management of emboli is crucial for medical-surgical nurses to effectively prevent postoperative complications.

One of the most common types of emboli is thromboembolism, which originates from a thrombus or blood clot. Thromboemboli often result from deep vein thrombosis (DVT), where clots form in the deep veins of the legs. If these clots dislodge, they can travel to the lungs and cause a pulmonary embolism (PE), a potentially life-threatening condition characterized by sudden shortness of breath, chest pain, and hypoxia.

Fat embolism syndrome (FES) is another type of embolic event that typically occurs after orthopedic trauma or surgery, especially involving long bones like the femur. Fat globules released into the circulation can obstruct pulmonary capillaries and systemic circulation, leading to respiratory distress, neurological symptoms, and a petechial rash.

Air embolism is less common but can occur during surgical procedures or intravenous therapy when air enters the venous or arterial system. In significant volumes, air emboli can obstruct blood flow and cause ischemia in critical organs.

The pathophysiology of emboli involves mechanical obstruction of blood vessels, leading to impaired perfusion and oxygenation of tissues distal to the site of occlusion. The severity of symptoms depends on the size and location of the embolus. For instance, cerebral embolism can result in a stroke, with symptoms ranging from mild neurological deficits to severe paralysis or death.

Prevention strategies for emboli are paramount in postoperative care. Medical-surgical nurses play a vital role in implementing prophylactic measures such as early mobilization of patients, the use of compression stockings or pneumatic devices, and the administration of anticoagulant medications like heparin or low-molecular-weight heparin (LMWH) as prescribed.

In cases where an embolic event is suspected, prompt recognition and intervention are crucial. Diagnostic tools such as Doppler ultrasound for DVT or computed tomography pulmonary angiography (CTPA) for PE are essential for confirming diagnoses. Treatment modalities may include anticoagulation therapy to prevent further clot formation or thrombolytic therapy to dissolve existing clots in severe cases.

Medical-surgical nurses must also be vigilant in monitoring patients for signs and symptoms indicative of embolic events. For instance, sudden onset dyspnea, tachypnea, pleuritic chest pain, hemoptysis, or unexplained hypoxemia may suggest pulmonary embolism. Neurological changes such as confusion, altered mental status, or focal deficits could indicate cerebral embolism.

In summary, emboli represent a significant risk factor for postoperative complications that require proactive prevention and management strategies. Medical-surgical nurses must be equipped with knowledge about different types of emboli, their pathophysiology, clinical manifestations, diagnostic approaches, and treatment options to ensure optimal patient outcomes. By maintaining vigilance and employing evidence-based interventions, nurses can effectively mitigate the risks associated with embolic events in surgical patients.

2.1.3 Patient Teaching:

Patient teaching is a fundamental component of medical-surgical nursing that involves educating patients and their families about health conditions, treatments, procedures, and self-care strategies. This process empowers patients to take an active role in their own healthcare, promoting better health outcomes, adherence to treatment plans, and an enhanced quality of life. Effective patient teaching requires the integration of communication skills, cultural competence, and evidence-based practice.

The primary goal of patient teaching is to ensure that patients understand their medical conditions and the necessary steps to manage them effectively. It involves explaining complex medical information in a way that is accessible and understandable to individuals with varying levels of health literacy. Nurses must assess each patient's learning needs, preferences, and potential barriers to learning, such as cognitive impairment or language differences.

One key aspect of patient teaching is the development of individualized education plans. These plans should be tailored to the specific needs and circumstances of each patient. For instance, a patient with diabetes may need education on blood glucose monitoring, dietary modifications, and insulin administration. In contrast, a patient recovering from surgery may require instructions on wound care, pain management, and activity restrictions.

Effective patient teaching also involves the use of various educational tools and resources. Visual aids, such as diagrams or videos, can enhance understanding for visual learners. Written materials should be clear and concise, avoiding medical jargon whenever possible. Interactive approaches, such as teach-back methods where patients repeat the information in their own words, can help reinforce learning and confirm comprehension.

Cultural competence plays a crucial role in patient teaching. Nurses must be aware of cultural beliefs and practices that may influence a patient's perception of illness and healthcare. Respecting these beliefs while providing accurate information is essential to building trust and ensuring effective communication. Additionally, involving family members or caregivers in the teaching process can provide additional support and reinforce learning.

Evaluation is an integral part of patient teaching. Nurses should assess the effectiveness of their teaching by observing changes in patient behavior or through direct feedback from the patient. If necessary, education plans should be adjusted to address any gaps in understanding or adherence.

Documentation of patient teaching is also critical. Accurate records ensure continuity of care by informing other healthcare team members about what has been taught and any identified learning needs or challenges. This documentation should include details about the content covered, the patient's response to the teaching session, and any follow-up actions required.

In summary, patient teaching is an essential responsibility for medical-surgical nurses that directly impacts patient outcomes. By providing clear, culturally sensitive education tailored to individual needs, nurses can empower patients to manage their health conditions effectively. This process requires ongoing assessment, adaptation, and evaluation to ensure that patients receive the support they need to navigate their healthcare journeys successfully. As such, mastery of patient teaching techniques is a critical competency for those preparing for the Medical-Surgical Nursing (MEDSURG-BC) certification exam.

2.1.3.1 Learning Preferences:

Learning preferences refer to the various ways in which individuals prefer to acquire, process, and retain information. In the context of medical-surgical nursing, understanding a patient's learning preferences is crucial for effective patient education, which is a significant component of nursing care. Recognizing these preferences allows nurses to tailor educational interventions, ensuring that patients understand their health conditions and the necessary self-care measures.

There are several models and theories regarding learning preferences, but one of the most widely recognized is the VARK model, which categorizes learning preferences into four main types: Visual, Auditory, Reading/Writing, and Kinesthetic.

1. Visual Learners: These individuals learn best through seeing. They prefer information presented in charts, graphs, diagrams, and other visual formats. For medical-surgical nurses, using visual aids such as anatomical models or videos can enhance understanding for visual learners. It's important to ensure that any visual materials are clear and directly related to the topic being taught.

2. Auditory Learners: Auditory learners absorb information more effectively when it is presented through listening. They benefit from discussions, lectures, and verbal instructions. Nurses can support auditory learners by engaging them in conversations about their condition or treatment plan and encouraging them to ask questions. Recording instructions or providing access to podcasts or audio resources can also be beneficial.

3. Reading/Writing Learners: These learners prefer information displayed as words. They thrive on reading texts and writing notes. For such patients, providing written materials like brochures, handouts, or detailed instructions will be most effective. Encouraging them to take notes during discussions can also reinforce their learning.

4. Kinesthetic Learners: Kinesthetic learners need to engage in physical activities to understand and remember information. They benefit from hands-on experiences such as demonstrations or practice sessions. In a medical-surgical setting, this might include allowing patients to practice wound care or use medical devices under supervision.

In addition to these primary learning preferences, it is essential for nurses to recognize that individuals may exhibit a combination of these styles rather than fitting neatly into one category. Therefore, a multimodal approach often proves effective in patient education.

To identify a patient's learning preferences, nurses can employ several strategies:

- Assessment Tools: Use formal assessment tools or questionnaires designed to determine learning preferences.

- Observation: Pay attention to how patients respond during teaching sessions; their engagement levels can provide clues about their preferred learning style.

- Patient Feedback: Encourage patients to express what methods they find most helpful when receiving new information.

Once learning preferences are identified, nurses should adapt their teaching strategies accordingly:

- Use diverse educational materials that cater to different learning styles.

- Provide opportunities for repetition and reinforcement of information through various modalities.

- Engage family members or caregivers who may also have distinct learning preferences but play a crucial role in supporting the patient's care plan.

Understanding and incorporating learning preferences into patient education not only enhances comprehension but also empowers patients by promoting self-efficacy and adherence to treatment regimens. As medical-surgical nurses prepare for the MEDSURG-BC exam, mastering this aspect of patient teaching is vital for delivering holistic and patient-centered care.

2.1.3.2 Barriers:

In the context of patient teaching, barriers refer to any obstacles that impede effective communication and understanding between healthcare professionals and patients. These barriers can significantly affect patients' ability to comprehend medical instructions, adhere to treatment plans, and make informed decisions about their healthcare. Understanding these barriers is crucial for medical-surgical nurses aiming to provide optimal patient education and care.

1. Language Barriers: Language differences are among the most common barriers in patient education. When patients do not speak the same language as their healthcare providers, it can lead to misunderstandings and miscommunications. Medical-surgical nurses must be aware of this barrier and utilize interpreters or translation services to ensure clear communication.

2. Cultural Barriers: Cultural differences can influence how patients perceive illness, treatment, and healthcare systems. Patients from diverse cultural backgrounds may have unique beliefs and practices that affect their acceptance of medical advice. Nurses should be culturally competent, respecting and integrating cultural considerations into patient education.

3. Literacy Barriers: Health literacy is the ability to understand health information and make informed decisions. Patients with low health literacy may struggle to comprehend medical jargon or instructions. Simplifying language, using visual aids, and confirming understanding through teach-back methods can help overcome this barrier.

4. Emotional Barriers: Patients experiencing anxiety, fear, or stress may have difficulty processing information effectively. Emotional distress can hinder concentration and memory retention. Nurses should create a supportive environment, address emotional concerns, and provide reassurance to facilitate learning.

5. Cognitive Barriers: Cognitive impairments due to conditions such as dementia or brain injury can limit a patient's ability to understand and retain information. Tailoring educational strategies to the patient's cognitive level and involving family members or caregivers in the teaching process can be beneficial.

6. Physical Barriers: Physical disabilities, such as hearing or vision impairments, can obstruct communication. Nurses should use adaptive communication techniques, such as providing written materials in large print for visually impaired patients or utilizing sign language interpreters for those who are deaf.

7. Environmental Barriers: The setting in which education takes place can also impact its effectiveness. A noisy or chaotic environment may distract patients from focusing on educational content. Ensuring a quiet, comfortable space for teaching sessions is essential.

8. Time Constraints: Limited time for patient interactions is a significant barrier in busy clinical settings. Nurses must prioritize key information and use efficient teaching strategies to maximize the effectiveness of brief encounters.

9. Motivational Barriers: A lack of motivation or interest in learning about their condition can prevent patients from engaging with educational efforts. Identifying personal motivators and emphasizing the benefits of adherence to treatment plans can enhance patient motivation.

10. Technological Barriers: With the increasing use of digital tools in healthcare education, some patients may face challenges related to technology use due to a lack of access or familiarity with digital devices. Providing alternative formats for educational materials ensures inclusivity.

Addressing these barriers requires a multifaceted approach tailored to each patient's unique needs and circumstances. Medical-surgical nurses must employ effective communication skills, cultural competence, empathy, and creativity in developing personalized educational plans that overcome these obstacles. By doing so, they enhance patient comprehension, adherence, and overall health outcomes, ultimately contributing to safer and more effective care delivery within the medical-surgical nursing practice.

2.1.3.3 Evaluation Of Learning:

Evaluation of learning in the context of patient teaching is a critical component of the nursing process that involves assessing the extent to which patients have acquired the intended knowledge, skills, and attitudes from educational interventions. This evaluation is essential for ensuring that patients understand their health conditions, treatment plans, and self-care responsibilities, which ultimately contributes to improved health outcomes and patient safety.

To begin with, the evaluation of learning should be an ongoing process that occurs throughout the patient education experience. It is not merely a final step but an integral part of each interaction between the nurse and the patient. This continuous assessment allows nurses to identify any gaps in understanding or barriers to learning early on, enabling timely adjustments to the teaching plan.

There are several methods nurses can use to evaluate learning effectively. One common approach is through direct observation of the patient's ability to perform specific tasks or procedures related to their care. For instance, a nurse might observe a patient administering insulin injections or performing wound care to assess their competency and confidence in these skills.

Another method is through verbal feedback and questioning. Nurses can engage patients in discussions about their condition and treatment regimen, asking open-ended questions that require more than yes or no answers. This technique helps gauge the depth of the patient's understanding and allows for clarification of any misconceptions.

Written assessments, such as quizzes or questionnaires, can also be useful tools for evaluating learning. These assessments can be tailored to the patient's literacy level and cultural background, ensuring they are accessible and relevant. Written evaluations provide a concrete measure of knowledge retention and can highlight areas needing further instruction.

Moreover, the teach-back method is a widely recommended strategy where patients are asked to repeat information in their own words. This method not only reinforces learning but also enables nurses to assess comprehension directly. If a patient struggles with the teach-back, it may indicate a need for revisiting or simplifying the information provided.

The evaluation process should also consider patient feedback regarding the education they received. Encouraging patients to express their thoughts about what was helpful or challenging in their learning experience provides valuable insights into the effectiveness of the teaching strategies and materials used.

It is important for nurses to document the outcomes of learning evaluations meticulously. Documentation should include details about what was taught, how it was taught, how understanding was assessed, and any follow-up actions taken as a result of the evaluation. This record serves as evidence of patient education efforts and facilitates continuity of care across healthcare providers.

Finally, cultural competence plays a vital role in evaluating learning. Nurses must be sensitive to cultural differences that may influence how patients perceive health information and education. Tailoring teaching methods to align with cultural values and beliefs enhances understanding and adherence to medical advice.

In conclusion, the evaluation of learning is an essential aspect of patient teaching that requires careful planning and execution. By employing various assessment techniques and maintaining cultural sensitivity, nurses can ensure that patients are well-informed about their health conditions and capable of managing their care effectively. This process not only empowers patients but also contributes significantly to achieving positive health outcomes, making it a fundamental responsibility for medical-surgical nurses preparing for certification exams like MEDSURG-BC.

2.1.4 Education Topics:

Education topics in the context of Medical-Surgical Nursing refer to the essential areas of knowledge and skills that nurses must master to provide high-quality care to adult patients with a wide range of medical conditions. These topics encompass both theoretical understanding and practical application, ensuring that nurses are well-equipped to handle the complexities of patient care in various healthcare settings.

One of the primary education topics is Pathophysiology, which involves understanding the physiological processes associated with disease states. This knowledge allows nurses to comprehend how diseases affect the body and aids in identifying clinical manifestations and potential complications. A strong grasp of pathophysiology is crucial for making informed clinical decisions and providing effective patient education.

Pharmacology is another critical area, focusing on the study of drugs and their effects on the human body. Nurses must be knowledgeable about different classes of medications, their mechanisms of action, therapeutic uses, side effects, and interactions. This topic also includes safe medication administration practices, dosage calculations, and monitoring for adverse reactions. Mastery of pharmacology ensures that nurses can safely manage medication regimens and educate patients about their treatments.

The Nursing Process is a fundamental framework used in medical-surgical nursing practice. It involves assessment, diagnosis, planning, implementation, and evaluation. Nurses use this systematic approach to deliver individualized patient care. Proficiency in the nursing process enables nurses to conduct thorough assessments, develop accurate nursing diagnoses, create effective care plans, implement interventions, and evaluate patient outcomes.

Patient Safety is an essential education topic that focuses on minimizing risks and preventing harm to patients during healthcare delivery. This includes understanding safety protocols, infection control measures, fall prevention strategies, and error reporting systems. Nurses play a vital role in maintaining a safe environment for patients by adhering to established guidelines and continuously monitoring for potential hazards.

Health Promotion and Disease Prevention are integral components of medical-surgical nursing education. Nurses must be equipped with strategies to promote healthy lifestyles, prevent illnesses, and manage chronic conditions. This involves educating patients about nutrition, exercise, stress management, vaccinations, and regular health screenings. By emphasizing health promotion and disease prevention, nurses contribute to improving overall patient outcomes and quality of life.

Cultural Competency is an important topic that addresses the need for nurses to provide culturally sensitive care. Understanding cultural differences in beliefs, values, and practices enables nurses to communicate effectively with diverse patient populations. Culturally competent care involves respecting patients' cultural preferences and incorporating them into the care plan whenever possible.

Legal and Ethical Considerations are crucial in guiding nursing practice within legal frameworks and ethical principles. Nurses must be familiar with laws governing healthcare practice, patient rights, confidentiality issues (such as HIPAA), informed consent processes, and ethical dilemmas they may encounter in clinical settings. Upholding legal standards and ethical principles ensures that nurses provide care that is both legally compliant and morally sound.

Finally, Professional Development emphasizes the importance of lifelong learning for medical-surgical nurses. This includes staying updated with current evidence-based practices through continuing education opportunities such as workshops or conferences; participating in professional organizations; seeking certification; engaging in reflective practice; pursuing advanced degrees if desired; mentoring new nurses; and contributing to research efforts when applicable—all aimed at enhancing personal growth while advancing the nursing profession collectively.

In summary, education topics in Medical-Surgical Nursing encompass a wide range of knowledge areas necessary for providing comprehensive patient care across diverse clinical settings while promoting safety standards alongside professional growth opportunities throughout one's career journey as a nurse practitioner specializing in this field, specifically tailored towards adult populations requiring acute or chronic management interventions based on individualized assessment findings obtained through systematic evaluation processes employed consistently over time during routine encounters in dynamic healthcare environments.

2.1.4.1 Self-management:

Self-management in the context of medical-surgical nursing refers to the active participation of patients in managing their own health and medical conditions. It encompasses a range of behaviors and skills that patients must acquire to effectively handle symptoms, treatment regimens, lifestyle changes, and the psychosocial impacts associated with chronic illnesses or post-surgical recovery. For medical-surgical nurses, understanding and facilitating self-management is crucial for promoting patient autonomy, improving health outcomes, and enhancing quality of life.

Comprehensive Definition: Self-management is a dynamic process in which patients take responsibility for their health by making informed decisions and adopting healthy behaviors. This involves not only adhering to prescribed treatments but also making lifestyle adjustments, monitoring symptoms, managing stress, and seeking timely medical assistance when necessary. It requires a collaborative approach in which healthcare providers empower patients with the knowledge, skills, and confidence needed to manage their health effectively.

In-depth Explanation:

1. Patient Education: A cornerstone of self-management is patient education. Nurses play a pivotal role in educating patients about their conditions, treatment options, potential side effects, and the importance of adherence to prescribed therapies. Education should be tailored to individual patient needs, taking into account their literacy levels, cultural backgrounds, and personal preferences. Providing clear instructions and using teach-back methods can ensure that patients understand how to manage their care.

2. Skill Development: Self-management involves developing specific skills such as medication management, symptom monitoring, and problem-solving. Nurses can teach patients how to use medical devices (e.g., glucometers for diabetes management), recognize warning signs of complications (e.g., shortness of breath in heart failure), and implement action plans (e.g., adjusting insulin doses based on blood sugar readings).

3. Behavioral Strategies: Encouraging healthy behaviors is essential for effective self-management. This includes promoting regular physical activity, balanced nutrition, smoking cessation, and stress reduction techniques. Nurses can support behavior change by setting realistic goals with patients, providing motivational interviewing, and connecting them with community resources or support groups.

4. Psychosocial Support: Chronic illnesses often have significant emotional and social impacts. Nurses should assess patients' mental health status and provide support or referrals as needed. Building a therapeutic relationship can help nurses identify barriers to self-management, such as depression or lack of social support, and address these challenges through counseling or collaboration with mental health professionals.

5. Technology Utilization: Advances in technology offer new avenues for supporting self-management. Mobile health applications, telehealth services, and electronic health records can facilitate communication between patients and healthcare providers, provide reminders for medication adherence, and track health metrics over time.

6. Collaborative Care: Self-management is most effective within a collaborative care framework where nurses work alongside other healthcare professionals to deliver comprehensive care. This includes coordinating with physicians for medication adjustments, dietitians for nutritional advice, physical therapists for exercise plans, and social workers for addressing socioeconomic barriers.

7. Evaluation and Feedback: Continuous evaluation of self-management strategies is vital. Nurses should regularly assess patients' progress toward their health goals and provide feedback to reinforce positive behaviors or adjust plans as needed.

In conclusion, self-management empowers patients by giving them control over their health while ensuring they have the necessary support from healthcare professionals. By fostering an environment of education, skill-building, behavioral change, psychosocial support, technology integration, collaborative care, and ongoing evaluation, medical-surgical nurses can significantly enhance patient outcomes through effective self-management practices.

2.1.4.2 Acute And Chronic Conditions:

Acute and chronic conditions represent two fundamental categories of health issues that medical-surgical nurses must understand thoroughly to provide effective patient care. These conditions differ primarily in their onset, duration, and the nature of the treatment required.

Acute conditions are characterized by a sudden onset and are typically short-lived. They often require immediate medical attention and can range from mild to severe. Examples include appendicitis, acute myocardial infarction, pneumonia, and fractures. The management of acute conditions focuses on rapid assessment, stabilization, and treatment to alleviate symptoms and prevent complications. Nurses play a critical role in monitoring vital signs, administering medications, providing wound care, and educating patients about lifestyle modifications to prevent recurrence.

In contrast, chronic conditions develop gradually and persist over an extended period, often for the remainder of the patient's life. They include diseases such as diabetes mellitus, hypertension, chronic obstructive pulmonary disease (COPD), and heart failure. Chronic conditions require long-term management strategies aimed at controlling symptoms, slowing disease progression, and improving quality of life. This involves regular monitoring, medication adherence, lifestyle changes, and routine follow-up care. Nurses are essential in coordinating care among different healthcare providers, educating patients about self-management techniques, and supporting them in adhering to treatment plans.

Understanding the pathophysiology of both acute and chronic conditions is crucial for nurses. Acute conditions often result from infections, injuries, or sudden exacerbations of underlying diseases. For instance, an acute asthma attack occurs due to a sudden narrowing of the airways triggered by allergens or irritants. In such cases, nurses must be adept at recognizing early signs of distress and administering bronchodilators promptly.

Chronic conditions typically involve complex pathophysiological processes that may affect multiple body systems. For example, in diabetes mellitus, there is an impairment in insulin production or utilization leading to hyperglycemia. Over time, this can cause damage to various organs, including the eyes (retinopathy), kidneys (nephropathy), and nerves (neuropathy). Nurses must understand these mechanisms to anticipate potential complications and educate patients on preventive measures.

The psychosocial aspects of living with chronic conditions also demand attention. Patients may experience anxiety, depression, or social isolation due to the illness's impact on daily life. Nurses should assess mental health regularly and provide resources for counseling or support groups when necessary.

Effective communication skills are vital when dealing with both acute and chronic conditions. In acute situations, clear instructions and calm reassurance can help alleviate patient anxiety during emergencies. For chronic conditions, ongoing dialogue about treatment goals and progress fosters trust and encourages patient engagement in their care plan.

Moreover, cultural competence is essential, as patients' beliefs about health and illness may influence their acceptance of medical interventions. Understanding cultural perspectives enables nurses to tailor education and support strategies that respect individual preferences while promoting health outcomes.

In conclusion, mastery of acute and chronic conditions is integral to the role of a medical-surgical nurse. By combining clinical knowledge with compassionate care delivery, nurses can significantly impact patients' recovery from acute episodes and their ability to manage chronic illnesses effectively over time. This comprehensive understanding not only enhances patient outcomes but also contributes to the overall efficiency of healthcare systems by reducing hospital readmissions and improving the quality of life for individuals with long-term health challenges.

2.1.4.3 Population Specific:

In the realm of medical-surgical nursing, understanding population-specific care is paramount for delivering patient-centered and effective healthcare. Population-specific refers to the tailored approach in nursing care that considers the unique characteristics, needs, and challenges of different patient populations. This encompasses recognizing variations in health conditions, cultural backgrounds, age groups, socioeconomic statuses, and other demographic factors that influence health outcomes and care delivery.

A comprehensive understanding of population-specific care involves several key components:

1. Demographic Awareness: Nurses must be knowledgeable about the demographics of the population they serve. This includes age distribution, gender, ethnicity, language preferences, and cultural practices. Such awareness helps in anticipating potential health risks and tailoring interventions accordingly.

2. Cultural Competence: Cultural competence is crucial in providing respectful and effective care. Nurses should be trained to understand and respect cultural differences, including beliefs about health and illness, dietary practices, and communication styles. This competence ensures that care plans are culturally sensitive and acceptable to patients.

3. Age-Specific Considerations: Different age groups have distinct physiological and psychological needs. For instance, pediatric patients require different communication strategies and dosing considerations compared to geriatric patients, who may present with multiple comorbidities and polypharmacy concerns. Understanding developmental stages is essential for appropriate assessment and intervention.

4. Chronic Disease Prevalence: Certain populations may have a higher prevalence of specific chronic diseases due to genetic predispositions or lifestyle factors. For example, African American populations have a higher incidence of hypertension and diabetes. Recognizing these patterns allows nurses to focus on preventive measures and early interventions tailored to these groups.

5. Socioeconomic Factors: Socioeconomic status significantly impacts access to healthcare resources, adherence to treatment plans, and overall health outcomes. Nurses must consider factors such as income level, education, employment status, and housing conditions when planning care. Addressing barriers like transportation or financial constraints is essential for ensuring equitable care.

6. Health Literacy: Health literacy varies widely among populations and affects the ability to understand health information and make informed decisions. Nurses should assess the health literacy levels of their patients and adjust their communication methods accordingly—using plain language, visual aids, or interpreters when necessary.

7. Risk Assessment: Population-specific risk assessments are crucial for identifying individuals at higher risk for certain conditions based on demographic factors. This includes screening for genetic disorders prevalent in certain ethnic groups or assessing environmental exposures common in particular communities.

8. Community Resources: Understanding the resources available within a community can enhance patient support systems. Nurses should be familiar with local healthcare facilities, social services, support groups, and educational programs that can aid in patient care.

9. Legal and Ethical Considerations: Different populations may have varying legal protections or ethical concerns related to healthcare access and treatment options. Nurses must be aware of these considerations to advocate effectively for their patients' rights.

10. Patient Advocacy: Finally, nurses play a critical role in advocating for population-specific needs within the healthcare system. This includes participating in policy development, research initiatives, and educational programs aimed at addressing disparities in healthcare delivery.

In summary, population-specific care in medical-surgical nursing requires a holistic approach that integrates demographic knowledge with clinical expertise to deliver personalized care that respects individual differences while addressing broader health determinants. By focusing on these aspects, nurses can significantly improve patient outcomes across diverse populations.

2.1.5 Patient Safety Measures:

Patient safety measures are systematic protocols and practices designed to prevent harm to patients during the provision of healthcare. These measures are fundamental in ensuring that patients receive care that is safe, effective, timely, efficient, equitable, and patient-centered. The primary goal of patient safety measures is to minimize the risk of errors and adverse events in healthcare settings, ultimately improving patient outcomes.

One of the core components of patient safety measures is the implementation of standardized procedures and checklists. These tools help ensure consistency in care delivery and reduce variability, which can lead to errors. For instance, surgical safety checklists are used to confirm patient identity, surgical site, and procedure before surgery begins. This practice has been shown to significantly reduce surgical complications and improve patient outcomes.

Infection prevention and control is another critical aspect of patient safety measures. Healthcare-associated infections (HAIs) are a significant concern in medical-surgical settings. Measures such as hand hygiene protocols, the use of personal protective equipment (PPE), sterilization of instruments, and isolation precautions are implemented to prevent the spread of infections. Adhering to these protocols is essential for protecting both patients and healthcare providers from infectious diseases.

Medication safety is a vital component of patient safety measures. Errors in medication administration can have severe consequences for patients. To mitigate this risk, healthcare facilities employ strategies such as medication reconciliation, barcoding systems for medication administration, and electronic prescribing. These measures help ensure that patients receive the correct medications at the right dosages and times.

Communication among healthcare providers is crucial for maintaining patient safety. Effective communication strategies include using standardized communication tools like SBAR (Situation-Background-Assessment-Recommendation) to ensure clear and concise information exchange during handoffs or shift changes. This reduces the likelihood of errors related to miscommunication.

Patient identification processes are also integral to patient safety measures. Ensuring that patients are correctly identified before receiving any treatment or procedure helps prevent errors such as wrong-site surgery or incorrect medication administration. Techniques such as using two identifiers (e.g., name and date of birth) and wristbands with barcodes enhance accuracy in patient identification.

Fall prevention strategies are important in minimizing injury risks for patients, particularly those who are elderly or have mobility impairments. Interventions include conducting fall risk assessments upon admission, implementing bed alarms, providing non-slip footwear, and ensuring that the environment is free from hazards.

Education and training for healthcare staff play a significant role in promoting patient safety. Continuous professional development ensures that staff members are up-to-date with the latest evidence-based practices and technologies related to patient care.

Simulation training is often used to enhance clinical skills and decision-making abilities in a controlled environment without risking patient harm.

Finally, fostering a culture of safety within healthcare organizations is essential for sustaining patient safety measures. This involves encouraging open communication about errors or near misses without fear of retribution, promoting teamwork, and engaging leadership support for safety initiatives.

In summary, patient safety measures encompass a wide range of strategies aimed at preventing harm to patients within healthcare settings. By implementing standardized procedures, infection control practices, medication safety protocols, effective communication techniques, accurate patient identification processes, fall prevention strategies, continuous staff education, and fostering a culture of safety, healthcare providers can significantly enhance the quality and safety of care delivered to patients.

2.1.5.1 Screening Tools:

Screening tools are standardized instruments or checklists used in healthcare settings to identify individuals at risk for certain conditions or complications, enabling early intervention and management. In the context of medical-surgical nursing, screening tools are vital for assessing patients' risks related to various factors such as falls, pressure ulcers, nutritional deficiencies, and mental health issues. These tools help ensure patient safety and improve outcomes by facilitating timely interventions.

One of the most commonly used screening tools in medical-surgical nursing is the Morse Fall Scale. This tool evaluates a patient's likelihood of falling by assessing factors such as history of falls, secondary diagnosis, use of ambulatory aids, intravenous therapy/heparin lock, gait, and mental status. Each factor is assigned a score, and the total score determines the patient's fall risk level. Nurses can then implement appropriate fall prevention strategies based on the risk level.

Another critical screening tool is the Braden Scale for Predicting Pressure Sore Risk. This tool assesses a patient's risk of developing pressure ulcers by examining six criteria: sensory perception, moisture, activity, mobility, nutrition, and friction/shear. Each category is scored from 1 to 4 (or 1 to 3 for friction/shear), with lower scores indicating a higher risk. Nurses use this information to implement preventive measures such as repositioning schedules, skin care regimens, and specialized support surfaces.

Nutritional screening tools like the Malnutrition Universal Screening Tool (MUST) are essential for identifying patients at risk of malnutrition. MUST considers body mass index (BMI), unintentional weight loss, and the acute disease effect on nutritional intake. Based on these parameters, patients are classified into low, medium, or high risk of malnutrition. Appropriate nutritional interventions can then be planned to address identified risks.

In addition to physical health risks, mental health screening tools are also employed in medical-surgical settings. The Patient Health Questionnaire-9 (PHQ-9) is a widely used tool for screening depression. It consists of nine questions that align with the diagnostic criteria for major depressive disorder. The total score indicates the severity of depressive symptoms and guides further psychiatric evaluation or intervention if necessary.

Pain assessment is another crucial aspect of patient care in medical-surgical nursing. Tools like the Numeric Pain Rating Scale (NPRS) or Visual Analog Scale (VAS) help quantify a patient's pain intensity. These scales enable nurses to monitor pain levels effectively and adjust pain management strategies accordingly.

Screening tools must be selected based on their validity and reliability within specific patient populations. They should be easy to administer and interpret while providing actionable data that can guide clinical decision-making. Moreover, ongoing education and training are essential for nurses to effectively utilize these tools and integrate them into routine patient assessments.

In summary, screening tools are indispensable in medical-surgical nursing practice for identifying patient risks early and implementing preventive measures to enhance safety and care quality. Understanding how to apply these tools effectively allows nurses to tailor interventions that address individual patient needs, ultimately leading to better health outcomes and improved patient satisfaction. As part of preparing for the MEDSURG-BC exam, nurses should familiarize themselves with various screening tools relevant to their practice area and develop competencies in their application and interpretation to ensure optimal patient care delivery.

2.1.5.2 Infection Prevention:

Infection prevention is a critical aspect of patient safety measures in medical-surgical nursing, aimed at minimizing the risk of healthcare-associated infections (HAIs) and ensuring optimal patient outcomes. It encompasses a series of systematic practices and protocols designed to reduce the transmission of infectious agents within healthcare settings. This approach is vital for protecting both patients and healthcare personnel from potential infectious threats.

The primary goal of infection prevention is to break the chain of infection by targeting each link, including the infectious agent, reservoir, portal of exit, mode of transmission, portal of entry, and susceptible host. Medical-surgical nurses play a pivotal role in implementing these preventive measures through adherence to established guidelines and protocols.

Hand hygiene is the cornerstone of infection prevention and is recognized as the most effective way to prevent the spread of infections. Nurses must perform hand hygiene before and after patient contact, after contact with potentially contaminated surfaces or equipment, and before performing any aseptic task. The use of alcohol-based hand sanitizers is recommended when hands are not visibly soiled; otherwise, soap and water should be used.

Personal protective equipment (PPE), such as gloves, gowns, masks, and eye protection, should be utilized appropriately based on the level of exposure risk. Correct donning and doffing procedures are essential to prevent self-contamination. Medical-surgical nurses must be proficient in selecting and using PPE according to the type of care being provided and the potential for exposure to infectious agents.

Environmental cleaning and disinfection are also crucial components of infection prevention. Regular cleaning schedules should be maintained for patient rooms, common areas, and medical equipment. High-touch surfaces require frequent disinfection to reduce microbial load. Nurses should collaborate with environmental services to ensure that cleaning protocols are strictly followed.

Isolation precautions are implemented based on the mode of transmission of specific pathogens. Standard precautions are applied universally to all patients, while transmission-based precautions—contact, droplet, or airborne—are used when certain infections are known or suspected. Medical-surgical nurses must be adept at recognizing when additional precautions are necessary and ensuring that they are effectively communicated and enforced.

The use of sterile techniques during invasive procedures is imperative to prevent infections. Sterility must be maintained throughout procedures such as catheter insertions, wound care, and surgical interventions. Nurses must be vigilant about maintaining aseptic conditions and promptly addressing any breaches in sterility.

Antimicrobial stewardship is another key aspect of infection prevention. It involves the judicious use of antibiotics to minimize resistance development while ensuring effective treatment for infections. Nurses contribute by monitoring for signs of infection, obtaining cultures before antibiotic initiation when appropriate, and educating patients about the importance of completing prescribed antibiotic courses.

Patient education plays a significant role in infection prevention efforts. Nurses should educate patients and their families about proper hand hygiene practices, respiratory etiquette (such as covering coughs), wound care techniques, and recognizing signs of infection that warrant medical attention.

In conclusion, infection prevention in medical-surgical nursing requires a comprehensive approach involving multiple strategies aimed at disrupting the transmission pathways of infectious agents. By adhering to evidence-based guidelines and maintaining vigilance in practice, medical-surgical nurses can significantly reduce the incidence of HAIs, thereby enhancing patient safety and promoting positive health outcomes. Through continuous education and adherence to best practices, nurses remain at the forefront of safeguarding against infections within healthcare environments.

2.1.5.3 Restraints:

In the context of medical-surgical nursing, restraints are defined as any physical or mechanical device, material, or equipment attached to or adjacent to the patient's body that the individual cannot easily remove and that restricts freedom of movement or normal access to one's body. Restraints are employed to prevent patients from harming themselves or others and to ensure the safety of both patients and healthcare providers.

The use of restraints in a healthcare setting is a critical issue, balancing patient safety with ethical considerations and patient rights. Restraints should only be used when absolutely necessary and when other, less restrictive measures have failed. The decision to apply restraints must be made with careful consideration and in accordance with established policies and procedures.

There are two main types of restraints: physical and chemical. Physical restraints include devices such as belts, vests, mittens, limb ties, or bedrails that restrict a patient's movement. Chemical restraints involve the use of medications to control behavior or restrict movement. These medications are not part of the standard treatment for the patient's medical or psychiatric condition.

The application of restraints must adhere strictly to legal and ethical guidelines. The Joint Commission and the Centers for Medicare & Medicaid Services (CMS) have set forth standards that require healthcare facilities to have policies in place regarding restraint use. These standards emphasize that restraints should only be used when necessary to ensure immediate physical safety and should be removed at the earliest possible time.

Before applying restraints, a comprehensive assessment must be conducted by a qualified healthcare professional. This assessment should evaluate the patient's physical and mental status, behavior patterns, underlying medical conditions, and potential risks associated with restraint use. Documentation of this assessment is crucial for legal purposes and for guiding future care decisions.

When restraints are deemed necessary, informed consent should be obtained from the patient or their legal representative whenever possible. This involves explaining the reason for restraint use, potential risks, benefits, and alternatives considered. Education about restraint use should also extend to family members to ensure understanding and support.

Once applied, continuous monitoring of the patient is essential. This includes regular checks on circulation, skin integrity, hydration, nutrition, elimination needs, comfort levels, and overall well-being. The frequency of monitoring should comply with institutional policies but generally occurs every 15 minutes for high-risk patients.

Healthcare providers must also document all aspects of restraint use meticulously. This documentation includes the rationale for restraint application, the type of restraint used, the duration of use, the patient's response to restraints, any adverse effects observed, and efforts made to remove restraints at the earliest possible time.

In addition to ensuring patient safety during restraint use, nurses play a crucial role in advocating for alternative measures before resorting to restraints. These alternatives may include environmental modifications (such as reducing noise levels), de-escalation techniques (such as verbal communication), or engaging patients in activities that promote relaxation.

In conclusion, while restraints can be necessary tools in certain situations within medical-surgical nursing practice, their use must always prioritize patient dignity and rights. Nurses must remain vigilant in assessing the need for restraints, implementing them safely when required, monitoring their effects diligently, and seeking alternatives whenever feasible. By adhering to these principles, nurses contribute significantly to maintaining a safe healthcare environment while respecting individual autonomy and promoting holistic care.

2.1.5.4 Medical Equipment:

Medical equipment refers to a broad range of devices, instruments, and machines used in the diagnosis, monitoring, treatment, and care of patients within a healthcare setting. As a medical-surgical nurse preparing for the MEDSURG-BC exam, it is crucial to have an in-depth understanding of various medical equipment to ensure patient safety and effective clinical outcomes.

Medical equipment can be categorized into several types based on its function and usage. Diagnostic equipment includes tools such as X-ray machines, MRI scanners, and ultrasound devices that help identify medical conditions. Monitoring equipment encompasses devices like cardiac monitors, blood pressure monitors, and pulse oximeters that track vital signs and other physiological parameters. Therapeutic equipment includes infusion pumps, ventilators, and dialysis machines that assist in the treatment of medical conditions. Lastly, life support equipment, such as defibrillators and incubators, is critical in maintaining life during emergencies or critical care situations.

The proper use and maintenance of medical equipment are paramount for ensuring patient safety. Nurses must be adept at operating these devices, understanding their functions, and recognizing any malfunctions or inaccuracies. Regular calibration and maintenance checks are essential to ensure the reliability and accuracy of medical equipment. Familiarity with the manufacturer's guidelines for operation and troubleshooting is necessary to prevent errors that could compromise patient care.

In addition to operational knowledge, nurses must also be aware of infection control practices related to medical equipment. Many devices come into direct contact with patients or bodily fluids, necessitating stringent cleaning and sterilization protocols to prevent cross-contamination and healthcare-associated infections (HAIs). Adhering to standard precautions and employing appropriate disinfection techniques are critical components of patient safety.

Nurses should also be knowledgeable about the legal and ethical considerations associated with the use of medical equipment. This includes understanding patient consent for procedures involving certain devices, maintaining confidentiality when handling electronic health records through computerized systems, and reporting any adverse events or device malfunctions through proper channels.

Furthermore, staying updated with technological advancements in medical equipment is crucial for modern nursing practice. Continuous education and training on new devices ensure that nurses remain competent in utilizing cutting-edge technology to enhance patient care. Participation in workshops, seminars, or online courses can provide valuable insights into emerging trends and innovations in medical equipment.

Effective communication among the healthcare team is vital when dealing with medical equipment. Nurses should collaborate with biomedical engineers, physicians, and other healthcare professionals to address any issues related to device functionality or patient safety concerns. Clear documentation of equipment usage, maintenance records, and incident reports is essential for ensuring accountability and quality assurance.

Lastly, nurses should advocate for patient education regarding the medical equipment used in their care. Providing clear explanations about how certain devices work and what patients can expect during procedures helps alleviate anxiety and fosters a sense of trust between patients and healthcare providers.

In summary, a comprehensive understanding of medical equipment is integral to the role of a medical-surgical nurse. Mastery of device operation, adherence to safety protocols, awareness of legal considerations, continuous professional development, effective communication, and patient education are all essential components in ensuring optimal patient outcomes while minimizing risks associated with the use of medical equipment. As you prepare for the MEDSURG-BC exam, focus on these aspects to enhance your proficiency in managing medical equipment safely and effectively within the clinical setting.

2.1.6 Non-pharmacologic Treatments:

Non-pharmacologic treatments refer to therapeutic interventions that do not involve medications. These treatments are integral to holistic patient care, particularly in medical-surgical nursing, where a comprehensive approach is often necessary to manage complex health conditions. Non-pharmacologic interventions can be used alone or in conjunction with pharmacologic treatments to enhance patient outcomes, reduce symptoms, and improve quality of life.

A key advantage of non-pharmacologic treatments is their ability to minimize the risk of medication-related side effects and interactions. This is especially important for patients with polypharmacy concerns or those who have contraindications to certain drugs. Moreover, these treatments often empower patients by actively involving them in their own care, promoting self-efficacy and adherence to treatment plans.

Several categories of non-pharmacologic treatments are commonly utilized in medical-surgical settings:

1. Physical Therapy and Exercise: These interventions aim to improve physical function, mobility, and strength. Physical therapy may include exercises tailored to the patient's specific needs, such as range-of-motion exercises, strengthening routines, and aerobic activities. Exercise has been shown to alleviate symptoms in conditions like arthritis, cardiovascular diseases, and postoperative recovery.

2. Cognitive-Behavioral Therapy (CBT): CBT is a structured psychological intervention that helps patients modify negative thought patterns and behaviors. It is effective in managing chronic pain, anxiety, depression, and insomnia. By addressing the psychological aspects of illness, CBT can reduce distress and enhance coping strategies.

3. Relaxation Techniques: Techniques such as deep breathing exercises, progressive muscle relaxation, guided imagery, and meditation are used to reduce stress and anxiety. These methods help lower physiological responses such as heart rate and blood pressure, contributing to overall well-being.

4. Dietary Modifications: Nutrition plays a critical role in managing many medical conditions. Dietary interventions may include reducing sodium intake for hypertension management or increasing fiber intake for gastrointestinal health. Nurses play a pivotal role in educating patients about healthy eating habits tailored to their specific health needs.

5. Acupuncture and Acupressure: These traditional Chinese medicine techniques involve stimulating specific points on the body to alleviate pain and promote healing. Acupuncture has been recognized for its effectiveness in treating chronic pain conditions such as migraines and osteoarthritis.

6. Massage Therapy: This involves manipulating soft tissues to relieve muscle tension, improve circulation, and promote relaxation. Massage therapy can be beneficial for patients experiencing musculoskeletal pain or stress-related disorders.

7. Music and Art Therapy: Engaging in creative activities can provide emotional relief and enhance mental health. Music therapy has been used effectively for pain management and improving mood among patients with chronic illnesses.

8. Environmental Modifications: Adjusting the physical environment can significantly impact patient comfort and safety. This might include optimizing lighting for patients with visual impairments or ensuring accessibility for those with mobility challenges.

9. Patient Education: Educating patients about their condition and self-care strategies is a cornerstone of non-pharmacologic treatment. Knowledge empowers patients to make informed decisions about their health and adhere to recommended lifestyle changes.

In conclusion, non-pharmacologic treatments are essential components of comprehensive care in medical-surgical nursing. They offer diverse options tailored to individual patient needs, focusing on enhancing physical function, psychological well-being, and overall quality of life without relying solely on medications. As healthcare providers, nurses must be adept at assessing patient needs and implementing appropriate non-pharmacologic interventions while educating patients about the benefits of these therapies in conjunction with traditional medical treatments.

2.1.6.1 Exploring Complementary and Alternative Medicine (CAM):

Complementary and Alternative Medicine (CAM) refers to a diverse range of medical and healthcare systems, practices, and products that are not traditionally considered part of conventional Western medicine. CAM is used alongside (complementary) or in place of (alternative) standard medical treatments. The goal of CAM is to enhance the body's natural healing processes, improve overall well-being, and provide holistic care by addressing physical, emotional, mental, and spiritual health.

CAM encompasses a wide array of practices and therapies, which can be broadly categorized into several groups:

1. Mind-Body Interventions: These techniques focus on the interactions between the brain, mind, body, and behavior. Examples include meditation, yoga, tai chi, qigong, and biofeedback. These practices aim to reduce stress and enhance relaxation, thereby improving health outcomes.

2. Biologically-Based Therapies: This category includes the use of natural substances such as herbs, vitamins, minerals, and dietary supplements. Herbal medicine utilizes plant-based products for therapeutic purposes. It is crucial for medical-surgical nurses to be aware of potential interactions between these supplements and prescribed medications.

3. Manipulative and Body-Based Practices: These therapies involve the movement or manipulation of body parts. Chiropractic care and osteopathic manipulation are common examples where practitioners use their hands to adjust or massage the musculoskeletal system to relieve pain or improve function.

4. Energy Therapies: These practices are based on the belief that energy fields exist within and around the body. Examples include Reiki, therapeutic touch, and electromagnetic therapy. Practitioners aim to balance or manipulate these energy fields to promote healing.

5. Whole Medical Systems: These are complete systems of theory and practice that have evolved independently from conventional medicine. Examples include Traditional Chinese Medicine (TCM), Ayurveda, homeopathy, and naturopathy. Each system has its own unique philosophy and approach to diagnosis and treatment.

Medical-surgical nurses should understand that CAM is increasingly being integrated into patient care plans due to growing evidence supporting its efficacy in certain conditions, such as chronic pain management, anxiety reduction, and improvement of quality of life in patients with chronic illnesses.

When incorporating CAM into patient care, it is essential for nurses to conduct thorough assessments that include asking patients about their use of CAM therapies. This information helps ensure safe practice by identifying potential interactions with conventional treatments and preventing adverse effects.

Nurses should also educate themselves about the evidence base for various CAM therapies so they can provide informed guidance to patients interested in exploring these options. This includes understanding both the benefits and limitations of each therapy.

Moreover, cultural competence plays a significant role in effectively integrating CAM into patient care. Nurses must respect patients' cultural beliefs and preferences regarding health practices while ensuring that any chosen CAM therapy does not compromise safety or efficacy.

In conclusion, Complementary and Alternative Medicine offers a broad spectrum of therapies that can complement conventional medical treatments by promoting holistic care. As a medical-surgical nurse preparing for the MEDSURG-BC exam, it is important to recognize the value CAM can bring to patient-centered care while maintaining a critical perspective on its application based on current evidence-based practice guidelines. Understanding CAM allows nurses to better support their patients' diverse healthcare needs within a multidisciplinary framework.

2.1.6.2 Diversional Activities:

Diversional activities are non-pharmacologic interventions utilized in medical-surgical nursing to enhance a patient's psychological and emotional well-being by providing mental stimulation, physical engagement, and social interaction. These activities are designed to divert the patient's attention away from pain, anxiety, or distressing symptoms, thereby promoting relaxation and improving overall quality of life during hospitalization or treatment.

The concept of diversional activities is rooted in the understanding that holistic care involves addressing not just the physical but also the emotional and psychological needs of patients. These activities can be tailored to individual patient preferences, abilities, and clinical conditions, ensuring that they are both enjoyable and therapeutic.

Diversional activities encompass a wide range of options, including, but not limited to, art therapy, music therapy, pet therapy, games, reading, gardening, and social interactions. Each activity serves to engage different senses and cognitive functions, providing a comprehensive approach to patient care.

Art therapy involves the use of creative processes such as drawing, painting, or sculpting to allow patients to express themselves emotionally and explore their feelings. This can be particularly beneficial for patients who find it difficult to articulate their emotions verbally. Engaging in art can lead to reduced stress levels and improved mood.

Music therapy employs listening to or creating music as a means of enhancing well-being. Music has been shown to reduce anxiety, lower blood pressure, and improve mood. It can be particularly effective for patients with cognitive impairments or those experiencing high levels of stress.

Pet therapy involves interactions with trained animals under the supervision of healthcare professionals. The presence of animals can provide comfort, reduce stress levels, and promote social interaction. It is especially beneficial for patients who may feel isolated or anxious.

Games and puzzles stimulate cognitive function and provide an enjoyable distraction from pain or discomfort. They encourage problem-solving skills and can be adapted to suit various ages and cognitive abilities. Board games, card games, and jigsaw puzzles are common examples used in diversional therapy.

Reading materials such as books or magazines offer mental stimulation and an escape from the hospital environment. Reading can be a solitary activity or shared with others through book clubs or group discussions, fostering social interaction.

Gardening activities involve planting seeds or caring for plants within a hospital garden or indoor setting. This activity connects patients with nature and provides a sense of accomplishment. Gardening can be particularly soothing for patients experiencing anxiety or depression.

Social interactions facilitated by nurses or volunteers include conversations, group activities, or support groups that encourage communication among patients. These interactions help build a sense of community and belonging within the healthcare setting.

In implementing diversional activities, nurses must assess each patient's interests, cognitive level, physical ability, cultural background, and medical condition to ensure appropriateness and safety. Tailoring these activities requires creativity and flexibility from healthcare providers.

The benefits of diversional activities are multifaceted; they promote relaxation, enhance coping mechanisms, reduce the perception of pain, decrease anxiety levels, improve mood states, foster patient autonomy through choice-making opportunities, and ultimately contribute to a more positive healthcare experience.

In summary, diversional activities are an integral component of holistic patient care in medical-surgical settings. By addressing the emotional and psychological needs through engaging non-pharmacologic interventions tailored to individual preferences, nurses can significantly enhance patient outcomes and satisfaction during their healthcare journey.

2.1.7 Medication Interactions & Adverse Effects:

In the realm of medical-surgical nursing, understanding medication interactions and adverse effects is crucial for ensuring patient safety and effective treatment outcomes. Medication interactions occur when the effects of one drug are altered by the presence of another drug, food, or substance. These interactions can enhance or diminish the effects of a medication, potentially leading to therapeutic failure or toxicity. Adverse effects, on the other hand, are unintended and harmful outcomes resulting from medication use. Both phenomena require vigilant monitoring and management by healthcare professionals.

Medication interactions can be classified into several types: pharmacokinetic, pharmacodynamic, and pharmaceutical. Pharmacokinetic interactions involve changes in the absorption, distribution, metabolism, or excretion of a drug. For instance, certain medications may compete for the same metabolic enzyme pathways in the liver, such as cytochrome P450 enzymes, leading to increased blood levels of one or both drugs and potential toxicity. Pharmacodynamic interactions occur when two drugs have additive, synergistic, or antagonistic effects on the same physiological process. An example is the concurrent use of anticoagulants like warfarin with nonsteroidal anti-inflammatory drugs (NSAIDs), which can increase the risk of bleeding due to their combined effects on platelet function and coagulation pathways.

Pharmaceutical interactions occur when drugs are physically or chemically incompatible outside the body, such as when mixed in an intravenous solution. This can lead to precipitation or inactivation of one or more components before administration.

Adverse effects are categorized based on their severity and predictability. Predictable adverse effects are often dose-dependent and related to the pharmacological action of the drug. For instance, opioids frequently cause constipation due to their effect on gastrointestinal motility. Unpredictable adverse effects include allergic reactions and idiosyncratic responses that are not dose-dependent and can vary among individuals.

Certain populations are at higher risk for medication interactions and adverse effects. Elderly patients often experience polypharmacy due to multiple comorbidities, increasing their risk for interactions. They also have altered pharmacokinetics due to age-related changes in organ function. Patients with renal or hepatic impairment may have reduced drug clearance, necessitating dosage adjustments to prevent toxicity.

Medical-surgical nurses play a critical role in identifying potential medication interactions and adverse effects through thorough patient assessment and history-taking. This includes reviewing all prescribed medications, over-the-counter drugs, herbal supplements, and dietary habits that could influence drug action. Nurses must also educate patients about potential interactions and adverse effects associated with their medications.

When an interaction or adverse effect is suspected, nurses should promptly report it to the prescribing healthcare provider for evaluation and possible intervention. This may involve adjusting dosages, discontinuing a drug, or substituting an alternative therapy with fewer interaction risks.

Documentation is vital in managing medication safety. Accurate recording of all administered medications, observed adverse effects, and patient responses ensures continuity of care and facilitates communication among healthcare team members.

In summary, understanding medication interactions and adverse effects is essential for medical-surgical nurses to safeguard patient health. Through vigilant assessment, education, monitoring, and collaboration with healthcare providers, nurses can minimize risks associated with drug therapy and optimize therapeutic outcomes for their patients.

2.1.7.1 Pain Management:

Pain management is a critical component of medical-surgical nursing, focusing on alleviating discomfort and enhancing the quality of life for patients experiencing pain due to various medical conditions, surgical interventions, or injuries. Pain is a subjective experience and can be classified into acute or chronic categories. Effective pain management requires a comprehensive approach that involves assessing the type, intensity, and source of pain, as well as implementing evidence-based interventions tailored to individual patient needs.

The assessment of pain is the first step in pain management. Nurses must utilize standardized tools such as the Numeric Rating Scale (NRS), Visual Analog Scale (VAS), or Wong-Baker FACES Pain Rating Scale to evaluate pain intensity accurately. Additionally, understanding the patient's description of pain—whether it is sharp, dull, throbbing, or burning—can provide insights into its etiology. It is also essential to consider factors such as the patient's emotional state, cultural background, and previous experiences with pain, as these can influence their perception and reporting of pain.

Pharmacological interventions are a cornerstone of pain management in medical-surgical settings. Analgesics are categorized into non-opioid analgesics (such as acetaminophen and NSAIDs), opioid analgesics (like morphine and oxycodone), and adjuvant medications (including antidepressants and anticonvulsants). Non-opioid analgesics are often used for mild to moderate pain and have anti-inflammatory properties that can be beneficial in conditions like arthritis. Opioids are reserved for moderate to severe pain but require careful monitoring due to the risks of side effects such as respiratory depression, constipation, and potential for addiction. Adjuvant medications can enhance analgesic effects or address specific types of pain, such as neuropathic pain.

Non-pharmacological interventions play a vital role in comprehensive pain management strategies. Techniques such as cognitive-behavioral therapy (CBT), relaxation exercises, acupuncture, transcutaneous electrical nerve stimulation (TENS), and physical therapy can complement pharmacological treatments. These methods aim to reduce pain perception by altering psychological responses to pain or enhancing physical function.

Patient education is another critical aspect of effective pain management. Nurses must educate patients about their pain management plan, including how to use medications correctly and recognize side effects. Patients should be encouraged to communicate openly about their pain levels and any concerns they have regarding their treatment plan.

Interdisciplinary collaboration is essential for optimizing pain management outcomes. Medical-surgical nurses often work alongside physicians, pharmacists, physical therapists, and other healthcare professionals to develop individualized care plans that address all aspects of a patient's health condition.

Continuous evaluation and adjustment of the pain management plan are necessary to ensure its effectiveness. This involves regular reassessment of pain levels, monitoring for adverse effects of medications, and making necessary modifications based on patient feedback and clinical judgment.

In summary, effective pain management in medical-surgical nursing involves a multidimensional approach that combines thorough assessment, appropriate pharmacological and non-pharmacological interventions, patient education, interdisciplinary collaboration, and ongoing evaluation. By employing these strategies, nurses can significantly improve patient comfort and facilitate recovery processes in diverse clinical settings.

2.1.7.2 Polypharmacy:

Polypharmacy is a term used to describe the concurrent use of multiple medications by a patient, typically defined as the regular use of five or more medications. This practice is particularly prevalent among older adults, who often have multiple chronic conditions requiring complex therapeutic regimens. Polypharmacy can lead to an increased risk of adverse drug interactions, medication non-adherence, and potential medication errors, making it a significant concern in medical-surgical nursing.

The phenomenon of polypharmacy arises from several factors. Firstly, the aging population often experiences multiple comorbidities such as hypertension, diabetes, and arthritis, each necessitating specific pharmacological interventions. Secondly, advancements in medical treatments have expanded the arsenal of available medications, encouraging more aggressive treatment strategies. Lastly, healthcare providers from different specialties may prescribe medications without fully coordinating with each other, leading to an accumulation of prescriptions.

The implications of polypharmacy are multifaceted. One major concern is the increased risk of adverse drug reactions (ADRs). The likelihood of ADRs escalates as the number of medications increases due to potential drug-drug interactions and the cumulative burden on metabolic pathways responsible for drug clearance. For example, certain medications may inhibit or induce cytochrome P450 enzymes, altering the metabolism of co-administered drugs and leading to either toxicity or therapeutic failure.

Moreover, polypharmacy can complicate medication adherence. Patients may struggle with complex dosing schedules and experience confusion over which medications to take and when. This complexity can lead to unintentional non-adherence, where patients skip doses or take incorrect amounts, potentially resulting in suboptimal therapeutic outcomes or exacerbation of disease states.

Additionally, polypharmacy poses challenges in accurately diagnosing new symptoms. Adverse effects from one medication may mimic symptoms of an underlying condition or be misattributed to another disease process. This diagnostic ambiguity can lead to a prescribing cascade, where new medications are added to treat side effects mistaken for new illnesses, further perpetuating polypharmacy.

To manage polypharmacy effectively, medical-surgical nurses play a crucial role in conducting thorough medication reconciliations during patient admissions and transitions of care. This process involves reviewing all current medications, including over-the-counter drugs and supplements, to identify potential duplications or interactions. Nurses must also educate patients about the purposes of their medications and potential side effects to enhance adherence and empower patients in their own care.

Interprofessional collaboration is essential in addressing polypharmacy. Nurses should work closely with pharmacists and prescribers to regularly review medication regimens for appropriateness and necessity. Deprescribing initiatives aim to systematically reduce unnecessary medications by evaluating each drug's risk-benefit profile concerning the patient's current health status and goals of care.

Furthermore, utilizing technology such as electronic health records (EHRs) with integrated clinical decision support systems can aid in identifying potentially inappropriate medications and alerting healthcare providers to possible interactions.

In conclusion, polypharmacy presents significant challenges in medical-surgical nursing due to its association with increased risks of adverse drug events and medication management complexities. By understanding the factors contributing to polypharmacy and employing strategies such as thorough medication reconciliation, patient education, interprofessional collaboration, and deprescribing efforts, nurses can help mitigate these risks and improve patient outcomes. Effective management of polypharmacy requires a comprehensive approach that prioritizes patient safety while optimizing therapeutic efficacy across diverse healthcare settings.

2.1.7.3 Drug-drug Interactions:

Drug-drug interactions occur when the effects of one drug are altered by the presence of another drug. These interactions can enhance or diminish the pharmacological effects of one or both drugs, potentially leading to therapeutic failure or an increased risk of adverse effects. Understanding drug-drug interactions is critical for medical-surgical nurses, as they play a vital role in medication administration and monitoring patient outcomes.

There are several mechanisms through which drug-drug interactions can occur:

1. Pharmacokinetic Interactions: These involve changes in the absorption, distribution, metabolism, or excretion of a drug due to the influence of another drug.

   - Absorption: One drug may alter the gastrointestinal environment, affecting the absorption rate of another. For example, antacids can increase gastric pH, reducing the absorption of certain antifungal medications.

- Distribution: Drugs that compete for protein binding sites can lead to increased free concentrations of one drug, enhancing its effects or toxicity. Warfarin and aspirin are classic examples where competition for albumin binding can increase the risk of bleeding.

- Metabolism: Enzyme induction or inhibition is a common cause of drug-drug interactions. For instance, rifampin induces CYP450 enzymes, accelerating the metabolism of drugs like oral contraceptives and reducing their efficacy. Conversely, inhibitors like ketoconazole can increase plasma levels of drugs metabolized by CYP3A4, such as statins.

- Excretion: Drugs that alter renal function can affect the excretion rates of other medications. Nonsteroidal anti-inflammatory drugs (NSAIDs) can reduce the renal clearance of lithium, raising its serum levels and increasing the risk of toxicity.

2. Pharmacodynamic Interactions: These occur when drugs have additive, synergistic, or antagonistic effects at their sites of action.

- Additive Effects: When two drugs with similar actions are used together, their combined effect equals the sum of their individual effects. For example, using two antihypertensive agents may result in better blood pressure control.

- Synergistic Effects: This occurs when the combined effect of two drugs is greater than the sum of their individual effects. A notable example is the use of beta-lactam antibiotics with aminoglycosides to treat certain bacterial infections more effectively.

- Antagonistic Effects: This happens when one drug reduces or opposes the effect of another. An example is using naloxone to reverse an opioid overdose.

3. Clinical Implications and Management:

- Assessment: Nurses should assess patient history for potential drug-drug interactions, including over-the-counter medications and supplements.

- Monitoring: Close monitoring for signs of toxicity or therapeutic failure is essential. Adjustments in dosage or alternative therapies may be necessary based on observed interactions.

- Patient Education: Educating patients about potential interactions and advising them to report new symptoms promptly can prevent adverse outcomes.

- Collaboration: Working closely with pharmacists and healthcare providers ensures that appropriate management strategies are implemented to mitigate interaction risks.

In summary, understanding drug-drug interactions involves recognizing how different drugs influence each other's pharmacokinetics and pharmacodynamics. Medical-surgical nurses must remain vigilant in identifying potential interactions to ensure safe and effective patient care. By integrating knowledge about these interactions into practice, nurses contribute significantly to optimizing therapeutic outcomes and minimizing harm from adverse effects associated with polypharmacy.

2.1.7.4 Food-drug Interactions:

Food-drug interactions occur when the food consumed by a patient affects the pharmacokinetics or pharmacodynamics of a medication, potentially altering its efficacy or causing adverse effects. Understanding these interactions is crucial for medical-surgical nurses, as they can significantly impact patient outcomes and medication management.

Pharmacokinetic interactions involve changes in drug absorption, distribution, metabolism, or excretion due to food intake. For instance, certain foods can alter the stomach's pH level, affecting drug solubility and absorption. A classic example is the interaction between calcium-rich foods, such as milk, and tetracycline antibiotics. Calcium binds to tetracycline, forming an insoluble complex that reduces the antibiotic's absorption and effectiveness.

Additionally, high-fat meals can delay gastric emptying, slowing the absorption of some medications while enhancing the absorption of others that are fat-soluble. Grapefruit juice is another well-known agent that affects drug metabolism. It inhibits cytochrome P450 3A4 enzymes in the liver and intestines, leading to increased blood levels of drugs like statins and certain antihypertensives, which can heighten their effects and risk of toxicity.

Pharmacodynamic interactions occur when food components directly influence a drug's action at its site of effect. For example, vitamin K found in leafy greens can antagonize the anticoagulant effects of warfarin, making it less effective in preventing blood clots. Patients on warfarin need to maintain a consistent dietary intake of vitamin K to ensure stable drug effects.

Moreover, tyramine-containing foods, such as aged cheese and cured meats, can interact with monoamine oxidase inhibitors (MAOIs), leading to hypertensive crises due to excessive accumulation of norepinephrine. This highlights the importance of dietary restrictions for patients on specific medications.

Medical-surgical nurses must educate patients about potential food-drug interactions to ensure safe medication administration. This involves assessing patients' dietary habits and providing tailored advice on the timing of medication relative to meals. For instance, some drugs should be taken on an empty stomach for optimal absorption, while others may require food to minimize gastrointestinal irritation or enhance absorption.

Furthermore, nurses should monitor for signs of altered drug efficacy or adverse effects stemming from food-drug interactions. This includes recognizing symptoms such as unexpected therapeutic failure or toxicity and adjusting patient care plans accordingly.

In clinical practice, collaboration with dietitians can enhance patient education and support adherence to dietary recommendations that minimize adverse food-drug interactions. Providing patients with written materials outlining potential interactions and encouraging open communication about their dietary habits can empower them to manage their medications effectively.

In summary, understanding food-drug interactions is essential for medical-surgical nurses in optimizing patient care. These interactions can significantly influence medication effectiveness and safety by altering drug pharmacokinetics or pharmacodynamics. Nurses play a vital role in educating patients about these interactions, monitoring for potential issues, and collaborating with other healthcare professionals to ensure comprehensive care. By doing so, they help prevent adverse outcomes and promote optimal therapeutic results for patients under their care.

2.1.8 Health And Wellness Promotion:

Health and wellness promotion in the context of medical-surgical nursing involves a proactive approach to healthcare aimed at enhancing the overall well-being of individuals, families, and communities. It encompasses strategies and interventions designed to prevent illness, manage existing health conditions, and promote optimal health outcomes. Medical-surgical nurses play a critical role in this process by integrating their clinical expertise with evidence-based practices to educate and empower patients.

At its core, health and wellness promotion is about encouraging positive lifestyle choices and behaviors that contribute to physical, mental, and social well-being. This includes promoting regular physical activity, balanced nutrition, adequate rest, stress management, and the avoidance of harmful substances such as tobacco and excessive alcohol. Nurses are instrumental in assessing patients' readiness for change, setting realistic goals, and providing the necessary support to achieve these goals.

A key component of health promotion is disease prevention. This involves identifying risk factors for chronic diseases such as hypertension, diabetes, and cardiovascular disease, and implementing strategies to mitigate these risks. Medical-surgical nurses are adept at conducting thorough assessments to identify these risk factors and developing individualized care plans that include preventive measures like screenings, vaccinations, and patient education.

Patient education is a cornerstone of health promotion. Nurses must possess excellent communication skills to effectively convey information about health risks and preventive measures. They educate patients on self-care practices, medication adherence, symptom management, and when to seek medical attention. By empowering patients with knowledge, nurses enable them to take an active role in managing their health.

In addition to individual patient care, medical-surgical nurses contribute to community health promotion efforts. This involves collaborating with other healthcare professionals and organizations to design and implement public health initiatives aimed at improving population health. These initiatives may include community screenings, health fairs, educational workshops, and advocacy for policies that promote healthy environments.

Health promotion also requires cultural competence. Nurses must be sensitive to the diverse cultural backgrounds of their patients and understand how cultural beliefs and practices influence health behaviors. By providing culturally appropriate care and education, nurses can build trust with their patients and improve health outcomes.

Furthermore, nurses must stay informed about current research and advancements in healthcare to provide evidence-based recommendations for health promotion. Continuous professional development through workshops, seminars, and certifications ensures that nurses are equipped with the latest knowledge and skills.

In summary, health and wellness promotion is an integral aspect of medical-surgical nursing that focuses on preventing illness and enhancing quality of life through education, empowerment, and evidence-based interventions. Nurses play a pivotal role in assessing risks, educating patients, promoting healthy lifestyles, preventing disease progression, advocating for community health initiatives, providing culturally competent care, and staying informed about healthcare innovations. By doing so, they contribute significantly to the overall goal of achieving optimal health outcomes for individuals and communities alike.

2.1.8.1 Screenings:

Screenings are a critical component of health and wellness promotion in medical-surgical nursing, serving as a proactive approach to identifying potential health issues before they manifest into more serious conditions. Screenings involve the systematic application of tests, examinations, or other procedures to asymptomatic individuals or populations to detect early signs of disease or risk factors for disease. The primary goal of screenings is to enable early intervention, thereby improving outcomes and reducing the burden of disease on individuals and healthcare systems.

In the context of medical-surgical nursing, screenings encompass a wide range of assessments tailored to various health conditions, including but not limited to cardiovascular diseases, cancers, diabetes, and infectious diseases. Nurses play a pivotal role in conducting these screenings, interpreting results, educating patients about the importance of early detection, and facilitating follow-up care when necessary.

One key aspect of screenings is understanding the different types: universal and selective. Universal screening refers to testing all individuals within a certain category or age group, regardless of their risk level. An example is mammography for breast cancer in women over a certain age. Selective screening targets individuals who have specific risk factors or belong to high-risk groups; for instance, screening for type 2 diabetes in individuals with obesity or a family history of diabetes.

The effectiveness of a screening program is determined by several factors: sensitivity, specificity, predictive values, and cost-effectiveness. Sensitivity refers to the test's ability to correctly identify those with the disease (true positive rate), while specificity indicates the test's ability to correctly identify those without the disease (true negative rate). High sensitivity and specificity are essential for minimizing false positives and negatives, which can lead to unnecessary anxiety or missed diagnoses.

Predictive values further refine the utility of screenings by indicating the likelihood that a positive or negative result correlates with the actual presence or absence of disease. Positive predictive value (PPV) is the probability that individuals with a positive screening test truly have the disease. Conversely, negative predictive value (NPV) is the probability that individuals with a negative test truly do not have the disease.

Cost-effectiveness analysis ensures that screening programs provide good value by balancing benefits, such as reduced morbidity and mortality, against costs incurred from testing and treatment. This analysis helps prioritize resource allocation in healthcare settings where resources may be limited.

In implementing screening programs, ethical considerations must also be addressed. Informed consent is paramount; patients should be fully aware of what the screening entails, including potential risks and benefits. Confidentiality must be maintained throughout the process to protect patient privacy.

Additionally, cultural competence is crucial in ensuring that screenings are accessible and acceptable to diverse populations. Nurses must be aware of cultural beliefs that may influence an individual's willingness to participate in screenings and adapt their approach accordingly.

In summary, screenings are an indispensable part of health promotion in medical-surgical nursing. They enable early detection and management of diseases, ultimately improving patient outcomes. As frontline healthcare providers, nurses must be adept at conducting screenings effectively while considering clinical efficacy, ethical principles, and cultural sensitivity. By doing so, they contribute significantly to preventive healthcare efforts and enhance the overall well-being of patients under their care.

2.1.8.2 Vaccinations:

Vaccinations, also known as immunizations, are a critical component of public health and individual wellness, serving as a primary preventive measure against infectious diseases. Vaccines work by stimulating the body's immune system to recognize and combat pathogens, such as viruses or bacteria, without causing the disease itself. This is achieved through the administration of an antigen, which is a substance that mimics the pathogen in a way that triggers an immune response.

The principle behind vaccinations is based on the body's natural ability to develop immunity. When a vaccine is introduced into the body, it prompts the immune system to produce antibodies. These antibodies are proteins that specifically target and neutralize foreign invaders. Additionally, vaccines help in the formation of memory cells that remember how to fight the pathogen if exposed in the future. This process ensures long-term immunity and protection against specific diseases.

There are several types of vaccines, each designed to elicit a protective immune response. These include:

1. Live-attenuated vaccines: These contain a weakened form of the germ that causes a disease. Examples include the measles, mumps, and rubella (MMR) vaccine. They provide strong and long-lasting immunity but are not suitable for individuals with weakened immune systems.

2. Inactivated vaccines: These contain killed pathogens or parts of them. They are stable and safe for immunocompromised individuals but may require booster shots for ongoing protection. The polio vaccine is an example.

3. Subunit, recombinant, polysaccharide, and conjugate vaccines: These use pieces of the pathogen, such as its protein, sugar, or capsid (a casing around the germ). Examples include the human papillomavirus (HPV) vaccine and the hepatitis B vaccine.

4. Toxoid vaccines: These contain toxins produced by bacteria that have been made harmless. They help protect against diseases like tetanus and diphtheria by teaching the immune system to fight off bacterial toxins.

5. mRNA vaccines: A newer type of vaccine used for COVID-19, these teach cells how to make a protein that triggers an immune response without using live virus particles.

Vaccinations play a crucial role in controlling and eradicating diseases. For instance, smallpox has been eradicated globally due to successful vaccination campaigns. Similarly, polio cases have significantly reduced worldwide because of extensive immunization efforts.

In medical-surgical nursing practice, understanding vaccinations involves not only knowing their types and mechanisms but also recognizing their importance in preventing disease outbreaks within healthcare settings and communities. Nurses must be knowledgeable about recommended immunization schedules provided by health organizations such as the Centers for Disease Control and Prevention (CDC) and the World Health Organization (WHO).

Moreover, nurses play an essential role in patient education regarding vaccinations. They must address concerns and misconceptions about vaccine safety and efficacy by providing evidence-based information. This includes explaining potential side effects—usually mild—and emphasizing that serious adverse reactions are rare compared to the benefits of vaccination.

Furthermore, nurses are responsible for ensuring the proper storage and handling of vaccines to maintain their effectiveness. This includes adhering to cold chain requirements—keeping vaccines at recommended temperatures from manufacturing until administration.

In summary, vaccinations are a cornerstone of preventive healthcare in medical-surgical nursing practice. They offer protection against numerous infectious diseases by harnessing the body's natural defense mechanisms to create lasting immunity while contributing significantly to public health through disease prevention and control efforts.

2.1.8.3 Healthy Lifestyle Modifications:

Healthy lifestyle modifications are a set of practices and behavioral changes aimed at improving overall health and well-being, reducing the risk of chronic diseases, and enhancing quality of life. For medical-surgical nurses, understanding these modifications is crucial, as they play a significant role in patient education and health promotion. Healthy lifestyle modifications encompass various aspects, such as diet, physical activity, stress management, sleep hygiene, and avoidance of harmful substances.

Dietary Modifications: A balanced diet is fundamental to maintaining health. Nurses should educate patients on the importance of consuming a variety of foods that provide essential nutrients. Emphasizing the intake of fruits, vegetables, whole grains, lean proteins, and healthy fats is vital. Reducing sodium, sugar, and saturated fat intake can help prevent conditions like hypertension, diabetes, and cardiovascular diseases. Nurses can guide patients in reading food labels and planning meals that align with dietary guidelines.

Physical Activity: Regular physical activity is essential for maintaining a healthy weight, improving cardiovascular health, and enhancing mental well-being. Nurses should encourage patients to engage in at least 150 minutes of moderate-intensity aerobic exercise per week, as recommended by health authorities. Activities such as walking, swimming, cycling, or strength training can be tailored to individual preferences and capabilities. Educating patients about the benefits of physical activity in managing chronic conditions like obesity and arthritis is crucial.

Stress Management: Chronic stress can adversely affect both physical and mental health. Teaching patients stress-reduction techniques such as mindfulness meditation, deep breathing exercises, yoga, or progressive muscle relaxation can be beneficial. Nurses should also emphasize the importance of social support networks and encourage patients to seek help when needed. Effective stress management can lead to improved immune function and a reduced risk of stress-related illnesses.

Sleep Hygiene: Adequate sleep is vital for physical recovery and cognitive function. Nurses should educate patients on establishing a regular sleep schedule, creating a conducive sleep environment, and avoiding stimulants like caffeine before bedtime. Addressing sleep disorders such as insomnia or sleep apnea through appropriate referrals or interventions is also important. Good sleep hygiene contributes to better mood regulation and overall health.

Avoidance of Harmful Substances: Educating patients on the risks associated with tobacco use, excessive alcohol consumption, and illicit drug use is critical. Nurses should provide resources for smoking cessation programs or substance abuse counseling when necessary. Highlighting the long-term benefits of quitting these harmful habits can motivate patients to make positive changes.

Patient-Centered Approach: It is essential for nurses to adopt a patient-centered approach when discussing lifestyle modifications. Understanding individual barriers to change and working collaboratively with patients to set realistic goals can enhance adherence to healthy behaviors. Cultural competence is also important in tailoring advice that respects diverse backgrounds and beliefs.

Monitoring and Support: Continuous monitoring of progress and providing support are key components in facilitating successful lifestyle modifications. Nurses should schedule follow-up appointments or check-ins to assess adherence and address any challenges faced by patients. Encouraging self-monitoring techniques, such as keeping food diaries or using fitness trackers, can empower patients to take charge of their health.

In conclusion, healthy lifestyle modifications are integral to disease prevention and health promotion in medical-surgical nursing practice. By equipping themselves with knowledge about these modifications, nurses can effectively guide patients toward healthier choices that lead to improved outcomes and enhanced quality of life.

3 Professional Role:

In the realm of medical-surgical nursing, the professional role encompasses a multifaceted set of responsibilities and expectations that a nurse must fulfill to provide optimal patient care. This role is integral to the healthcare system, requiring a combination of clinical expertise, ethical practice, and effective communication.

At its core, the professional role of a medical-surgical nurse involves being a competent caregiver. This entails possessing a thorough understanding of pathophysiology, pharmacology, and nursing interventions to manage a wide range of medical conditions. Nurses must be adept at conducting comprehensive assessments, developing and implementing care plans, and evaluating patient outcomes. They are expected to apply evidence-based practices to ensure high-quality care.

A key component of the professional role is advocacy. Medical-surgical nurses serve as advocates for their patients, ensuring that their rights and needs are respected and addressed. This involves communicating effectively with other members of the healthcare team to coordinate care, as well as educating patients and their families about treatment options and health maintenance strategies. Advocacy also extends to participating in policy development and improvement initiatives within healthcare settings to enhance patient care standards.

Ethical practice is another cornerstone of the professional role. Medical-surgical nurses must adhere to ethical principles such as autonomy, beneficence, non-maleficence, and justice. They are responsible for maintaining patient confidentiality, obtaining informed consent, and delivering care that respects cultural diversity and individual preferences. Nurses must also be prepared to address ethical dilemmas that may arise in clinical practice, using critical thinking and ethical frameworks to guide decision-making.

Professional development is crucial in maintaining competence in the dynamic field of medical-surgical nursing. Nurses are expected to engage in lifelong learning through continuing education opportunities, certification programs like MEDSURG-BC, and participation in professional organizations. This commitment to ongoing education ensures that nurses remain current with advancements in medical knowledge and technology.

Collaboration is essential in fulfilling the professional role. Medical-surgical nurses work as part of interdisciplinary teams that include physicians, pharmacists, therapists, social workers, and other healthcare professionals. Effective collaboration requires strong communication skills, mutual respect, and an understanding of each team member's contributions to patient care. Nurses often take on leadership roles within these teams, coordinating care delivery and advocating for quality improvement initiatives.

The professional role also encompasses leadership responsibilities. Whether formally or informally, medical-surgical nurses are leaders who influence practice standards and mentor peers. Leadership involves demonstrating accountability, integrity, and professionalism in all aspects of nursing practice. It includes participating in quality improvement projects, contributing to policy development, and fostering a culture of safety within healthcare environments.

Finally, self-care is an important aspect of the professional role that cannot be overlooked. Medical-surgical nurses must manage stress effectively to prevent burnout and maintain personal well-being. This includes setting boundaries between work and personal life, seeking support when needed, and engaging in activities that promote physical and mental health.

In summary, the professional role of a medical-surgical nurse is comprehensive and demands a balance of clinical expertise, ethical practice, advocacy, collaboration, leadership, continuous learning, and self-care. By embodying these elements, nurses contribute significantly to patient outcomes and the overall effectiveness of healthcare delivery systems.

3.1.1 Therapeutic Communication:

Therapeutic communication is a fundamental skill in medical-surgical nursing that involves the use of specific strategies to encourage patients to express their feelings and thoughts, thereby promoting patient well-being and enhancing the nurse-patient relationship. This form of communication is intentional and goal-directed, aiming to understand the patient's perspective and provide support, comfort, and education.

At its core, therapeutic communication is centered around empathy, active listening, and respect for the patient's autonomy. It requires the nurse to be fully present and engaged with the patient, demonstrating an understanding of their needs and concerns. This is achieved through both verbal and non-verbal communication techniques that facilitate an open dialogue.

Key components of therapeutic communication include:

1. Active Listening: This involves giving full attention to the patient, acknowledging their message, and responding appropriately. It requires the nurse to be attentive, avoid interrupting, and use verbal affirmations such as I understand or Tell me more about that. Active listening helps build trust and encourages patients to share more openly.

2. Empathy: Demonstrating empathy involves putting oneself in the patient's shoes to understand their feelings and experiences. This can be communicated through statements like That sounds really difficult or I can see why you're feeling upset. Empathy validates the patient's emotions and fosters a supportive environment.

3. Open-Ended Questions: These questions encourage patients to elaborate on their thoughts and feelings rather than providing yes or no answers. For example, asking How do you feel about your treatment plan? invites a more detailed response compared to Are you okay with your treatment?

4. Clarification: Nurses should seek clarification when they do not fully understand a patient's message. Phrases like Can you explain what you mean by that? or I'm not sure I understand; could you tell me more? help ensure accurate understanding and prevent miscommunication.

5. Reflection: Reflecting involves repeating or paraphrasing what the patient has said to show understanding and encourage further discussion. For instance, if a patient says they are worried about surgery, a reflective response might be, You're feeling anxious about your upcoming procedure.

6. Silence: The strategic use of silence allows patients time to think and process their thoughts without feeling rushed. It can be a powerful tool in encouraging patients to continue speaking when they are ready.

7. Non-Verbal Communication: Body language, facial expressions, eye contact, and gestures all play significant roles in conveying empathy and understanding. Maintaining an open posture and making appropriate eye contact can reinforce verbal messages.

8. Providing Information: Educating patients about their condition or treatment options in a clear, concise manner empowers them to make informed decisions about their care.

9. Summarization: Summarizing key points of a conversation helps ensure mutual understanding between the nurse and patient. It also provides an opportunity for patients to correct any misunderstandings before concluding the interaction.

In medical-surgical nursing practice, therapeutic communication is essential for effective patient assessment, intervention planning, and evaluation of outcomes. It enhances patient satisfaction by ensuring that their needs are met holistically—addressing not only physical health but also emotional well-being.

Therapeutic communication is not merely a set of techniques but an ongoing process requiring continuous self-reflection and development on the part of the nurse. By mastering these skills, medical-surgical nurses can significantly improve the quality of patient care while fostering meaningful connections with those they serve.

3.1.1.1 Patient- And Family-centered Care:

Patient- and family-centered care (PFCC) is a holistic approach to healthcare that emphasizes collaboration among patients, families, and healthcare providers. It recognizes the vital role that families play in ensuring the health and well-being of patients, especially in the context of medical-surgical nursing. This model of care is built upon four core concepts: respect and dignity, information sharing, participation, and collaboration.

Respect and dignity are fundamental to PFCC. In this context, healthcare providers honor the perspectives and choices of patients and their families. This means acknowledging the unique needs, values, beliefs, and cultural backgrounds of each patient. By doing so, medical-surgical nurses can create a supportive environment where patients feel valued and understood. Respectful interactions foster trust and enhance the therapeutic relationship between nurses and their patients.

Information sharing is another critical component of PFCC. Effective communication is essential for ensuring that patients and families are well-informed about the patient's condition, treatment options, and care plans. Medical-surgical nurses must provide clear, comprehensive information using language that is understandable to patients and families. This transparency empowers patients to make informed decisions about their care. Additionally, it encourages family members to actively participate in the patient's healthcare journey.

Participation refers to the active involvement of patients and their families in the decision-making process regarding the patient's care. In a PFCC model, medical-surgical nurses encourage patients to express their preferences and concerns openly. They also invite family members to contribute their insights, as they often have valuable knowledge about the patient's history and needs. By facilitating participation, nurses ensure that care plans are tailored to meet the specific goals and desires of each patient.

Collaboration is the final core concept of PFCC. It involves healthcare providers working together with patients and families as partners in the care process. In medical-surgical settings, this means involving interdisciplinary teams to address complex patient needs comprehensively. Nurses play a pivotal role in coordinating care among different specialists while keeping patients and families informed about each step of the process. Collaborative efforts lead to more efficient and effective care delivery that aligns with patient-centered goals.

Implementing PFCC in medical-surgical nursing requires a shift from traditional provider-centric models to one where patients and families are at the center of all healthcare activities. This transformation involves training nurses in communication skills that promote empathy, active listening, and shared decision-making. It also necessitates creating hospital policies that support family presence during rounds or procedures when appropriate.

Research has shown that PFCC improves patient outcomes by enhancing satisfaction levels, reducing anxiety, decreasing hospital readmissions, and improving adherence to treatment plans. When patients feel respected and involved in their care decisions, they are more likely to engage positively with healthcare providers.

In conclusion, patient- and family-centered care is an integral aspect of medical-surgical nursing that prioritizes the needs and preferences of both patients and their families. By focusing on respect, information sharing, participation, and collaboration, medical-surgical nurses can deliver compassionate care that not only addresses clinical needs but also supports emotional well-being. As healthcare continues to evolve towards more personalized approaches, PFCC remains a cornerstone for achieving optimal patient outcomes while fostering meaningful partnerships between caregivers and those they serve.

3.1.1.2 Cultural Competence:

Cultural competence in medical-surgical nursing is the ability of healthcare providers to understand, respect, and effectively interact with patients from diverse cultural backgrounds. It involves recognizing the influence of culture on health behaviors and outcomes and integrating this understanding into patient care. This competence is not just about awareness but also about applying this knowledge in clinical practice to improve patient outcomes and provide equitable care.

Cultural competence encompasses several key components: cultural awareness, cultural knowledge, cultural skills, cultural encounters, and cultural desire. Cultural awareness involves self-examination and in-depth exploration of one's own cultural and professional background. It requires nurses to recognize their own biases, prejudices, and assumptions about individuals who are different from themselves.

Cultural knowledge refers to the process of seeking and obtaining a solid educational foundation about diverse cultural groups. This includes understanding the health-related beliefs, practices, and values of different cultures. For example, some cultures may prefer traditional healing practices over conventional medicine, or there may be specific dietary restrictions that must be considered when planning care.

Cultural skills involve the ability to collect relevant cultural data regarding the patient's presenting problem and accurately perform a culturally-based physical assessment. This means asking appropriate questions that respect the patient's cultural beliefs while gathering necessary health information. For instance, understanding how certain symptoms are described within different cultures can aid in accurate diagnosis and treatment.

Cultural encounters are interactions that provide opportunities for healthcare providers to engage directly with patients from culturally diverse backgrounds. These encounters help refine or modify existing beliefs about a cultural group and prevent stereotyping. Through these interactions, nurses can develop better communication strategies that are culturally sensitive.

Cultural desire is the motivation of healthcare providers to want to become culturally aware, knowledgeable, and skillful. It is an intrinsic quality that drives one to be open-minded and accepting of cultural differences, showing a genuine interest in learning about other cultures.

In practice, cultural competence involves using therapeutic communication techniques that respect the patient's cultural norms. For example, understanding non-verbal cues such as eye contact or personal space can vary significantly across cultures. In some cultures, direct eye contact may be seen as disrespectful or confrontational, while in others, it is expected as a sign of attentiveness.

Moreover, language barriers can pose significant challenges. Employing professional interpreters rather than relying on family members ensures accuracy in communication and maintains patient confidentiality. Nurses should also be aware of health literacy levels, which can vary widely among patients from different cultural backgrounds.

Incorporating cultural competence into nursing practice enhances patient satisfaction and compliance with treatment plans. It reduces misunderstandings and potential conflicts between healthcare providers and patients. Additionally, it fosters a more inclusive healthcare environment where patients feel valued and understood.

For medical-surgical nurses preparing for the MEDSURG-BC exam, mastering cultural competence is essential not only for passing the certification but also for delivering high-quality care in a diverse society. It requires ongoing education and reflection to continually improve one's ability to provide culturally competent care.

In summary, cultural competence is an integral part of nursing practice that ensures effective communication and care delivery across diverse populations. By embracing this approach, nurses can better meet the needs of their patients and contribute to positive health outcomes within their communities.

3.1.2 <u>Interdisciplinary Healthcare Team Collaboration:</u>

Interdisciplinary healthcare team collaboration is a critical aspect of medical-surgical nursing, encompassing the integration of diverse healthcare professionals working together toward a common goal: optimizing patient outcomes. This collaborative approach involves the coordinated efforts of various disciplines, such as physicians, nurses, pharmacists, social workers, physical therapists, and dietitians, each contributing their specialized knowledge and skills to deliver comprehensive care.

The foundation of interdisciplinary collaboration is built on open communication, mutual respect, and shared decision-making among team members. Effective communication is paramount; it ensures that all team members are informed about the patient's condition, treatment plans, and any changes in their status. This involves regular meetings, discussions, and the use of electronic health records to maintain up-to-date information accessible to all involved.

Mutual respect among team members acknowledges the unique expertise each discipline brings to patient care. Recognizing and valuing these contributions fosters a supportive environment where each professional feels empowered to voice their insights and concerns. This respect is crucial for resolving conflicts and maintaining a harmonious working relationship.

Shared decision-making is another cornerstone of interdisciplinary collaboration. It involves engaging all relevant team members in the planning and implementation of patient care strategies. This collaborative decision-making process ensures that care plans are comprehensive and consider multiple perspectives, leading to more holistic patient management.

In practice, interdisciplinary collaboration can manifest in various forms. Case conferences or multidisciplinary rounds are common methods where team members gather to discuss complex cases, share insights, and develop integrated care plans. These meetings facilitate real-time communication and allow for immediate input from different specialties.

The benefits of effective interdisciplinary collaboration are numerous. For patients, it often results in improved health outcomes due to the comprehensive nature of care provided. The pooling of expertise allows for more accurate diagnoses, effective treatment plans, and timely interventions. Patients also benefit from a more seamless healthcare experience as transitions between different levels of care are better coordinated.

For healthcare providers, collaboration reduces the risk of burnout by distributing the workload among team members and providing emotional support through shared responsibilities. It also enhances professional satisfaction as providers work together toward successful patient outcomes.

Despite its advantages, interdisciplinary collaboration can face challenges, such as hierarchical structures within healthcare settings that may inhibit open communication or cultural differences among team members that can lead to misunderstandings. Overcoming these barriers requires a commitment to fostering an inclusive culture that promotes equality and understanding across disciplines.

To enhance interdisciplinary collaboration, ongoing education and training are essential. Programs focusing on teamwork skills, conflict resolution, and communication techniques can equip healthcare professionals with the necessary tools to work effectively in a collaborative environment. Leadership plays a crucial role in facilitating this process by modeling collaborative behaviors and supporting initiatives that promote teamwork.

In conclusion, interdisciplinary healthcare team collaboration is an integral component of medical-surgical nursing practice that significantly impacts the quality of patient care. By leveraging the collective expertise of diverse healthcare professionals through effective communication, mutual respect, and shared decision-making, medical-surgical nurses can contribute to achieving optimal health outcomes for their patients. As healthcare continues to evolve toward more integrated models of care delivery, mastering the principles of interdisciplinary collaboration will remain vital for medical-surgical nurses aiming to excel in their field.

3.1.2.1 **Delegation:**

Delegation in the context of medical-surgical nursing is a critical skill that involves the transfer of responsibility for the performance of a task from one individual to another while retaining accountability for the outcome. It is an essential component of effective team collaboration in healthcare settings, allowing nurses to manage their workload efficiently while ensuring patient safety and quality care.

In medical-surgical nursing, delegation involves assigning tasks to unlicensed assistive personnel (UAP), licensed practical nurses (LPNs), or other team members who are competent to perform specific duties. The nurse must assess the complexity of the task, the skill level of the delegatee, and the patient's condition before delegating any task. This process requires a clear understanding of each team member's scope of practice, as defined by state laws and institutional policies.

Effective delegation relies on several key principles. Firstly, the nurse must ensure that the task is appropriate for delegation. This means that the task should be routine, have a predictable outcome, and not require nursing judgment or critical decision-making. For instance, tasks like taking vital signs, assisting with activities of daily living, or performing basic wound care can often be delegated.

Secondly, it is crucial to select the right person for the task. The nurse must consider the delegatee's training, experience, and current workload. It is important to verify that the delegatee understands how to perform the task and is aware of any specific instructions or precautions. Communication plays a vital role here; clear instructions and expectations should be provided to ensure that the delegatee knows what is required.

Thirdly, supervision and evaluation are integral parts of delegation. The nurse must provide appropriate supervision based on the nature of the task and the experience level of the delegatee. This may involve direct observation or periodic check-ins to ensure that tasks are being performed correctly and safely. After the completion of the task, evaluation is necessary to assess outcomes and provide feedback. This helps identify areas for improvement and ensures continuous learning for both parties involved.

Accountability remains with the delegating nurse even after a task has been delegated. This means that if a delegated task is not performed correctly or results in an adverse outcome, it is ultimately the responsibility of the nurse who delegated it. Therefore, thorough documentation of all aspects of delegation—task assigned, instructions given, and supervision provided—is essential for legal protection and quality assurance.

Delegation also plays a strategic role in enhancing team collaboration within interdisciplinary healthcare teams. By effectively delegating tasks, nurses can focus on more complex patient care needs that require their specialized skills and knowledge. This optimizes resource utilization within healthcare settings and contributes to improved patient outcomes.

However, challenges in delegation can arise due to factors such as unclear communication, lack of trust among team members, or resistance from staff who may feel overburdened or undervalued. Addressing these challenges requires fostering an environment of mutual respect and open communication within healthcare teams.

In summary, delegation is a vital skill in medical-surgical nursing that enhances efficiency and teamwork while maintaining high standards of patient care. By understanding its principles and implementing them effectively, nurses can ensure safe practice environments where all team members contribute optimally to patient care outcomes.

3.1.2.2 **Consults:**

In the context of medical-surgical nursing, consults refer to the process by which healthcare professionals seek the expertise or opinion of another specialist or department to enhance patient care. This interdisciplinary approach ensures that patients receive comprehensive evaluations and treatments tailored to their specific needs. Consults are integral to managing complex cases where multiple health issues intersect, necessitating input from various specialties.

Consults typically begin with a primary healthcare provider identifying a need for additional expertise. This need may arise due to the complexity of a patient's condition, the necessity for specialized diagnostic tests, or therapeutic interventions that fall outside the primary provider's scope. The process involves formally requesting input from another healthcare professional, often documented in the patient's medical record to ensure clarity and continuity of care.

The consult process is crucial for several reasons. First, it enhances patient safety by ensuring that all aspects of a patient's health are considered. For instance, a surgical patient with cardiac issues may require a cardiology consult to assess perioperative risks and manage any underlying heart conditions. Similarly, a patient with diabetes undergoing surgery might benefit from an endocrinology consult to optimize blood glucose control pre- and postoperatively.

Second, consults facilitate evidence-based practice by integrating diverse expert opinions into patient care plans. This collaboration can lead to more accurate diagnoses, effective treatment plans, and improved patient outcomes. For example, in a case of complex wound management, a consult with a wound care specialist can provide advanced techniques and products that promote healing and prevent infection.

Third, consults foster professional development and learning among healthcare providers. By engaging with specialists from different fields, nurses and other practitioners can expand their knowledge base and stay updated on the latest advancements in medical science and technology. This continuous learning is essential for maintaining high standards of care in an ever-evolving healthcare landscape.

For medical-surgical nurses preparing for the MEDSURG-BC exam, understanding the role of consults is vital. Nurses often play a pivotal role in initiating and coordinating consults. They are typically the first to recognize changes in a patient's condition that may warrant additional expertise. Effective communication skills are essential for conveying pertinent clinical information to consulting teams and ensuring that recommendations are implemented promptly.

Furthermore, nurses must be adept at managing the logistics of consults. This includes scheduling appointments, facilitating communication between different departments, and ensuring that all relevant documentation is complete and accessible. Nurses also act as advocates for their patients during this process, ensuring that their needs and preferences are considered when developing interdisciplinary care plans.

In summary, consults are a fundamental component of interdisciplinary healthcare team collaboration in medical-surgical settings. They ensure comprehensive patient assessments, enhance safety through expert input, promote evidence-based practice, and contribute to professional development among healthcare providers. For medical-surgical nurses preparing for certification exams like MEDSURG-BC, mastering the intricacies of consults is crucial for delivering high-quality patient care and excelling in their roles within multidisciplinary teams. Understanding how to effectively initiate, coordinate, and implement consult recommendations will not only improve patient outcomes but also reinforce the nurse's role as a central figure in the collaborative healthcare environment.

3.1.3 Nursing Ethics:

Nursing ethics is a branch of applied ethics that focuses on the activities within the field of nursing. It comprises a set of moral principles, values, and standards that guide the behavior and decision-making processes of nurses in their professional practice. Nursing ethics ensures that nurses provide care that respects the dignity, rights, and autonomy of patients while promoting health and well-being.

At its core, nursing ethics is guided by several fundamental principles: autonomy, beneficence, non-maleficence, justice, fidelity, and veracity. Autonomy refers to respecting patients' rights to make informed decisions about their own healthcare. Nurses must ensure that patients receive all necessary information to make choices regarding their treatment options without coercion or undue influence.

Beneficence involves acting in the best interest of the patient by promoting good and preventing harm. Nurses are expected to provide care that benefits the patient while considering their individual needs and circumstances. Non-maleficence is closely related and emphasizes the obligation to do no harm. This principle requires nurses to avoid actions that could cause unnecessary harm or suffering to patients.

Justice in nursing ethics pertains to fairness and equality in the distribution of healthcare resources. Nurses are responsible for ensuring that all patients receive fair treatment, regardless of their background or socioeconomic status. This principle also involves advocating for vulnerable populations and addressing disparities in healthcare access.

Fidelity refers to being faithful to the commitments made to patients and upholding professional responsibilities. Nurses must maintain trust by being reliable, honest, and accountable in their interactions with patients. Veracity involves truthfulness and transparency in communication with patients. Nurses are expected to provide accurate information and avoid misleading or deceiving patients.

In addition to these principles, nursing ethics encompasses confidentiality and privacy. Nurses must protect patient information and ensure it is only shared with authorized individuals involved in the patient's care. This obligation extends to both verbal communication and electronic health records.

Nursing ethics also addresses issues such as informed consent, end-of-life care, cultural competence, and professional boundaries. Informed consent requires nurses to ensure that patients understand the risks and benefits of proposed treatments before agreeing to them. End-of-life care involves ethical considerations related to palliative care, advance directives, and decisions about life-sustaining treatments.

Cultural competence requires nurses to respect diverse cultural beliefs and practices while providing care that is sensitive to individual patient needs. This includes understanding how cultural factors may influence health behaviors and decision-making processes.

Professional boundaries are essential in maintaining appropriate nurse-patient relationships. Nurses must avoid conflicts of interest or situations where personal interests could compromise professional judgment.

Ethical dilemmas are common in nursing practice due to complex patient situations, resource limitations, or conflicting values between healthcare providers and patients. Nurses must use critical thinking skills and ethical reasoning frameworks to navigate these challenges effectively.

The American Nurses Association (ANA) Code of Ethics for Nurses provides a foundational guide for ethical practice in nursing. It outlines the ethical obligations of nurses across various settings and serves as a reference for resolving ethical issues.

In conclusion, nursing ethics is an integral component of professional practice that ensures nurses deliver compassionate, respectful, and equitable care while upholding moral principles. Understanding these ethical foundations prepares medical-surgical nurses for the complexities they may encounter during their careers while promoting patient advocacy and quality care delivery.

3.1.3.1 Advocacy:

Advocacy in nursing is a fundamental aspect of professional practice, particularly for medical-surgical nurses who are often at the forefront of patient care. Advocacy involves the nurse's role in supporting and promoting the interests and well-being of patients, ensuring that their rights are respected and that they receive appropriate care. It is a critical component of nursing ethics, emphasizing the nurse's responsibility to act as a liaison between patients and the healthcare system.

At its core, advocacy means being a voice for patients who may not be able to speak for themselves due to illness, lack of knowledge, or other barriers. It requires nurses to possess a deep understanding of patients' needs, preferences, and values, and to use this understanding to guide clinical decision-making and communication with other healthcare professionals. Nurses must be vigilant in recognizing when patients' rights are at risk or when their care might be compromised, taking action to address these issues promptly.

An essential element of advocacy is informed consent. Medical-surgical nurses play a crucial role in ensuring that patients understand their treatment options, including potential risks and benefits. This involves providing clear, concise information and verifying that the patient comprehends this information before consenting to procedures or treatments. Nurses must ensure that consent is obtained voluntarily and without coercion, respecting the patient's autonomy in making healthcare decisions.

Advocacy also extends to safeguarding patient privacy and confidentiality. Nurses must adhere to legal and ethical standards, such as the Health Insurance Portability and Accountability Act (HIPAA) in the United States, which protects patient information. This involves careful handling of medical records and being cautious about discussions regarding patient care in public or unsecured settings.

In situations where there is a conflict between a patient's wishes and the recommendations of healthcare providers, nurses serve as mediators. They must facilitate open communication between all parties involved, striving to reach a resolution that honors the patient's preferences while ensuring safe and effective care. This may involve advocating for alternative treatment plans or seeking second opinions when necessary.

Furthermore, advocacy encompasses addressing social determinants of health that may impact patient outcomes. Medical-surgical nurses should be aware of factors such as socioeconomic status, cultural background, and access to resources that can influence health disparities. By identifying these issues, nurses can work towards connecting patients with community resources or support services that address these broader determinants.

Professional advocacy is another dimension where nurses advocate for improvements within the healthcare system itself. This can involve participating in policy development, engaging with professional organizations, or contributing to research that aims to enhance the quality and safety of patient care. By advocating for systemic changes, nurses help shape an environment conducive to optimal patient outcomes.

Lastly, self-advocacy is crucial for nurses to maintain their own well-being and professional integrity. This involves seeking opportunities for continuing education, advocating for safe staffing levels, and ensuring a healthy work-life balance. By prioritizing their own health and professional development, nurses are better equipped to advocate effectively for their patients.

In summary, advocacy in medical-surgical nursing is multifaceted, encompassing direct patient support, adherence to ethical practices, mediation in conflicts, addressing social determinants of health, influencing healthcare policy, and self-care. It requires a proactive approach where nurses are committed to upholding ethical standards while championing the needs and rights of their patients within an ever-evolving healthcare landscape.

3.1.4 Evidence-based Practice:

Evidence-based Practice (EBP) is a systematic approach to clinical decision-making that integrates the best available research evidence with clinical expertise and patient preferences. It is a cornerstone of modern healthcare, ensuring that patient care is grounded in the most current and robust scientific knowledge. For medical-surgical nurses, EBP is crucial for delivering high-quality care, improving patient outcomes, and enhancing healthcare efficiency.

The foundation of EBP lies in its three core components: the best available evidence, clinical expertise, and patient values and preferences. The best available evidence refers to data derived from rigorous research studies, such as randomized controlled trials, cohort studies, and meta-analyses. These studies provide reliable information on the effectiveness and safety of various interventions. Clinical expertise involves the skills and experience that nurses accumulate over time, allowing them to interpret evidence in the context of individual patient situations. Patient values and preferences emphasize the importance of considering patients' unique needs, desires, and cultural contexts when making clinical decisions.

The process of implementing EBP involves several steps. First, it begins with formulating a clear clinical question using the PICO(T) framework—Population/Patient problem, Intervention, Comparison, Outcome, and Timeframe. This structured approach helps in identifying specific information needs. For instance, a medical-surgical nurse might askIn post-operative patients (Population), does early ambulation (Intervention) compared to delayed ambulation (Comparison) reduce the incidence of deep vein thrombosis (Outcome) within 30 days post-surgery (Timeframe)?

Once the question is defined, the next step is to search for relevant evidence. This involves conducting a thorough literature review using databases like PubMed, CINAHL, or the Cochrane Library to find high-quality studies related to the clinical question. After gathering evidence, it must be critically appraised to assess its validity, reliability, and applicability to the specific clinical scenario.

After appraising the evidence, it is integrated with clinical expertise and patient preferences to make informed decisions about patient care. This integration is essential because even robust evidence may not be applicable if it does not align with an individual patient's circumstances or if it contradicts professional judgment based on experience.

The final step in EBP is evaluating the outcomes of the implemented intervention. This involves assessing whether the desired health outcomes were achieved and whether any adjustments are necessary for future practice. Continuous evaluation helps refine nursing practices and contributes to ongoing professional development.

For medical-surgical nurses preparing for the MEDSURG-BC exam, understanding EBP is vital as it reflects their ability to provide care that meets contemporary standards. It also demonstrates a commitment to lifelong learning and adaptability in a rapidly evolving healthcare environment.

EBP not only improves patient outcomes but also enhances nurse satisfaction by fostering a sense of professional competence and empowerment. Nurses who engage in EBP are better equipped to advocate for their patients and contribute meaningfully to interdisciplinary teams.

In summary, Evidence-based Practice is an essential framework that guides medical-surgical nurses in delivering optimal care through informed decision-making processes that incorporate research evidence, clinical expertise, and patient preferences. Mastery of EBP principles is crucial for certification candidates, as it underpins effective nursing practice and aligns with the professional standards expected by the Medical-Surgical Nursing Certification Board (MSNCB).

3.1.4.1 Education:

In the context of medical-surgical nursing, education is a critical component that encompasses both the continuous professional development of nurses and the patient education they provide. It is a multifaceted process aimed at enhancing knowledge, skills, and competencies to ensure high-quality patient care and improve health outcomes.

For medical-surgical nurses, professional education involves ongoing learning and development activities that keep them abreast of the latest evidence-based practices, technological advancements, and emerging trends in healthcare. This continuous professional development is essential for maintaining certification and ensuring that nurses are equipped to deliver safe, effective, and patient-centered care.

Professional education for medical-surgical nurses includes formal educational programs such as workshops, seminars, conferences, and online courses. These programs are designed to enhance clinical skills, promote critical thinking, and foster a deeper understanding of complex medical conditions and their management. Additionally, professional education may involve participating in research activities, which not only contribute to personal growth but also advance the nursing profession by generating new knowledge.

Moreover, medical-surgical nurses are encouraged to engage in interprofessional education opportunities. Collaborating with other healthcare professionals through interdisciplinary training sessions can enhance communication skills, promote teamwork, and lead to more coordinated and comprehensive patient care.

Equally important is the role of medical-surgical nurses in patient education. Educating patients is a fundamental nursing responsibility that empowers individuals to participate actively in their own care. Effective patient education involves assessing the patient's learning needs, preferences, and readiness to learn. Nurses must use clear, concise language and tailor their teaching methods to accommodate different learning styles.

Patient education covers a wide range of topics, including disease processes, treatment plans, medication management, lifestyle modifications, and self-care strategies. For instance, a nurse may educate a patient with diabetes on how to monitor blood glucose levels, recognize signs of hypoglycemia or hyperglycemia, and understand the importance of adhering to dietary recommendations.

Furthermore, patient education should be an ongoing process that begins at admission and continues throughout the hospital stay and after discharge. Discharge planning is a critical component where nurses provide patients with written instructions and resources to ensure continuity of care at home. This includes teaching about follow-up appointments, signs of complications that require immediate attention, and whom to contact for questions or concerns.

To effectively educate patients, medical-surgical nurses must possess strong communication skills and cultural competence. Understanding cultural differences in health beliefs and practices enables nurses to deliver more personalized education that respects the patient's values and preferences.

In conclusion, education in medical-surgical nursing is a dual-faceted endeavor involving both the continuous professional development of nurses and comprehensive patient education. For nurses, it ensures they remain competent practitioners capable of delivering evidence-based care. For patients, it empowers them with the knowledge needed to manage their health conditions effectively. By prioritizing education in both these areas, medical-surgical nurses play a pivotal role in enhancing healthcare quality and improving patient outcomes.

3.1.4.2 Supporting Materials:

Supporting materials in the context of evidence-based practice (EBP) for medical-surgical nursing are resources and tools that provide the necessary information, data, and guidelines to facilitate informed decision-making in clinical practice. These materials serve as a foundation for integrating research evidence with clinical expertise and patient preferences to deliver high-quality care.

Supporting materials encompass a wide range of resources, including research articles, clinical guidelines, systematic reviews, meta-analyses, textbooks, policy statements, expert opinions, and patient care protocols. Each type of supporting material plays a unique role in enhancing the nurse's ability to apply evidence-based principles effectively.

Research articles are primary sources of evidence that report on original studies conducted to investigate specific clinical questions. These articles provide detailed information about study design, methodology, results, and conclusions. They are essential for understanding the latest advancements and findings in medical-surgical nursing.

Clinical guidelines are systematically developed statements that assist practitioners in making decisions about appropriate healthcare for specific clinical circumstances. They are based on a thorough review of existing evidence and are often developed by professional organizations or government agencies. Clinical guidelines offer recommendations that can be adapted to individual patient needs and local contexts.

Systematic reviews and meta-analyses synthesize existing research on a particular topic to provide a comprehensive overview of the available evidence. Systematic reviews involve a rigorous process of identifying, appraising, and summarizing studies, while meta-analyses statistically combine results from multiple studies to determine overall trends. These resources are invaluable for understanding the breadth and depth of evidence on specific interventions or outcomes.

Textbooks offer foundational knowledge and comprehensive coverage of medical-surgical nursing concepts. They provide context and background information that support the understanding and application of EBP principles. Textbooks often include references to key studies and guidelines, serving as a bridge between theoretical knowledge and practical application.

Policy statements from reputable organizations outline positions on important healthcare issues and provide guidance on best practices. These statements reflect consensus among experts and are grounded in evidence. They help nurses align their practice with current standards and address broader healthcare challenges.

Expert opinions fill gaps where high-quality evidence may be lacking or where emerging issues require immediate attention. While not as robust as other forms of evidence, expert opinions offer valuable insights based on clinical experience and expertise.

Patient care protocols are standardized procedures designed to ensure consistent and effective care delivery. These protocols incorporate evidence-based recommendations and are tailored to specific clinical settings or patient populations. They provide clear instructions for nurses to follow in routine practice or emergency situations.

In summary, supporting materials are integral components of evidence-based practice in medical-surgical nursing. They empower nurses with the knowledge needed to make informed clinical decisions, improve patient outcomes, and maintain professional competence. By critically appraising and applying these resources, medical-surgical nurses can bridge the gap between research findings and practical implementation, ultimately enhancing the quality of care provided to patients. Understanding how to effectively utilize supporting materials is crucial for success in the Medical-Surgical Nursing (MEDSURG-BC) certification exam and in everyday clinical practice.

MEDSURG-BC Practice Questions [SET 1]

Question 1: David, a 65-year-old male with type 2 diabetes, seeks guidance on enhancing his wellness. Which evidence-based intervention should you recommend?
A) Encouraging him to take vitamin D supplements daily.
B) Advising him to participate in a structured diabetes self-management education program.
C) Recommending he increase his water intake to at least eight glasses per day.
D) Suggesting he incorporate more lean proteins into his diet.

Question 2: During a multidisciplinary team meeting, the team is discussing the care plan for Mr. Johnson, a 68-year-old patient with congestive heart failure. The nurse notices that Mr. Johnson has been non-compliant with his medication regimen. Which action should the nurse take to address this issue within the interdisciplinary team?
A) Inform the primary care physician about the non-compliance.
B) Discuss the issue with the pharmacist to explore alternative medication options.
C) Collaborate with the social worker to identify potential barriers to compliance.
D) Schedule an educational session with Mr. Johnson and his family.

Question 3: In the context of adult learning theory, which principle should be prioritized when designing an educational program for medical-surgical nurses?
A) Self-directed learning
B) Rote memorization
C) Standardized testing
D) Passive observation

Question 4: When taking a health history from Mr. Lee, a 45-year-old patient with hypertension, which question would best help identify lifestyle factors contributing to his condition?
A) "Do you have a family history of hypertension?"
B) "What medications are you currently taking?"
C) "Can you describe your typical daily diet?"
D) "Have you experienced any recent weight changes?"

Question 5: David, a 35-year-old male recovering from major surgery, shows signs of withdrawal and irritability during his hospital stay. He denies any history of substance abuse but admits feeling stressed about returning to work. What is the most appropriate nursing action based on this psychosocial assessment?
A) Arrange for David to speak with a social worker about workplace stress.
B) Suggest relaxation techniques such as deep breathing exercises.
C) Monitor David closely for signs of postoperative complications.
D) Refer David to an occupational therapist for work-related adjustments.

Question 6: In the context of diversional activities for elderly patients with dementia, which activity is most likely to enhance cognitive function and social interaction?
A) Playing card games
B) Gardening
C) Solving puzzles
D) Participating in group singing sessions

Question 7: In evaluating cognitive impairment, why is it essential to conduct a thorough medication review?
A) To identify potential drug interactions
B) To assess adherence to prescribed medications
C) To detect medications that may cause or exacerbate cognitive impairment
D) To ensure accurate dosage of all medications

Question 8: Which intervention is most appropriate for a patient with acute decompensated heart failure to improve cardiac output?
A) Administering a beta-blocker
B) Administering an ACE inhibitor
C) Administering intravenous diuretics
D) Administering digoxin

Question 9: A 72-year-old patient named Mr. Lee has been admitted with confusion and an elevated temperature. You suspect sepsis as a potential diagnosis. Which clinical skill should you prioritize to confirm your suspicion?
A) Blood culture collection
B) Urine analysis
C) Chest X-ray interpretation
D) Neurological examination

Question 10: John, a 45-year-old male, presents to the emergency department with complaints of severe depression and feelings of hopelessness. During the assessment, he mentions that he has been having thoughts about ending his life but has not made any plans. Which of the following is the most appropriate initial nursing intervention?
A) Initiate a no-suicide contract.
B) Conduct a detailed psychosocial assessment.
C) Place John on one-to-one observation.
D) Refer John to a psychiatrist for medication management.

Question 11: Mr. Garcia, a 45-year-old male with end-stage renal disease (ESRD), is preparing for discharge after initiating dialysis treatment. What is the primary educational focus for his discharge plan?
A) Teaching him how to recognize signs of infection at the dialysis access site.
B) Instructing him on dietary restrictions specific to ESRD.
C) Educating him on fluid intake limitations.
D) Ensuring he understands the importance of medication adherence.

Question 12: For postoperative patients experiencing mild depression, which diversional activity is most effective in promoting physical recovery and emotional well-being?
A) Light exercise such as walking
B) Journaling their experiences
C) Watching motivational videos
D) Practicing mindfulness meditation

Question 13: John, a 45-year-old male, presents to the emergency department with confusion, tremors, and hallucinations. He has a history of chronic alcohol use and reports that he stopped drinking abruptly three days ago. What is the most likely diagnosis?
A) Alcohol intoxication
B) Alcohol withdrawal delirium
C) Wernicke-Korsakoff syndrome
D) Hepatic encephalopathy

Question 14: For a postoperative patient with an indwelling urinary catheter, which intervention is most effective in preventing catheter-associated urinary tract infections (CAUTIs)?
A) Daily cleansing of the perineal area with antiseptic solution
B) Maintaining a closed drainage system
C) Regularly changing the catheter every 72 hours
D) Administering prophylactic antibiotics

Question 15: A patient named Mr. Lee with a history of hypertension is considering complementary therapies to help manage his blood pressure alongside conventional treatment. Which CAM approach is best supported by current research for this purpose?
A) Yoga
B) Chiropractic Care
C) Herbal Supplements
D) Cupping Therapy

Question 16: In the context of cultural competence, which approach is most effective when planning care for a patient from a diverse background?
A) Assuming cultural practices based on ethnicity
B) Encouraging adherence to Western medical practices
C) Conducting a cultural assessment with the patient
D) Avoiding discussions about cultural beliefs

Question 17: Robert, a 70-year-old male post-colon resection surgery patient, has not passed gas or had a bowel movement by postoperative day four. He reports abdominal discomfort and bloating. What should be the nurse's initial action?
A) Administer prescribed laxatives immediately.
B) Encourage ambulation and increased oral fluids.
C) Insert a nasogastric tube for decompression.
D) Perform an abdominal assessment including auscultation.

Question 18: David, a 45-year-old male recovering from abdominal surgery, reports severe pain despite receiving analgesics. What is the most appropriate nursing intervention?
A) Reassessing pain level and medication effectiveness
B) Increasing the dose of current analgesics
C) Consulting with the pain management team
D) Implementing non-pharmacological pain relief methods

Question 19: During her physical assessment of Mr. Patel, who has been experiencing dizziness and lightheadedness, Nurse Laura performs orthostatic vital signs measurement. She observes that his blood pressure drops significantly upon standing from a supine position. What condition does this finding most likely indicate?
A) Hypovolemia
B) Essential hypertension
C) Postural orthostatic tachycardia syndrome (POTS)
D) Vasovagal syncope

Question 20: Which of the following interventions is most appropriate for managing a postoperative patient experiencing signs of internal bleeding?
A) Administering intravenous fluids and monitoring vital signs
B) Applying pressure to the surgical site
C) Elevating the patient's legs above heart level
D) Initiating a blood transfusion immediately

Question 21: Maria, a 67-year-old female with type 2 diabetes mellitus and chronic kidney disease stage 3, presents with worsening edema and shortness of breath. Which intervention is most appropriate for managing her fluid overload?
A) Initiating hemodialysis immediately
B) Administering intravenous furosemide
C) Restricting fluid intake strictly
D) Prescribing a low-sodium diet

Question 22: Jane, a medical-surgical nurse, is caring for Mr. Smith, who has expressed concerns about the side effects of his prescribed medication. Jane believes that Mr. Smith's concerns are valid and decides to advocate on his behalf. Which action best demonstrates effective advocacy in this scenario?
A) Encouraging Mr. Smith to research the medication online.
B) Discussing Mr. Smith's concerns with the prescribing physician.
C) Reassuring Mr. Smith that the side effects are normal and temporary.
D) Advising Mr. Smith to refuse the medication until further notice.

Question 23: Mr. Smith, a 45-year-old patient with chronic pain due to rheumatoid arthritis, reports feeling isolated and depressed. Which diversional activity would best address both his emotional and physical needs?
A) Encouraging participation in a group exercise class
B) Suggesting he read a self-help book on chronic pain management
C) Providing access to an online support group for arthritis patients
D) Recommending he take up knitting or another craft activity

Question 24: James, a 45-year-old male with a history of hypertension and coronary artery disease, presents with chest pain radiating to his left arm and jaw. Which diagnostic test should be performed first?
A) Echocardiogram
B) Cardiac enzyme levels
C) Electrocardiogram (ECG)
D) Chest X-ray

Question 25: In managing polypharmacy for patients with chronic diseases, which approach should be prioritized to ensure medication safety and efficacy?
A) Simplifying the medication regimen
B) Regularly monitoring renal function
C) Increasing patient education on each drug
D) Ensuring adherence through pill organizers

Question 26: Nurse John is assigned to care for Mrs. Garcia, a 55-year-old Latina woman recovering from surgery who primarily speaks Spanish and has limited English proficiency. What is the most culturally competent approach Nurse John can take to ensure effective communication?
A) Use medical jargon as much as possible since it is universally understood.
B) Rely on Mrs. Garcia's family members to translate complex medical information.
C) Utilize a professional medical interpreter to facilitate communication.
D) Speak slowly and loudly in English assuming she might understand better.

Question 27: Which non-pharmacologic treatment has shown significant efficacy in managing symptoms of fibromyalgia?
A) Aerobic exercise
B) Biofeedback
C) Herbal supplements
D) Chiropractic care

Question 28: Mrs. Garcia, who has a history of chronic obstructive pulmonary disease (COPD), requires non-invasive ventilation support at home. Which device should be recommended for her condition?
A) Nasal cannula
B) Bi-level Positive Airway Pressure (BiPAP)
C) Venturi mask
D) Simple face mask

Question 29: During a follow-up visit, Nurse Sam needs to evaluate the learning outcomes of patient John, who

recently received education on hypertension management. Which approach should Nurse Sam use to ensure comprehensive evaluation?
A) Reviewing John's self-reported blood pressure log
B) Discussing John's dietary changes and exercise routine
C) Asking John to explain the importance of medication adherence
D) Combining review of self-reported logs, discussion on lifestyle changes, and explanation of medication adherence

Question 30: Mrs. Smith, a 58-year-old female with a history of hypertension and diabetes, presents with sudden onset of shortness of breath and chest pain radiating to her left arm. Which assessment skill is paramount to determine if she is experiencing a myocardial infarction?
A) Electrocardiogram interpretation
B) Blood pressure measurement
C) Heart rate monitoring
D) Respiratory rate assessment

Question 31: During a health history collection, Nurse Lisa is interviewing Mr. Johnson, a 55-year-old male with a history of hypertension and diabetes. He mentions experiencing intermittent chest pain. Which question should Nurse Lisa prioritize to further investigate his symptom?
A) "Can you describe the nature of your chest pain?"
B) "Do you have a family history of heart disease?"
C) "Have you experienced any recent weight gain or loss?"
D) "How often do you monitor your blood sugar levels?"

Question 32: Which factor is most likely to enhance the effectiveness of an interdisciplinary consult in improving patient outcomes?
A) The frequency of consults
B) The hierarchical structure of the healthcare team
C) The presence of a dedicated case manager
D) The use of evidence-based guidelines

Question 33: Which communication technique is most effective in establishing a therapeutic relationship with a patient experiencing acute anxiety?
A) Providing reassurance
B) Active listening
C) Offering advice
D) Reflective questioning

Question 34: Robert, a 70-year-old male with chronic obstructive pulmonary disease (COPD), presents with increased dyspnea, productive cough with green sputum, and fever. His arterial blood gas shows pH 7.30, PaCO2 55 mmHg, PaO2 60 mmHg on room air. What is the most likely diagnosis?
A) Acute Asthma Exacerbation
B) Acute Respiratory Distress Syndrome (ARDS)
C) Community-Acquired Pneumonia
D) COPD Exacerbation

Question 35: Maria, a 60-year-old patient with a history of atrial fibrillation, presents with sudden onset of left leg pain, pallor, and pulselessness after undergoing abdominal surgery. What is the most appropriate initial diagnostic test?
A) Venous Doppler ultrasound
B) Arterial blood gas analysis
C) CT angiography
D) MRI of the lower extremities

Question 36: Sarah, a 55-year-old woman with a family history of breast cancer, visits the clinic for her annual check-up. Considering her age and family history, which screening test is most appropriate for Sarah to undergo?
A) Mammography
B) Breast MRI
C) Genetic testing for BRCA1/BRCA2 mutations
D) Clinical breast exam

Question 37: Which physical assessment finding is most indicative of early-stage right-sided heart failure?
A) Jugular venous distension
B) Peripheral edema
C) Hepatomegaly
D) Ascites

Question 38: Mr. Smith, a patient with diabetes, is struggling to manage his condition despite attending multiple education sessions. What approach should the nurse take to enhance Mr. Smith's self-management skills?
A) Repeating the same educational content
B) Utilizing teach-back method to confirm understanding
C) Increasing the frequency of education sessions
D) Providing additional written materials

Question 39: Nurse Tom is caring for Ms. Garcia, who is hesitant about undergoing a recommended surgical procedure due to potential complications she read about online. How should Tom advocate for Ms. Garcia while respecting her autonomy?
A) Telling Ms. Garcia that her fears are unfounded.
B) Providing Ms. Garcia with evidence-based information about the surgery.
C) Insisting that Ms. Garcia proceed with the surgery as recommended.
D) Suggesting that Ms. Garcia seek a second opinion from another surgeon.

Question 40: Which of the following assessments is most indicative of increased intracranial pressure (ICP) in a patient with a traumatic brain injury?
A) Unequal pupil size
B) Decreased deep tendon reflexes
C) Bilateral motor weakness
D) Altered level of consciousness

Question 41: In evaluating a patient postoperatively for potential development of an embolism, which diagnostic test provides definitive confirmation?
A) D-dimer test
B) Ventilation-perfusion (V/Q) scan
C) Computed tomography pulmonary angiography (CTPA)
D) Electrocardiogram (ECG)

Question 42: In managing a postoperative patient with a suspected infection, which diagnostic test provides the most rapid and specific information to guide initial treatment?
A) Complete blood count (CBC)
B) Blood cultures
C) C-reactive protein (CRP)
D) Procalcitonin levels

Question 43: During postoperative care, which laboratory value is most critical to monitor for early detection of bleeding complications?
A) Hemoglobin level
B) White blood cell count
C) Platelet count
D) Prothrombin time (PT)

Question 44: Nurse Alex is developing a discharge plan for Mrs. Thompson, who has been hospitalized for heart failure exacerbation. Which skill-based intervention should he prioritize to ensure effective self-management

at home?
A) Educating the patient on recognizing early signs of heart failure exacerbation.
B) Scheduling regular follow-up appointments with her cardiologist.
C) Ensuring the patient understands her medication regimen.
D) Arranging home health visits for ongoing monitoring.

Question 45: While collecting a health history from a 55-year-old patient named Mr. Johnson, who presents with chronic cough and shortness of breath, which aspect of his history is most crucial to assess to identify potential occupational hazards?
A) Family history of respiratory diseases
B) Duration and nature of the cough
C) Past occupational exposure to dust or chemicals
D) Recent travel history

Question 46: Nurse Emily is caring for Mr. Johnson, a 65-year-old patient with chronic obstructive pulmonary disease (COPD). She notices that he is struggling to understand the importance of using his inhaler regularly. Which approach should Nurse Emily use to effectively educate Mr. Johnson about his medication regimen?
A) Provide a detailed pamphlet and ask him to read it.
B) Use a teach-back method to confirm his understanding.
C) Show him an instructional video on inhaler use.
D) Schedule a follow-up appointment for further education.

Question 47: In terms of supporting materials for clinical decision-making in medical-surgical nursing, which type of resource provides the highest level of evidence?
A) Randomized controlled trials (RCTs)
B) Case studies
C) Expert opinion articles
D) Cohort studies

Question 48: Mrs. Johnson, a 65-year-old diabetic patient, is admitted for a knee replacement surgery. As part of infection prevention strategies, which intervention should the nurse prioritize to reduce the risk of postoperative infection?
A) Administering prophylactic antibiotics within one hour before the surgical incision
B) Applying a topical antiseptic to the surgical site immediately after surgery
C) Ensuring the patient fasts for at least 12 hours before surgery
D) Using chlorhexidine wipes on the surgical site daily postoperatively

Question 49: Which of the following assessment tools is most appropriate for evaluating a patient's ability to perform Activities of Daily Living (ADLs) independently?
A) Barthel Index
B) Mini-Mental State Examination (MMSE)
C) Braden Scale
D) Glasgow Coma Scale

Question 50: Which assessment skill is most crucial for a nurse to accurately identify early signs of sepsis in a postoperative patient?
A) Palpation
B) Auscultation
C) Temperature monitoring
D) Blood pressure measurement

Question 51: A 55-year-old male named Mr. Davis presents with fatigue, decreased deep tendon reflexes, and hypotension. His lab results reveal a serum magnesium level of 1.0 mg/dL. What is the best initial treatment for his condition?
A) Oral magnesium supplements.
B) Intravenous magnesium sulfate.
C) Increase dietary magnesium intake.
D) Intravenous normal saline.

Question 52: Mr. Johnson, a 58-year-old patient with Type 2 Diabetes, has been struggling to manage his blood glucose levels despite being on medication. During a follow-up visit, the nurse emphasizes the importance of self-management strategies. Which of the following strategies is most effective in improving Mr. Johnson's self-management of his diabetes?
A) Attending monthly diabetes education classes
B) Using a continuous glucose monitor (CGM)
C) Maintaining a daily food and exercise journal
D) Scheduling bi-weekly visits with a dietitian

Question 53: What blood product should be administered to a patient with severe hypofibrinogenemia?
A) Cryoprecipitate
B) Fresh Frozen Plasma (FFP)
C) Platelets
D) Albumin

Question 54: In a review of systems, which symptom would most likely warrant further evaluation for a gastrointestinal disorder?
A) Night sweats
B) Abdominal bloating after meals
C) Shortness of breath during activity
D) Increased urinary frequency

Question 55: John, a 67-year-old patient with chronic obstructive pulmonary disease (COPD), is admitted with an acute exacerbation. Which intervention should the nurse prioritize to improve John's oxygenation status?
A) Administering bronchodilators as prescribed
B) Initiating high-flow oxygen therapy
C) Encouraging deep breathing exercises
D) Positioning the patient in a high Fowler's position

Question 56: During a family meeting about Mr. Johnson's post-operative care plan, his daughter expresses concern about the lack of communication from the healthcare team. As a nurse, what is the most appropriate response to ensure patient- and family-centered care?
A) "We have been very busy, but I will make sure to update you more frequently."
B) "I apologize for any inconvenience; let's schedule regular updates with the team."
C) "It's important for you to trust us; we are doing our best."
D) "You can always ask the doctor directly for updates."

Question 57: A patient on monoamine oxidase inhibitors (MAOIs) should avoid consuming which type of food due to the risk of hypertensive crisis?
A) Aged cheese
B) Fresh fruits
C) Lean meats
D) Whole grains

Question 58: In the context of evaluating ADLs, why is it important to assess both basic and instrumental activities?
A) To determine overall physical health
B) To understand social engagement levels
C) To evaluate comprehensive functional status
D) To diagnose specific medical conditions

Question 59: Ms. Garcia, a 45-year-old patient with fibromyalgia, is exploring non-pharmacologic

treatments to manage her widespread musculoskeletal pain and fatigue. Which intervention should be considered first based on current guidelines?**
A) Tai Chi
B) Chiropractic Care
C) Meditation
D) Heat Therapy

Question 60: A 55-year-old patient named Mr. Johnson, who has been experiencing chronic lower back pain, is interested in exploring complementary and alternative medicine (CAM) options. He asks the nurse about the most evidence-based CAM therapy for his condition. Which of the following should the nurse recommend?
A) Acupuncture
B) Aromatherapy
C) Homeopathy
D) Reflexology

Question 61: Nurse Alex is evaluating the effectiveness of a diabetes management teaching session with patient Maria. Which method would provide the most accurate assessment of Maria's understanding and ability to manage her condition?
A) Asking Maria to verbally repeat the information taught
B) Having Maria demonstrate blood glucose monitoring and insulin administration
C) Providing a written test on diabetes management concepts
D) Observing Maria during a follow-up visit without direct interaction

Question 62: According to Erikson's stages of psychosocial development, which developmental challenge is most relevant for a middle-aged adult?
A) Identity vs. Role Confusion
B) Generativity vs. Stagnation
C) Intimacy vs. Isolation
D) Integrity vs. Despair

Question 63: Maria, a 68-year-old patient, is recovering from a hip replacement surgery. During her postoperative assessment, she expresses concerns about her ability to return to her gardening hobby. Which developmental stage is Maria most likely experiencing according to Erikson's psychosocial theory?
A) Integrity vs. Despair
B) Generativity vs. Stagnation
C) Intimacy vs. Isolation
D) Identity vs. Role Confusion

Question 64: Which approach best exemplifies a medical-surgical nurse's role in promoting interprofessional collaboration?
A) Leading team meetings to discuss patient care plans
B) Delegating tasks based on each team member's expertise
C) Encouraging open communication among all team members
D) Evaluating team performance regularly

Question 65: For a patient with diabetes mellitus, which modification in their exercise regimen should be prioritized to prevent hypoglycemia?
A) Engage in high-intensity interval training.
B) Exercise immediately after insulin administration.
C) Monitor blood glucose levels before and after exercise.
D) Avoid carbohydrate intake before exercise.

Question 66: Mrs. Johnson, a 68-year-old patient with type 2 diabetes, is being discharged after a hospitalization for hyperglycemia. As part of her discharge teaching, which of the following strategies should the nurse prioritize to ensure Mrs. Johnson effectively manages her condition at home?
A) Provide a detailed pamphlet on diabetes management.
B) Schedule a follow-up appointment with her endocrinologist.
C) Teach her how to monitor her blood glucose levels and administer insulin.
D) Advise her to join a diabetes support group.

Question 67: During a routine physical examination, Mr. Lee, a 45-year-old male with no significant medical history, reports experiencing occasional palpitations. Which physical assessment finding would most likely suggest that these palpitations are due to atrial fibrillation?
A) Regularly irregular pulse
B) Irregularly irregular pulse
C) Bradycardia
D) Tachycardia

Question 68: Mr. Johnson, a 65-year-old male with a history of hypertension and diabetes, presents to the emergency department with complaints of dizziness and fatigue. His vital signs are as follows: BP 90/60 mmHg, HR 110 bpm, RR 20 breaths/min, Temp 98.6°F. Which of the following interventions should be prioritized?
A) Administer IV fluids to address potential hypovolemia.
B) Start an antihypertensive medication to manage blood pressure.
C) Provide oxygen therapy to improve oxygen saturation.
D) Administer insulin to control blood glucose levels.

Question 69: In the context of health promotion among older adults, which intervention has been shown to significantly reduce the risk of falls?
A) Strength training exercises
B) Vitamin D supplementation
C) Home safety assessments
D) Balance training exercises

Question 70: Nurse Taylor is managing a team on a medical-surgical floor and needs to delegate medication administration for Mr. Lee, who requires routine oral medications but has a history of dysphagia (difficulty swallowing). Who should Nurse Taylor assign this task to?
A) Another registered nurse (RN)
B) A certified nursing assistant (CNA)
C) A licensed practical nurse (LPN)
D) The patient's family member under guidance

Question 71: In evaluating the outcomes of a nursing care plan for a diabetic patient, which criterion is most indicative of successful management?
A) Reduction in HbA1c levels over three months
B) Patient's adherence to dietary recommendations
C) Consistent monitoring of blood glucose levels
D) Absence of diabetic complications

Question 72: Mr. Smith, a 65-year-old male with a history of hypertension and diabetes, has been prescribed metformin and lisinopril. He is now starting on a new medication, furosemide, for edema. Which potential adverse effect should the nurse monitor for due to the interaction between these medications?
A) Hyperkalemia
B) Hypokalemia
C) Hyperglycemia
D) Hypoglycemia

Question 73: In evaluating the effectiveness of an educational program on medication adherence, which outcome measure is considered the most reliable?

A) Patient self-reports
B) Pill count
C) Pharmacy refill records
D) Clinical outcomes

Question 74: In diagnosing deep vein thrombosis (DVT), which skill should a nurse prioritize?
A) Inspection for redness and swelling
B) Palpation for tenderness along the vein
C) Measurement of calf circumference
D) Assessment of Homan's sign

Question 75: In assessing a patient for fluid volume deficit, which clinical sign is most indicative of this condition?
A) Jugular venous distention
B) Orthostatic hypotension
C) Peripheral edema
D) Hypertension

Question 76: Sarah, a 45-year-old woman, presents to the emergency department with multiple bruises and a fractured rib. She seems anxious and avoids eye contact. During the assessment, she mentions that she "fell down the stairs." What should be the nurse's priority action in this scenario?
A) Document her statement and proceed with the physical examination.
B) Report the injury to law enforcement immediately.
C) Assess for additional signs of abuse and ensure Sarah's safety.
D) Refer Sarah to a social worker for further evaluation.

Question 77: In managing postoperative care for elderly patients, which intervention is most effective in preventing delirium?
A) Administering routine sedatives
B) Ensuring adequate hydration
C) Limiting nighttime disturbances
D) Providing high-protein meals

Question 78: When considering multimodal analgesia for postoperative pain management, which combination of medications would be most effective?
A) Acetaminophen and ibuprofen
B) Morphine and codeine
C) Gabapentin and acetaminophen
D) Fentanyl and oxycodone

Question 79: A 65-year-old patient, Mr. Smith, is recovering from a total hip replacement surgery. As the medical-surgical nurse, you are responsible for planning his discharge. Which of the following steps should be prioritized in developing his discharge plan?
A) Schedule a follow-up appointment with his orthopedic surgeon.
B) Provide education on postoperative exercises and mobility aids.
C) Coordinate with physical therapy for home visits.
D) Assess his home environment for potential hazards.

Question 80: Mr. Garcia, a 65-year-old male with chronic obstructive pulmonary disease (COPD), has been prescribed multiple medications by different specialists. He reports new symptoms of confusion and muscle weakness. What is the most appropriate initial nursing intervention?
A) Assess for potential adverse effects of his medications.
B) Suggest a comprehensive vitamin panel test.
C) Refer him to a neurologist for further evaluation.
D) Advise him to increase physical activity to strengthen muscles.

Question 81: Which drug combination is most likely to cause a significant increase in potassium levels?
A) Lisinopril and Spironolactone
B) Atorvastatin and Ezetimibe
C) Levothyroxine and Calcium Carbonate
D) Omeprazole and Clopidogrel

Question 82: Which clinical manifestation is most characteristic of left-sided heart failure?
A) Peripheral edema
B) Jugular venous distension
C) Pulmonary congestion
D) Hepatomegaly

Question 83: Nurse Alex is developing an educational program for heart failure patients aimed at reducing readmission rates. Which component should be prioritized to achieve this goal?
A) Detailed pathophysiology of heart failure
B) Medication adherence strategies
C) Lifestyle modification tips
D) Symptom recognition and management

Question 84: Which of the following strategies is most effective for a nurse to use when addressing cultural competence in patient care?
A) Using a standardized care plan for all patients
B) Incorporating cultural assessments into patient evaluations
C) Relying on personal cultural experiences to guide care
D) Avoiding discussions about cultural differences to prevent discomfort

Question 85: Nurse Emily is preparing to administer intravenous medication to a patient with severe dehydration. Which medical equipment should she use to ensure precise control over the infusion rate?
A) Gravity drip set
B) Syringe pump
C) Elastomeric pump
D) Infusion pump

Question 86: Ms. Smith, a 45-year-old woman recovering from abdominal surgery, reports inadequate pain relief despite receiving morphine via PCA (patient-controlled analgesia). What should be the next step in her pain management plan?
A) Increase the basal rate of morphine infusion.
B) Add a non-opioid adjuvant such as gabapentin.
C) Switch to a different opioid like fentanyl.
D) Assess and address potential psychological factors contributing to her pain.

Question 87: During a busy shift, Nurse Alex notices that he accidentally administered a higher dose of medication than prescribed to Mrs. Thompson. What should be Nurse Alex's immediate ethical response?
A) Monitor Mrs. Thompson closely for adverse effects without reporting the error.
B) Inform Mrs. Thompson about the error and monitor her condition.
C) Report the medication error to his supervisor and document it accurately.
D) Consult with another nurse before deciding whether to report it.

Question 88: Mr. Smith, a 55-year-old male with diabetes mellitus, presents with a non-healing ulcer on his left foot. Upon assessment, you note erythema, warmth, and purulent drainage from the wound site. What is the most critical diagnostic test to perform initially?
A) Blood glucose level
B) Wound culture and sensitivity

C) Complete blood count (CBC)
D) X-ray of the foot

Question 89: Nurse Alex is caring for Mr. Johnson, a post-operative patient who has developed unexpected complications. The surgical team has requested a consult from the infectious disease specialist due to a suspected infection. What is the primary responsibility of Nurse Alex in this scenario?
A) Ensure that all relevant patient information and documentation are available for the consultant.
B) Perform an independent assessment to confirm the need for the consult.
C) Inform the patient's family about the consult before it takes place.
D) Administer prescribed antibiotics before the consultant arrives.

Question 90: When assessing a patient's fluid balance, which skill is paramount to ensure accurate evaluation?
A) Daily weight measurement
B) Urine output monitoring
C) Skin turgor assessment
D) Blood urea nitrogen (BUN) levels

Question 91: Nurse Sarah is caring for Mr. Johnson, a 75-year-old patient with severe dementia who has been attempting to remove his IV line and wander off the unit. Which of the following actions should Nurse Sarah take first before applying physical restraints?
A) Obtain a physician's order for restraints.
B) Assess Mr. Johnson's need for toileting and pain relief.
C) Explain the need for restraints to Mr. Johnson's family.
D) Document Mr. Johnson's behavior in the medical record.

Question 92: In assessing a child for potential abuse, which finding would be most concerning for physical abuse?
A) Chronic absenteeism from school
B) Frequent urinary tract infections
C) Multiple bruises at various stages of healing
D) Developmental delays without medical explanation

Question 93: For women aged 21-29, which cervical cancer screening method is currently recommended?
A) Pap smear every year
B) Pap smear every three years
C) HPV testing alone every five years
D) Co-testing with Pap smear and HPV test every five years

Question 94: For patients with insomnia, which CAM approach has demonstrated the highest efficacy according to randomized controlled trials?
A) Melatonin supplementation
B) Cognitive Behavioral Therapy for Insomnia (CBT-I)
C) Tai Chi
D) Progressive Muscle Relaxation

Question 95: While caring for Mr. Ahmed, a 60-year-old Muslim man who observes fasting during Ramadan, Nurse Lisa notices that he is becoming increasingly fatigued due to his fasting schedule conflicting with medication administration times. How should Nurse Lisa address this situation?
A) Advise Mr. Ahmed to break his fast for the sake of his health.
B) Disregard the fasting practice and continue administering medications as scheduled.
C) Collaborate with Mr. Ahmed and his healthcare provider to adjust medication times around fasting periods.
D) Provide additional nutritional supplements without altering medication times.

Question 96: When collecting a health history from an elderly patient, which factor is most important to consider to ensure accurate information?
A) Cognitive function
B) Family support system
C) Previous hospitalizations
D) Nutritional status

Question 97: According to contemporary research, which learning preference is most effective for teaching a patient with low health literacy about postoperative care?
A) Visual learning
B) Auditory learning
C) Kinesthetic learning
D) Reading/writing learning

Question 98: Which of the following strategies is most effective in enhancing communication within an interdisciplinary healthcare team to improve patient outcomes?
A) Regularly scheduled team meetings
B) Use of standardized communication tools like SBAR
C) Informal hallway conversations
D) Individual email updates

Question 99: In a patient presenting with acute abdominal pain, which physical examination finding suggests peritonitis?
A) Rebound tenderness
B) Murphy's sign
C) McBurney's point tenderness
D) Rovsing's sign

Question 100: Nurse Alex is working with a patient, Mrs. Johnson, who has expressed concerns about her upcoming surgery. Which approach should Nurse Alex take to fulfill his professional role effectively?
A) Providing detailed technical information about the surgery.
B) Encouraging Mrs. Johnson to discuss her fears and concerns.
C) Reassuring Mrs. Johnson that everything will be fine without further discussion.
D) Referring Mrs. Johnson to a psychologist immediately.

Question 101: During a post-operative visit, Mr. Johnson expresses anxiety about his upcoming physical therapy sessions, fearing they will be too painful. Which therapeutic communication technique should the nurse use to best address his concerns?
A) Reassure him that the pain will be minimal.
B) Share a personal story about overcoming pain.
C) Encourage him to express his feelings and fears.
D) Distract him with unrelated conversation.

Question 102: Emily, a 9-year-old girl with suspected learning disabilities, struggles with memory retention and problem-solving in school. Which developmental age-appropriate cognitive assessment should be used?
A) Wechsler Intelligence Scale for Children (WISC)
B) Stanford-Binet Intelligence Scales
C) Kaufman Assessment Battery for Children (KABC)
D) Bayley Scales of Infant Development

Question 103: When providing discharge instructions to a non-English-speaking patient, what is the best practice for ensuring understanding?
A) Speaking slowly and loudly in English
B) Using professional medical interpreters
C) Giving written instructions in English only
D) Asking family members to translate

Question 104: Which cognitive assessment tool is most

appropriate for evaluating executive function in a patient with suspected early-stage dementia?
A) Mini-Mental State Examination (MMSE)
B) Montreal Cognitive Assessment (MoCA)
C) Clock Drawing Test (CDT)
D) Trail Making Test Part B (TMT-B)

Question 105: Mr. Smith, a 68-year-old patient with chronic obstructive pulmonary disease (COPD), is admitted for worsening respiratory symptoms. During your initial assessment, you notice he struggles with short-term memory and problem-solving tasks. Which factor should be prioritized in assessing his cognitive impairment?
A) Oxygen saturation levels
B) Blood glucose levels
C) Medication review
D) Nutritional status

Question 106: In managing a patient with suspected sepsis, which piece of equipment is crucial for early goal-directed therapy?
A) Central venous catheter
B) Pulmonary artery catheter
C) Non-invasive cardiac output monitor
D) Peripheral intravenous line

Question 107: In the context of therapeutic communication, what is the most effective strategy for a medical-surgical nurse to build trust with a patient?
A) Providing detailed explanations of medical procedures
B) Listening actively to the patient's concerns
C) Offering reassurance about treatment outcomes
D) Maintaining professional boundaries at all times

Question 108: John, a 60-year-old male with a history of smoking, presents with chronic cough, hemoptysis, and unintentional weight loss. On physical examination, you notice clubbing of the fingers. What is the most likely diagnosis?
A) Chronic Obstructive Pulmonary Disease (COPD)
B) Tuberculosis
C) Lung Cancer
D) Pneumonia

Question 109: Which finding during a review of systems is most concerning for a potential neurological disorder?
A) Intermittent joint pain
B) Sudden onset of severe headache
C) Occasional dizziness when standing quickly
D) Chronic fatigue

Question 110: Mrs. Lee, a 60-year-old diabetic patient, is being educated on insulin administration. What educational strategy should the nurse prioritize to ensure Mrs. Lee can independently manage her insulin injections at home?
A) Providing detailed written instructions with diagrams
B) Demonstrating the injection technique on an orange
C) Allowing Mrs. Lee to practice injections under supervision
D) Showing an instructional video during the teaching session

Question 111: Mr. Smith, a 70-year-old patient with COPD, is hospitalized with pneumonia. To prevent hospital-acquired infections, which measure should be implemented first?
A) Placing Mr. Smith in a private room with contact precautions
B) Encouraging early ambulation and deep breathing exercises
C) Performing hand hygiene before and after patient contact
D) Providing Mr. Smith with an incentive spirometer

Question 112: When performing a cardiovascular assessment on a patient with suspected heart failure, which finding would most strongly suggest left-sided heart failure?
A) Jugular venous distention (JVD)
B) Peripheral edema
C) Pulmonary crackles
D) Hepatomegaly

Question 113: John, a 65-year-old male, underwent abdominal surgery. On the second postoperative day, he complains of sudden shortness of breath and chest pain. What is the most appropriate immediate nursing intervention?
A) Administer oxygen and notify the physician.
B) Perform a full respiratory assessment.
C) Encourage deep breathing exercises and ambulation.
D) Check for signs of infection at the surgical site.

Question 114: Sarah, a 78-year-old woman, presents with confusion and difficulty completing tasks she previously found simple. Her family reports that she has become increasingly forgetful over the past six months. Which cognitive assessment tool is most appropriate for evaluating Sarah's developmental age-related cognitive decline?
A) Mini-Mental State Examination (MMSE)
B) Montreal Cognitive Assessment (MoCA)
C) Clock Drawing Test
D) Geriatric Depression Scale (GDS)

Question 115: Nurse Taylor receives an order for an endocrinology consult for Mr. Lee, who has poorly controlled diabetes despite current treatment plans. Which action should Nurse Taylor take first to ensure an effective consult?
A) Review Mr. Lee's blood glucose logs and medication adherence history.
B) Educate Mr. Lee about potential changes in his treatment regimen post-consult.
C) Schedule follow-up appointments with other specialists preemptively.
D) Prepare educational materials about diabetes management for Mr. Lee.

Question 116: Maria, a 45-year-old woman with no family history of breast cancer but dense breast tissue on mammography, seeks advice on additional screening tools. Which tool should be recommended to further evaluate her breast health?
A) Breast MRI
B) Ultrasound
C) Digital Mammography
D) Clinical Breast Exam

Question 117: Which diversional activity is most effective in reducing anxiety and improving mood in hospitalized patients with chronic pain?
A) Watching television
B) Engaging in art therapy
C) Reading books
D) Listening to music

Question 118: A 55-year-old patient named John is recovering from a hip replacement surgery. On the third postoperative day, he suddenly experiences shortness of breath, chest pain, and a rapid heart rate. Which of the following interventions should be prioritized to manage his condition?
A) Administering IV fluids to maintain blood pressure
B) Initiating anticoagulant therapy immediately

C) Performing a chest X-ray to confirm pneumonia
D) Providing supplemental oxygen via nasal cannula

Question 119: Maria, a 32-year-old female, is admitted for severe agitation and paranoia. She admits to recent methamphetamine use. Which immediate intervention is most appropriate?
A) Administering benzodiazepines
B) Initiating antipsychotic medication
C) Providing a quiet environment with reassurance
D) Starting methadone therapy

Question 120: Mrs. Thompson, a 75-year-old patient with a history of hypertension and diabetes, is brought to the emergency department by her daughter, who reports that her mother has been increasingly forgetful and disoriented over the past week. Upon assessment, you observe that Mrs. Thompson is unable to recall recent events and has difficulty following simple instructions. Which cognitive assessment tool would be most appropriate to evaluate Mrs. Thompson's cognitive impairment?
A) Mini-Mental State Examination (MMSE)
B) Montreal Cognitive Assessment (MoCA)
C) Clock Drawing Test (CDT)
D) Confusion Assessment Method (CAM)

Question 121: Which educational strategy is most effective for enhancing patient adherence to a complex medication regimen in a medical-surgical setting?
A) Lecture-based education
B) Interactive workshops
C) Written handouts
D) Individualized teaching sessions

Question 122: Which of the following strategies is most effective in preventing catheter-associated urinary tract infections (CAUTIs) in hospitalized patients?
A) Routine use of antimicrobial-coated catheters
B) Implementing a closed drainage system
C) Regularly changing the catheter every 48 hours
D) Ensuring proper hand hygiene before and after catheter manipulation

Question 123: Mrs. Smith, a 72-year-old patient with chronic kidney disease, presents with muscle cramps and an irregular heartbeat. Her lab results show a potassium level of 6.5 mEq/L. Which of the following treatments should be initiated first?
A) Administer intravenous calcium gluconate.
B) Administer sodium polystyrene sulfonate.
C) Initiate hemodialysis immediately.
D) Administer loop diuretics.

Question 124: Mrs. Johnson, a 65-year-old female with a history of chronic kidney disease (CKD), presents with fatigue and swelling in her legs. Her recent laboratory results show elevated serum creatinine and blood urea nitrogen (BUN) levels. Which additional diagnostic test is most appropriate to assess her kidney function?
A) Urinalysis
B) Serum electrolytes
C) Glomerular filtration rate (GFR)
D) Complete blood count (CBC)

Question 125: John, a 65-year-old patient with chronic atrial fibrillation, is prescribed warfarin for anticoagulation. He is also taking amiodarone for rhythm control. What should the nurse monitor closely in John due to the potential drug-drug interaction between warfarin and amiodarone?
A) Blood glucose levels
B) Serum potassium levels
C) International Normalized Ratio (INR)
D) Liver function tests

ANSWER WITH DETAILED EXPLANATION SET [1]

Question 1: Correct Answer: B) Advising him to participate in a structured diabetes self-management education program.
Rationale: Participation in a structured diabetes self-management education program is strongly supported by evidence for improving glycemic control, reducing complications, and enhancing quality of life for individuals with type 2 diabetes. Vitamin D supplementation (Option A), increasing water intake (Option C), and incorporating lean proteins into the diet (Option D) can be beneficial but are not as impactful as comprehensive education programs that empower patients through knowledge and self-care skills specific to diabetes management. Therefore, Option B provides the most holistic approach for David's wellness enhancement.
Question 2: Correct Answer: C) Collaborate with the social worker to identify potential barriers to compliance.
Rationale: Collaborating with the social worker helps identify underlying barriers such as financial issues or lack of understanding, which can be addressed comprehensively. Informing the primary care physician (A) may not directly address barriers, discussing alternatives with the pharmacist (B) doesn't tackle root causes, and scheduling an educational session (D) might not be effective if barriers are not identified first. Hence, option C is correct as it addresses potential root causes through interdisciplinary collaboration.
Question 3: Correct Answer: A) Self-directed learning
Rationale: Adult learning theory emphasizes self-directed learning (A), where learners take responsibility for their education, enhancing motivation and engagement. Rote memorization (B) and standardized testing (C) do not align with adult learners' need for practical application and critical thinking. Passive observation (D) lacks active participation, crucial for adult learners. Contemporary research shows that self-directed learning fosters deeper understanding and retention in professional settings.
Question 4: Correct Answer: C) "Can you describe your typical daily diet?"
Rationale: Asking about Mr. Lee's typical daily diet (Option C) helps identify lifestyle factors such as sodium intake that contribute significantly to hypertension management. While family history (Option A), current medications (Option B), and recent weight changes (Option D) provide valuable information, understanding dietary habits offers direct insight into modifiable risk factors that can be addressed through lifestyle changes and dietary interventions.
Question 5: Correct Answer: A) Arrange for David to speak with a social worker about workplace stress.
Rationale: Addressing David's stress related to returning to work by arranging a meeting with a social worker (A) is crucial as it directly targets his expressed concern. Suggesting relaxation techniques (B), while helpful, does not address the root cause. Monitoring for complications (C), though important, overlooks his psychological needs. An occupational therapist referral (D) focuses more on physical adjustments rather than addressing stress management directly.
Question 6: Correct Answer: D) Participating in group singing sessions
Rationale: Group singing sessions have been shown to enhance cognitive function and social interaction in elderly patients with dementia by stimulating memory, language skills, and social engagement. Playing card games (A), gardening (B), and solving puzzles (C) are beneficial but may not provide the same level of social interaction or cognitive stimulation as group singing, which involves both mental engagement and communal participation.
Question 7: Correct Answer: C) To detect medications that may cause or exacerbate cognitive impairment
Rationale: Certain medications, especially anticholinergics and benzodiazepines, can impair cognition. Identifying these helps differentiate between drug-induced and true cognitive decline. While drug interactions, adherence, and dosage are critical, they do not directly address the root cause of cognitive symptoms as effectively as identifying offending medications.
Question 8: Correct Answer: C) Administering intravenous diuretics
Rationale: Intravenous diuretics are the most effective intervention for acute decompensated heart failure as they rapidly reduce preload and pulmonary congestion, thereby improving cardiac output. Beta-blockers (A) and ACE inhibitors (B) are important in chronic management but not ideal for acute settings due to their slower onset of action. Digoxin (D), while beneficial in certain chronic heart failure cases, does not provide the immediate relief needed in acute decompensation.
Question 9: Correct Answer: A) Blood culture collection
Rationale: Blood culture collection is pivotal in confirming sepsis by identifying the causative pathogen in the bloodstream, guiding appropriate antibiotic therapy. While urine analysis (Option B), chest X-ray interpretation (Option C), and neurological examination (Option D) can provide additional information about infection sources or complications, they do not directly confirm bloodstream infection essential for diagnosing sepsis. Timely blood culture results are critical for effective treatment and improving patient outcomes in suspected sepsis cases.
Question 10: Correct Answer: C) Place John on one-to-one observation.
Rationale: The most immediate concern with a patient expressing suicidal ideation is ensuring their safety. Placing John on one-to-one observation ensures continuous monitoring, which is critical in preventing self-harm. A no-suicide contract (A) is less effective and not recommended as the sole intervention. Conducting a detailed psychosocial assessment (B) and referring to a psychiatrist (D) are important but secondary to ensuring immediate safety.
Question 11: Correct Answer: A) Teaching him how to recognize signs of infection at the dialysis access site.
Rationale: The primary educational focus should be teaching Mr. Garcia how to recognize signs of infection at the dialysis access site because infections are a common and serious complication in patients undergoing dialysis. While dietary restrictions (B), fluid intake limitations (C), and medication adherence (D) are critical components of managing ESRD, immediate recognition and management of infections take precedence due to their potential severity.
Question 12: Correct Answer: A) Light exercise such as walking
Rationale: Light exercise such as walking promotes physical recovery by enhancing circulation, reducing the risk of complications, and improving mood through the release of endorphins. Journaling (B), while helpful for emotional expression, does not provide physical benefits. Watching motivational videos (C) can uplift mood but lacks physical engagement. Practicing mindfulness meditation (D), although beneficial for emotional well-being, does not contribute directly to physical recovery like light exercise does.
Question 13: Correct Answer: B) Alcohol withdrawal delirium
Rationale: Alcohol withdrawal delirium (delirium tremens) typically occurs within 48-96 hours after cessation of heavy alcohol use and is characterized by confusion, tremors, and hallucinations. Alcohol intoxication (A) would present with recent consumption symptoms like slurred speech and incoordination. Wernicke-Korsakoff syndrome (C) involves chronic thiamine deficiency leading to neurological symptoms but not acute withdrawal signs. Hepatic

encephalopathy (D) results from liver dysfunction causing cognitive impairment but lacks the specific timeline and withdrawal context seen here.

Question 14: Correct Answer: B) Maintaining a closed drainage system

Rationale: Maintaining a closed drainage system minimizes contamination risk, effectively preventing CAUTIs. Daily cleansing with antiseptic solution (A), while beneficial for hygiene, does not specifically prevent CAUTIs. Regularly changing catheters every 72 hours (C) increases infection risk due to frequent manipulation. Prophylactic antibiotics (D), although potentially reducing infections short-term, contribute to resistance and are not recommended for CAUTI prevention without symptoms.

Question 15: Correct Answer: A) Yoga

Rationale: Yoga has demonstrated significant benefits in lowering blood pressure through stress reduction and improved cardiovascular health, supported by numerous studies. Chiropractic care primarily focuses on musculoskeletal issues rather than systemic conditions like hypertension. Herbal supplements can interact with medications and lack consistent regulation or robust evidence for hypertension management. Cupping therapy is more commonly used for musculoskeletal pain rather than blood pressure control, making yoga the most supported CAM approach in this context.

Question 16: Correct Answer: C) Conducting a cultural assessment with the patient

Rationale: Conducting a cultural assessment with the patient ensures that care plans are tailored to individual needs and respect their cultural beliefs and practices. Assuming cultural practices based on ethnicity (A) can lead to stereotyping and ineffective care. Encouraging adherence to Western medical practices (B) may disregard important cultural values and preferences. Avoiding discussions about cultural beliefs (D) can result in misunderstandings and decreased patient satisfaction and compliance with treatment plans.

Question 17: Correct Answer: D) Perform an abdominal assessment including auscultation.

Rationale: The initial action should be to perform an abdominal assessment to determine if there are signs of paralytic ileus or other complications before intervening further. Administering laxatives (Option A) without assessment could exacerbate issues if there's an obstruction. Encouraging ambulation and fluids (Option B) supports bowel motility but must follow an assessment. Inserting a nasogastric tube (Option C) might be necessary but only after confirming findings through an assessment.

Question 18: Correct Answer: A) Reassessing pain level and medication effectiveness

Rationale: Reassessing pain level and medication effectiveness ensures that any changes in David's condition are promptly identified and managed appropriately. Increasing analgesic dose (Option B), consulting with the pain management team (Option C), and implementing non-pharmacological methods (Option D) may be necessary steps following reassessment but are not initial interventions without proper evaluation of current treatment efficacy.

Question 19: Correct Answer: A) Hypovolemia

Rationale: A significant drop in blood pressure upon standing indicates orthostatic hypotension, often due to hypovolemia—an insufficient volume of blood in circulation causing reduced perfusion when changing positions. Essential hypertension (Option B) generally presents as persistently elevated blood pressure without significant postural changes. Postural orthostatic tachycardia syndrome (POTS; Option C), although involving postural changes, primarily features an excessive increase in heart rate rather than a significant BP drop. Vasovagal syncope (Option D), while involving fainting episodes related to sudden drops in heart rate and blood pressure, is typically triggered by specific stressors rather than simple positional changes.

Question 20: Correct Answer: A) Administering intravenous fluids and monitoring vital signs

Rationale: Administering intravenous fluids and monitoring vital signs are crucial initial steps in managing internal bleeding, as they help maintain hemodynamic stability and assess the severity of blood loss. Applying pressure to the surgical site (Option B) is not effective for internal bleeding. Elevating the patient's legs (Option C) may temporarily improve circulation but does not address the root cause. Initiating a blood transfusion (Option D) may be necessary later but requires confirmation of significant blood loss and cross-matching, making Option A the most immediate and appropriate intervention.

Question 21: Correct Answer: B) Administering intravenous furosemide

Rationale: Intravenous furosemide is effective for rapid diuresis in fluid overload situations, making it the best choice here. Option A may be necessary if diuretics fail but isn't first-line. Option C is supportive but insufficient alone for acute management. Option D helps prevent future overload but does not address the immediate issue.

Question 22: Correct Answer: B) Discussing Mr. Smith's concerns with the prescribing physician.

Rationale: Effective advocacy involves communicating the patient's concerns to the appropriate healthcare provider to ensure their voice is heard and their needs are addressed. Option A may lead to misinformation, Option C dismisses the patient's concerns, and Option D could compromise patient care without professional consultation. Therefore, discussing with the prescribing physician (Option B) is the most appropriate action as it ensures professional evaluation and consideration of Mr. Smith's concerns.

Question 23: Correct Answer: A) Encouraging participation in a group exercise class

Rationale: Group exercise classes offer both physical benefits through movement and emotional benefits through social interaction, addressing Mr. Smith's feelings of isolation and depression. Reading a self-help book (B), while informative, does not provide social interaction. An online support group (C) offers emotional support but lacks the physical activity component. Knitting or crafting (D), though beneficial for fine motor skills, might not sufficiently address the need for social engagement and physical exercise.

Question 24: Correct Answer: C) Electrocardiogram (ECG)

Rationale: An ECG is the first diagnostic test for suspected myocardial infarction due to its ability to quickly identify ischemic changes. Option B provides essential information but follows ECG. Option A offers detailed structural information but isn't as immediate. Option D can rule out other causes but isn't specific for ischemia detection.

Question 25: Correct Answer: A) Simplifying the medication regimen

Rationale: Simplifying the medication regimen should be prioritized as it reduces complexity, minimizes the risk of errors, and improves adherence. While monitoring renal function (Option B), increasing patient education (Option C), and using pill organizers (Option D) are beneficial, they do not directly address reducing potential confusion and errors associated with complex regimens. Simplification leads to better management and fewer adverse effects.

Question 26: Correct Answer: C) Utilize a professional medical interpreter to facilitate communication.

Rationale: Utilizing a professional medical interpreter ensures accurate and effective communication, which is crucial for patient safety and understanding (Option C). Medical jargon (Option A) can be confusing even for native speakers, let alone non-English speakers. Relying on family members (Option B) may lead to misinterpretation of medical information due to lack of medical knowledge or biases, while speaking slowly and loudly in English (Option D) can be perceived as disrespectful and ineffective if the patient does not understand the language.

Question 27: Correct Answer: A) Aerobic exercise

Rationale: Aerobic exercise is well-documented to significantly alleviate fibromyalgia symptoms by improving cardiovascular health, reducing fatigue, and enhancing overall well-being. Biofeedback (B), while helpful for stress management, lacks strong evidence for symptom reduction. Herbal supplements (C) have inconsistent efficacy and potential side effects. Chiropractic care (D), although beneficial for musculoskeletal issues, does not have robust evidence supporting its use specifically for fibromyalgia symptom management.

Question 28: Correct Answer: B) Bi-level Positive Airway Pressure (BiPAP)

Rationale: BiPAP provides non-invasive ventilation support by delivering two levels of pressure – higher during inhalation and lower during exhalation – which is particularly beneficial for patients with COPD like Mrs. Garcia. A nasal cannula delivers low-flow oxygen, insufficient for her needs; a Venturi mask offers controlled oxygen concentration but lacks pressure support; and a simple face mask provides basic oxygen delivery without the benefits of positive airway pressure provided by BiPAP.

Question 29: Correct Answer: D) Combining review of self-reported logs, discussion on lifestyle changes, and explanation of medication adherence

Rationale: A comprehensive evaluation involves multiple facets of hypertension management. By combining review of logs (A), discussing lifestyle changes (B), and explaining medication adherence (C), Nurse Sam ensures all aspects are covered. Each individual method alone may miss critical components; together, they provide a holistic view of John's understanding and application.

Question 30: Correct Answer: A) Electrocardiogram interpretation

Rationale: Electrocardiogram (ECG) interpretation is essential in diagnosing myocardial infarction (MI), as it reveals ischemic changes like ST-segment elevation or T-wave inversion. Blood pressure measurement (Option B), heart rate monitoring (Option C), and respiratory rate assessment (Option D) provide vital signs that may indicate distress but do not specifically diagnose MI. Accurate ECG interpretation allows prompt identification and treatment of MI, critical for patient outcomes.

Question 31: Correct Answer: A) "Can you describe the nature of your chest pain?"

Rationale: The priority in this scenario is to gather detailed information about the chest pain, which could indicate a cardiac issue. Option A helps in understanding the characteristics of the pain, crucial for differential diagnosis. While B), C), and D) are relevant to his overall health history, they do not immediately address the acute symptom that could signify a serious condition like angina or myocardial infarction.

Question 32: Correct Answer: D) The use of evidence-based guidelines

Rationale: The use of evidence-based guidelines enhances consult effectiveness by ensuring that recommendations are grounded in current best practices, leading to improved patient outcomes. Although frequent consults (A), hierarchical structures (B), and dedicated case managers (C) play roles in coordination and management, they do not guarantee that decisions are based on the latest research. Evidence-based guidelines provide standardized approaches that reduce variability in care and support optimal clinical decision-making across interdisciplinary teams.

Question 33: Correct Answer: B) Active listening

Rationale: Active listening is the most effective communication technique for establishing a therapeutic relationship with an anxious patient. It involves fully concentrating, understanding, responding, and remembering what the patient says. This helps build trust and shows empathy. Providing reassurance (Option A) may minimize the patient's feelings. Offering advice (Option C) can seem dismissive if not solicited. Reflective questioning (Option D) is useful but may increase anxiety if overused. Active listening stands out because it validates the patient's feelings and promotes a sense of safety.

Question 34: Correct Answer: D) COPD Exacerbation

Rationale: Robert's symptoms of increased dyspnea and productive cough with green sputum suggest a COPD exacerbation often triggered by infection. The ABG showing respiratory acidosis (pH 7.30, PaCO2 55 mmHg), typical in COPD exacerbations due to hypoventilation. Acute asthma exacerbation (A) would present differently in ABG values and patient history. ARDS (B) involves more severe hypoxemia and different clinical settings. Community-acquired pneumonia (C), while possible, would not explain the chronic hypercapnia seen here.

Question 35: Correct Answer: C) CT angiography

Rationale: The clinical presentation suggests an arterial embolism, likely originating from her atrial fibrillation. CT angiography provides detailed images of blood vessels and is the gold standard for diagnosing arterial emboli. Venous Doppler ultrasound (A) is used for venous thromboembolism but not arterial emboli. Arterial blood gas analysis (B) can assess tissue perfusion but won't identify the embolus location. MRI (D), though useful for soft tissue imaging, is less effective than CT angiography for vascular assessment.

Question 36: Correct Answer: A) Mammography

Rationale: Mammography is the most appropriate screening test for Sarah given her age and family history of breast cancer. It is recommended annually for women aged 50-74. While Breast MRI (B) and genetic testing (C) are useful in specific high-risk cases, they are not standard screening tools. A clinical breast exam (D), although important, is not as effective as mammography in early detection. The key difference lies in mammography's proven efficacy in reducing mortality through early detection.

Question 37: Correct Answer: A) Jugular venous distension

Rationale: Jugular venous distension (JVD) is a hallmark sign of early-stage right-sided heart failure due to increased central venous pressure. Peripheral edema (B), hepatomegaly (C), and ascites (D) are also associated with right-sided heart failure but typically present in more advanced stages. JVD occurs earlier as the right atrium struggles to accommodate increased blood volume, causing visible neck vein distention. Peripheral edema, hepatomegaly, and ascites develop later as fluid accumulates in tissues and organs due to prolonged elevated venous pressure.

Question 38: Correct Answer: B) Utilizing teach-back method to confirm understanding

Rationale: The teach-back method ensures that patients understand the information by having them explain it back in their own words. This technique identifies gaps in knowledge and allows for immediate clarification. Option A may not address comprehension issues; Option C might overwhelm without ensuring understanding; Option D alone may not be sufficient if literacy or comprehension barriers exist.

Question 39: Correct Answer: B) Providing Ms. Garcia with evidence-based information about the surgery.

Rationale: Advocacy involves supporting patient autonomy by providing accurate and comprehensive information to help them make informed decisions (Option B). Telling her fears are unfounded (Option A) dismisses her concerns, insisting on surgery (Option C) undermines her autonomy, and suggesting a second opinion (Option D), though supportive, does not directly address her need for reliable information from her current care team.

Question 40: Correct Answer: D) Altered level of consciousness

Rationale: Altered level of consciousness is the most sensitive and early indicator of increased ICP. While unequal pupil size (A) and bilateral motor weakness (C) can also occur, they are typically later signs. Decreased deep tendon reflexes (B) are less specific for ICP and can result from various other conditions. Monitoring consciousness provides immediate insight into cerebral function, making it a crucial assessment.

Question 41: Correct Answer: C) Computed tomography pulmonary angiography (CTPA)

Rationale: CTPA is the gold standard for definitively diagnosing pulmonary embolism due to its high sensitivity and specificity. The D-dimer test (A), while useful in ruling out PE when negative, lacks specificity. A V/Q scan (B), though helpful, has lower accuracy compared to CTPA. An ECG (D), although it can show changes suggestive of PE, cannot confirm the diagnosis definitively. CTPA directly visualizes clots in pulmonary arteries, providing clear evidence of embolism presence.

Question 42: Correct Answer: B) Blood cultures

Rationale: Blood cultures provide specific information about the causative organism and its antibiotic sensitivities, guiding targeted therapy. CBC (A) indicates infection presence but lacks specificity. CRP (C) and procalcitonin levels (D) are inflammatory markers that suggest infection severity but do not identify pathogens or guide specific treatment. Blood cultures offer rapid identification and susceptibility data essential for effective management.

Question 43: Correct Answer: A) Hemoglobin level

Rationale: Hemoglobin level is critical for detecting bleeding complications as it directly reflects the oxygen-carrying capacity of the blood, which decreases with significant blood loss. White blood cell count (Option B) indicates infection or inflammation but not bleeding. Platelet count (Option C) is important for clotting but does not indicate active bleeding. Prothrombin time (PT, Option D) measures clotting ability but does not directly reflect blood volume or oxygen-carrying capacity. Therefore, hemoglobin level provides the most direct indication of potential hemorrhage.

Question 44: Correct Answer: A) Educating the patient on recognizing early signs of heart failure exacerbation.

Rationale: Educating the patient on recognizing early signs of heart failure exacerbation empowers her to seek timely medical intervention, preventing hospital readmissions. While scheduling follow-up appointments (Option B), ensuring understanding of medication regimen (Option C), and arranging home health visits (Option D) are important, they are secondary to the patient's ability to self-identify worsening symptoms. Early recognition skills directly contribute to better self-management and prompt response to changes in condition.

Question 45: Correct Answer: C) Past occupational exposure to dust or chemicals

Rationale: Assessing past occupational exposure to dust or chemicals (Option C) is crucial for identifying potential occupational hazards that could contribute to Mr. Johnson's chronic cough and shortness of breath. While family history (Option A) can provide insight into genetic predispositions, it doesn't directly address environmental exposures. The duration and nature of the cough (Option B) are important but do not pinpoint the cause. Recent travel history (Option D) may identify infectious causes but is less relevant for chronic symptoms linked to long-term exposure.

Question 46: Correct Answer: B) Use a teach-back method to confirm his understanding.

Rationale: The teach-back method ensures that the patient understands the information by asking them to repeat it in their own words. This approach confirms comprehension and allows for immediate clarification, making it highly effective for patient education. Providing a pamphlet (A) or showing a video (C) might not ensure understanding, while scheduling a follow-up (D) delays immediate learning reinforcement. The teach-back method directly involves the patient in their care, promoting better adherence and outcomes.

Question 47: Correct Answer: A) Randomized controlled trials (RCTs)

Rationale: Randomized controlled trials (RCTs) provide the highest level of evidence due to their design, which minimizes bias by randomly assigning subjects to intervention or control groups. This allows for a clear comparison of outcomes directly attributable to the intervention. Case studies offer detailed insights but lack generalizability. Expert opinion articles provide valuable perspectives but are subjective. Cohort studies follow groups over time and offer strong evidence but can be affected by confounding variables. Therefore, RCTs are considered the gold standard in clinical research for decision-making.

Question 48: Correct Answer: A) Administering prophylactic antibiotics within one hour before the surgical incision

Rationale: Administering prophylactic antibiotics within one hour before the surgical incision is crucial as it significantly reduces the risk of postoperative infections by ensuring adequate tissue levels of the antibiotic during surgery. Option B (topical antiseptics post-surgery) is less effective than preoperative antibiotics. Option C (fasting) is not directly related to infection prevention. Option D (chlorhexidine wipes postoperatively) helps but is not as critical as timely antibiotic administration.

Question 49: Correct Answer: A) Barthel Index

Rationale: The Barthel Index is specifically designed to measure a patient's ability to perform ADLs independently, such as feeding, bathing, and dressing. The MMSE assesses cognitive function, which can indirectly affect ADLs but does not directly measure them. The Braden Scale evaluates pressure ulcer risk, and the Glasgow Coma Scale assesses consciousness levels. While these tools are useful in clinical settings, they do not directly evaluate the performance of ADLs as effectively as the Barthel Index.

Question 50: Correct Answer: C) Temperature monitoring

Rationale: Temperature monitoring is the most critical skill for identifying early signs of sepsis, as fever or hypothermia can be an early indicator. While palpation (A) can detect localized infection, auscultation (B) may reveal abnormal lung sounds, and blood pressure measurement (D) can indicate hypotension, these are typically later signs. Early detection relies heavily on recognizing changes in temperature, making it the most essential skill.

Question 51: Correct Answer: B) Intravenous magnesium sulfate.

Rationale: For symptomatic hypomagnesemia with levels as low as 1.0 mg/dL, intravenous magnesium sulfate (Option B) is the best initial treatment due to its rapid effect on correcting deficiencies and alleviating symptoms such as hypotension and decreased reflexes. Oral magnesium supplements (Option A), while useful for mild deficiencies, are insufficient for acute management. Increasing dietary magnesium intake (Option C) would not provide immediate relief from symptoms. Intravenous normal saline (Option D), although helpful in some electrolyte imbalances, does not address the specific need for magnesium replacement in this scenario.

Question 52: Correct Answer: C) Maintaining a daily food and exercise journal

Rationale: Maintaining a daily food and exercise journal is most effective because it provides real-time feedback and helps identify patterns that affect blood glucose levels. This self-monitoring tool encourages accountability and allows for adjustments in diet and activity. While attending education classes (A) and using CGM (B) are beneficial, they do not provide the immediate, personalized feedback that journaling does. Bi-weekly visits with a dietitian (D), though helpful, lack the daily tracking necessary for effective self-management.

Question 53: Correct Answer: A) Cryoprecipitate

Rationale: Cryoprecipitate contains high levels of fibrinogen and is specifically used to treat hypofibrinogenemia. FFP also contains fibrinogen but in lower concentrations compared to cryoprecipitate. Platelets are irrelevant as they address platelet count, not fibrinogen levels. Albumin is a volume expander and does not contain fibrinogen or other clotting factors. Hence, cryoprecipitate is the best choice for severe hypofibrinogenemia.

Question 54: Correct Answer: B) Abdominal bloating after

meals
Rationale: Abdominal bloating after meals is a common symptom that can indicate gastrointestinal disorders such as irritable bowel syndrome (IBS), food intolerances, or other digestive issues. Night sweats (Option A) are more commonly associated with infections or hormonal imbalances, shortness of breath during activity (Option C) points towards cardiovascular or pulmonary problems, and increased urinary frequency (Option D) suggests urological concerns. The specificity of abdominal bloating post-meals directly relates to digestive function, necessitating further GI evaluation.
Question 55: Correct Answer: D) Positioning the patient in a high Fowler's position
Rationale: High Fowler's position maximizes lung expansion and facilitates easier breathing, which is crucial during an acute COPD exacerbation. Administering bronchodilators (Option A) and initiating high-flow oxygen therapy (Option B) are important but secondary to positioning for immediate relief. Encouraging deep breathing exercises (Option C) can be beneficial long-term but may not provide immediate improvement in oxygenation like positioning can.
Question 56: Correct Answer: B) "I apologize for any inconvenience; let's schedule regular updates with the team."
Rationale: Scheduling regular updates ensures consistent communication and involves the family in the care process, aligning with patient- and family-centered care principles. Option A acknowledges busyness but lacks a proactive solution. Option C emphasizes trust but doesn't address communication needs. Option D places the burden on the family rather than facilitating structured communication.
Question 57: Correct Answer: A) Aged cheese
Rationale: Aged cheese contains high levels of tyramine, which can cause a hypertensive crisis when consumed with MAOIs. Fresh fruits, lean meats, and whole grains do not contain significant amounts of tyramine and are generally safe for patients on MAOIs. The critical factor is the tyramine content, which is particularly high in aged cheeses.
Question 58: Correct Answer: C) To evaluate comprehensive functional status
Rationale: Assessing both basic (e.g., bathing, dressing) and instrumental (e.g., managing finances, using transportation) activities provides a complete picture of a patient's functional status. This evaluation helps identify areas where the patient may need support or intervention. While physical health (Option A), social engagement (Option B), and specific medical diagnoses (Option D) are important aspects of care, they do not provide a holistic view of functional abilities like a comprehensive assessment of both basic and instrumental ADLs does.
Question 59: Correct Answer: A) Tai Chi
Rationale: Tai Chi is recommended by contemporary guidelines for fibromyalgia due to its combination of gentle physical activity, mindfulness, and relaxation techniques that collectively address both musculoskeletal pain and fatigue. Chiropractic care (B), while potentially helpful for localized musculoskeletal issues, lacks comprehensive evidence for fibromyalgia management. Meditation (C), though beneficial for stress reduction and mental health, does not directly target physical symptoms as effectively as Tai Chi. Heat therapy (D), although it provides temporary relief from muscle stiffness and soreness, does not offer the holistic benefits of Tai Chi in managing fibromyalgia symptoms comprehensively.
Question 60: Correct Answer: A) Acupuncture
Rationale: Acupuncture has been extensively studied and shown to be effective for chronic lower back pain, supported by numerous clinical trials and systematic reviews. Aromatherapy, while beneficial for relaxation, lacks strong evidence for pain management. Homeopathy's efficacy remains controversial and is not well-supported by rigorous scientific research. Reflexology can help with general well-being but lacks specific evidence for chronic back pain relief. Therefore, acupuncture is the most evidence-based recommendation.
Question 61: Correct Answer: B) Having Maria demonstrate blood glucose monitoring and insulin administration
Rationale: Demonstrating skills such as blood glucose monitoring and insulin administration is a practical method that directly assesses Maria's understanding and ability to manage her condition. This hands-on approach ensures she can apply what she has learned in real-life situations. While verbal repetition (A) and written tests (C) can gauge knowledge, they do not confirm practical competence. Observing without interaction (D) may miss critical errors or misunderstandings.
Question 62: Correct Answer: B) Generativity vs. Stagnation
Rationale: Erikson's theory posits that middle adulthood (ages 40-65) involves the challenge of Generativity vs. Stagnation, focusing on contributing to society and helping guide the next generation. Identity vs. Role Confusion pertains to adolescence, Intimacy vs. Isolation is relevant to young adulthood, and Integrity vs. Despair applies to older adults reflecting on life. The correct answer addresses the specific psychosocial task of middle adulthood, distinguishing it from other life stages.
Question 63: Correct Answer: A) Integrity vs. Despair
Rationale: According to Erikson's psychosocial theory, individuals in late adulthood (65 years and older) are typically in the "Integrity vs. Despair" stage. This stage involves reflecting on one's life and accomplishments, leading to feelings of integrity or despair. Maria's concern about returning to her hobby reflects her desire to maintain a sense of purpose and satisfaction in life. "Generativity vs. Stagnation" applies to middle adulthood (40-65 years), focusing on contributing to society and helping the next generation. "Intimacy vs. Isolation" pertains to young adulthood (20-40 years), emphasizing forming intimate relationships. "Identity vs. Role Confusion" is relevant during adolescence (12-18 years), focusing on developing a personal identity.
Question 64: Correct Answer: C) Encouraging open communication among all team members
Rationale: Encouraging open communication ensures that all team members can contribute their expertise, leading to comprehensive care plans. While leading meetings (Option A), delegating tasks (Option B), and evaluating performance (Option D) are important, fostering open communication directly enhances collaboration by ensuring everyone's input is considered.
Question 65: Correct Answer: C) Monitor blood glucose levels before and after exercise.
Rationale: Monitoring blood glucose levels before and after exercise helps prevent hypoglycemia by allowing timely adjustments in diet or insulin dosage. High-intensity interval training (A), while beneficial for fitness, can unpredictably affect glucose levels. Exercising immediately after insulin administration (B) increases the risk of hypoglycemia. Avoiding carbohydrate intake before exercise (D) could lead to low blood sugar during physical activity.
Question 66: Correct Answer: C) Teach her how to monitor her blood glucose levels and administer insulin.
Rationale: Teaching Mrs. Johnson how to monitor her blood glucose levels and administer insulin is crucial for immediate self-management of her condition. This empowers her with the skills necessary to maintain glycemic control and prevent complications. Option A provides information but lacks hands-on training. Option B ensures continuity of care but does not equip her with immediate skills. Option D offers emotional support but does not directly impact daily management. Thus, C is the most critical initial teaching strategy.
Question 67: Correct Answer: B) Irregularly irregular pulse
Rationale: An irregularly irregular pulse is characteristic of atrial fibrillation (AF), where there is no consistent rhythm

due to erratic electrical activity in the atria. A regularly irregular pulse (A) suggests patterns like premature ventricular contractions but not AF. Bradycardia (C), defined as a slow heart rate, does not align with typical AF presentation unless medication-induced or secondary to another condition. Tachycardia (D), while common in AF episodes, lacks specificity without accompanying irregular rhythm details essential for AF diagnosis.

Question 68: Correct Answer: A) Administer IV fluids to address potential hypovolemia.

Rationale: The priority intervention is to administer IV fluids to address potential hypovolemia, as indicated by the low blood pressure (90/60 mmHg). Hypovolemia can cause dizziness and fatigue due to decreased perfusion. Starting an antihypertensive medication (Option B) is inappropriate because the patient's BP is already low. Providing oxygen therapy (Option C) may not address the primary issue of hypovolemia. Administering insulin (Option D) is not urgent unless hyperglycemia is confirmed and contributing to symptoms.

Question 69: Correct Answer: D) Balance training exercises

Rationale: Balance training exercises are specifically designed to improve stability and coordination, directly addressing the primary cause of falls in older adults. Strength training (A) can enhance muscle mass but may not sufficiently improve balance. Vitamin D supplementation (B) can support bone health but does not directly impact balance. Home safety assessments (C) help identify hazards but do not improve physical stability. Therefore, balance training is the most effective intervention for fall prevention.

Question 70: Correct Answer: C) A licensed practical nurse (LPN)

Rationale: LPNs are qualified to administer medications, including oral medications, and can monitor patients with conditions like dysphagia effectively. While an RN could also administer medications, it is more efficient for RNs to handle tasks requiring higher-level critical thinking skills. CNAs are not authorized to administer medications, and relying on a family member even under guidance is inappropriate due to potential safety risks and lack of professional training in medication administration.

Question 71: Correct Answer: A) Reduction in HbA1c levels over three months

Rationale: Reduction in HbA1c levels over three months is a reliable indicator of long-term blood glucose control and successful diabetes management. It reflects sustained improvements rather than short-term fluctuations. While adherence to dietary recommendations (B), consistent monitoring (C), and absence of complications (D) are crucial components, they are intermediate steps or outcomes that contribute to achieving lower HbA1c levels. Therefore, HbA1c reduction provides a more comprehensive measure of overall effectiveness in managing diabetes over time.

Question 72: Correct Answer: B) Hypokalemia

Rationale: Furosemide, a loop diuretic, can cause potassium loss leading to hypokalemia. Metformin and lisinopril do not typically cause significant potassium loss, but the addition of furosemide increases this risk. Hyperkalemia (Option A) is more likely with potassium-sparing diuretics or ACE inhibitors alone. Hyperglycemia (Option C) and hypoglycemia (Option D) are related to diabetes management but are not direct interactions between these medications.

Question 73: Correct Answer: D) Clinical outcomes

Rationale: Clinical outcomes are the most reliable measure of an educational program's effectiveness on medication adherence because they directly reflect the impact on patient health. Patient self-reports can be biased or inaccurate, pill counts may not account for proper medication use, and pharmacy refill records do not confirm ingestion. Clinical outcomes provide concrete evidence of adherence through measurable health improvements or stabilization, making them the gold standard in evaluation.

Question 74: Correct Answer: C) Measurement of calf circumference

Rationale: Measurement of calf circumference is essential in diagnosing DVT as it quantifies swelling, a key indicator. Inspection for redness and swelling (A), palpation for tenderness (B), and Homan's sign assessment (D) are useful but less specific. Calf circumference offers an objective measure that correlates strongly with DVT presence, providing more reliable diagnostic information.

Question 75: Correct Answer: B) Orthostatic hypotension

Rationale: Orthostatic hypotension is a hallmark sign of fluid volume deficit due to decreased blood volume affecting vascular tone when changing positions. Jugular venous distention indicates fluid overload rather than deficit. Peripheral edema also suggests excess fluid accumulation in tissues rather than depletion. Hypertension typically results from increased fluid volume or other factors unrelated to volume deficit. Therefore, orthostatic hypotension directly correlates with decreased intravascular volume, making it the most indicative clinical sign of fluid volume deficit.

Question 76: Correct Answer: C) Assess for additional signs of abuse and ensure Sarah's safety.

Rationale: The nurse's priority action is to assess for additional signs of abuse and ensure Sarah's safety. This step is crucial as it helps identify if there is an immediate threat to her well-being. While documenting her statement (Option A) and referring her to a social worker (Option D) are important steps, they do not address the immediate concern of ensuring her safety. Reporting to law enforcement (Option B) may be necessary but should follow a thorough assessment and confirmation of abuse. Ensuring safety first allows for appropriate interventions based on the assessment findings.

Question 77: Correct Answer: B) Ensuring adequate hydration

Rationale: Ensuring adequate hydration is crucial in preventing delirium in elderly postoperative patients. Dehydration can lead to electrolyte imbalances and reduced cerebral perfusion, increasing the risk of delirium. Administering routine sedatives (A) may exacerbate confusion and is not recommended. Limiting nighttime disturbances (C) is helpful but not as directly impactful as hydration. High-protein meals (D) are beneficial for recovery but do not specifically address the primary risk factor of dehydration linked to delirium.

Question 78: Correct Answer: C) Gabapentin and acetaminophen

Rationale: Multimodal analgesia aims to target different pain pathways using various medications. Gabapentin (neuropathic pain modulator) combined with acetaminophen (nociceptive pain reliever) provides effective postoperative pain relief by addressing both types of pain pathways. Acetaminophen and ibuprofen (A), while both useful for nociceptive pain, do not provide the same breadth of analgesia. Morphine and codeine (B), both opioids, increase risk of side effects without enhancing multimodal benefits. Fentanyl and oxycodone (D), also both opioids, similarly fail to cover multiple mechanisms effectively. Research supports gabapentin's role in reducing postoperative opioid requirements when used in combination with acetaminophen.

Question 79: Correct Answer: D) Assess his home environment for potential hazards.

Rationale: Assessing Mr. Smith's home environment for potential hazards is crucial to prevent falls and ensure a safe recovery post-discharge. While scheduling follow-ups (A), providing education (B), and coordinating with physical therapy (C) are important, ensuring a hazard-free environment directly impacts his immediate safety and recovery at home.

Question 80: Correct Answer: A) Assess for potential adverse effects of his medications.

Rationale: Assessing for adverse effects is essential as polypharmacy can lead to confusion and muscle weakness due to drug interactions or side effects. Suggesting a vitamin panel (B) may be useful later but doesn't immediately address polypharmacy concerns. Referring to a neurologist (C) may be necessary if symptoms persist but isn't the first step. Increasing physical activity (D) without understanding medication effects could worsen symptoms.

Question 81: Correct Answer: A) Lisinopril and Spironolactone

Rationale: Lisinopril (an ACE inhibitor) and Spironolactone (a potassium-sparing diuretic) both increase potassium levels, risking hyperkalemia. Atorvastatin and Ezetimibe lower cholesterol without affecting potassium. Levothyroxine absorption is reduced by Calcium Carbonate but does not affect potassium. Omeprazole reduces Clopidogrel's effectiveness but does not impact potassium.

Question 82: Correct Answer: C) Pulmonary congestion

Rationale: Pulmonary congestion is a hallmark of left-sided heart failure due to fluid backing up into the lungs when the left ventricle fails to pump effectively. Peripheral edema (Option A), jugular venous distension (Option B), and hepatomegaly (Option D) are more indicative of right-sided heart failure, where fluid backs up into the systemic circulation. Therefore, pulmonary congestion specifically points to left-sided heart failure, differentiating it from right-sided manifestations.

Question 83: Correct Answer: D) Symptom recognition and management

Rationale: Prioritizing symptom recognition and management empowers patients to identify early warning signs of deterioration and seek timely intervention, thus reducing readmissions. While Options A, B, and C are important, they do not directly address the immediate need for recognizing symptoms that can prevent rehospitalization as effectively as symptom management does.

Question 84: Correct Answer: B) Incorporating cultural assessments into patient evaluations

Rationale: Incorporating cultural assessments into patient evaluations is essential as it allows the nurse to understand the patient's unique cultural background and preferences, leading to more personalized and effective care. Standardized care plans (A) fail to account for individual differences. Personal experiences (C) may introduce bias, and avoiding discussions (D) can lead to misunderstandings and inadequate care. Cultural competence requires recognizing and integrating patients' cultural values and beliefs into their care plans.

Question 85: Correct Answer: D) Infusion pump

Rationale: An infusion pump allows for precise control over the infusion rate, which is crucial for administering intravenous medication accurately, especially in cases of severe dehydration. A gravity drip set lacks precision, a syringe pump is typically used for smaller volumes and specific medications, and an elastomeric pump delivers medication at a pre-set rate without the flexibility needed for adjusting infusion rates as accurately as an infusion pump.

Question 86: Correct Answer: D) Assess and address potential psychological factors contributing to her pain.

Rationale: Psychological factors can significantly influence pain perception and response to treatment. Addressing these factors ensures comprehensive pain management. Increasing the basal rate of morphine (A) might not address underlying issues and could lead to overdose. Adding gabapentin (B), while useful for neuropathic pain, may not be immediately effective post-surgery. Switching opioids (C) should be considered only after other factors are evaluated; psychological assessment is less invasive and can provide critical insights into her pain experience.

Question 87: Correct Answer: C) Report the medication error to his supervisor and document it accurately.

Rationale: Transparency in reporting medication errors ensures patient safety and allows for corrective measures to be taken promptly. Monitoring without reporting (Option A), informing only Mrs. Thompson (Option B), or consulting another nurse first (Option D), fail to address institutional protocols for handling medication errors and compromise overall patient safety standards by not initiating immediate corrective actions through proper channels.

Question 88: Correct Answer: B) Wound culture and sensitivity

Rationale: Performing a wound culture and sensitivity test is crucial for identifying the causative organism and determining appropriate antibiotic therapy. While monitoring blood glucose levels (Option A) is essential for diabetic patients, it does not directly address the infection. A CBC (Option C) can provide information on systemic infection but does not identify specific pathogens. An X-ray (Option D) may be necessary to rule out osteomyelitis but should follow after identifying the infection source.

Question 89: Correct Answer: A) Ensure that all relevant patient information and documentation are available for the consultant.

Rationale: Nurse Alex's primary responsibility is to ensure that all relevant patient information and documentation are available for the consultant. This ensures that the consultant can make an informed assessment. Option B is incorrect because confirming the need for a consult is not within Nurse Alex's independent scope of practice. Option C, while important, is not the primary responsibility in this context. Option D may interfere with the consultant's ability to accurately diagnose and should only be done if explicitly ordered by the primary team.

Question 90: Correct Answer: A) Daily weight measurement

Rationale: Daily weight measurement is the most reliable method for assessing fluid balance as it provides direct information about fluid gain or loss. Urine output monitoring (B), skin turgor assessment (C), and BUN levels (D) are also important but can be influenced by other factors such as renal function and skin elasticity. Weight changes reflect overall fluid status more precisely.

Question 91: Correct Answer: B) Assess Mr. Johnson's need for toileting and pain relief.

Rationale: Before applying physical restraints, it is crucial to assess and address any underlying causes of agitation, such as the need for toileting or pain relief (Option B). This aligns with contemporary research emphasizing non-restraint interventions first. While obtaining a physician's order (Option A), explaining to the family (Option C), and documenting behavior (Option D) are important steps, they follow after immediate assessment of basic needs which may resolve the issue without restraints.

Question 92: Correct Answer: C) Multiple bruises at various stages of healing

Rationale: Multiple bruises at various stages of healing are highly indicative of physical abuse as they suggest repeated trauma over time. Chronic absenteeism from school (A), frequent urinary tract infections (B), and developmental delays without medical explanation (D) can be associated with neglect or other forms of maltreatment but are less specific to physical abuse. Bruises at different healing stages point directly to ongoing physical harm, making it the most concerning finding in this context.

Question 93: Correct Answer: B) Pap smear every three years

Rationale: For women aged 21-29, a Pap smear every three years is recommended as it effectively detects precancerous changes without over-screening. Annual Pap smears (A) are no longer advised due to potential harms from overtreatment. HPV testing alone (C), while effective in older age groups, is not recommended for this age range due to transient infections that often resolve spontaneously. Co-testing with Pap smear and HPV test (D) is more appropriate for women aged 30-65, where combined testing enhances detection rates.

Question 94: Correct Answer: B) Cognitive Behavioral Therapy for Insomnia (CBT-I)

Rationale: Randomized controlled trials indicate that CBT-I is highly effective for treating insomnia by addressing behavioral and cognitive factors contributing to sleep disturbances. Melatonin supplementation (A), while useful, often shows variable effectiveness across different populations. Tai Chi (C), although beneficial for overall health, does not specifically target insomnia as effectively as CBT-I. Progressive Muscle Relaxation (D), though helpful, typically offers less comprehensive benefits compared to CBT-I's structured approach. Hence, CBT-I stands out as the most efficacious CAM approach for insomnia based on current evidence.

Question 95: Correct Answer: C) Collaborate with Mr. Ahmed and his healthcare provider to adjust medication times around fasting periods.

Rationale: Cultural competence involves respecting patients' religious practices while ensuring their health needs are met (Option C). Adjusting medication times demonstrates respect for Mr. Ahmed's beliefs while maintaining therapeutic effectiveness. Advising him to break his fast (Option A) may not respect his religious commitment; disregarding the fasting practice (Option B) fails to consider patient-centered care principles; providing supplements without adjusting medication times (Option D) does not address the primary issue of medication adherence during fasting periods.

Question 96: Correct Answer: A) Cognitive function

Rationale: Cognitive function (A) is essential to assess because it directly impacts the accuracy of the health history provided by an elderly patient. If cognitive impairments are present, they may affect memory and understanding, leading to incomplete or inaccurate information. While family support system (B), previous hospitalizations (C), and nutritional status (D) are significant aspects of health history, they do not directly influence the accuracy of the patient's self-reported information like cognitive function does.

Question 97: Correct Answer: A) Visual learning

Rationale: Visual learning is most effective for patients with low health literacy because it utilizes images, diagrams, and videos to convey information, making complex concepts easier to understand. Auditory learning (B) relies on verbal instructions, which may be difficult for such patients to follow. Kinesthetic learning (C), while engaging, may not provide the clear step-by-step guidance needed. Reading/writing learning (D) is less effective due to the patient's low literacy level. Visual aids can bridge comprehension gaps better than other methods.

Question 98: Correct Answer: B) Use of standardized communication tools like SBAR

Rationale: Standardized communication tools like SBAR (Situation, Background, Assessment, Recommendation) are designed to ensure clear, concise, and structured communication among healthcare professionals. While regular meetings (A) and informal conversations (C) can aid in communication, they lack the structured approach provided by SBAR. Individual emails (D), although useful for documentation, do not facilitate immediate interactive dialogue necessary for urgent patient care decisions. The use of SBAR has been shown to reduce errors and improve patient outcomes by ensuring that critical information is accurately conveyed.

Question 99: Correct Answer: A) Rebound tenderness

Rationale: Rebound tenderness is a key sign of peritonitis, indicating irritation of the peritoneum. Murphy's sign (B), McBurney's point tenderness (C), and Rovsing's sign (D) are associated with specific conditions like cholecystitis and appendicitis but do not universally indicate peritonitis. Rebound tenderness is elicited by pressing down on the abdomen and then releasing quickly, causing pain due to peritoneal inflammation, thus making it a crucial finding for diagnosing peritonitis.

Question 100: Correct Answer: B) Encouraging Mrs. Johnson to discuss her fears and concerns.

Rationale: Encouraging open communication (Option B) demonstrates therapeutic communication and respects the patient's autonomy and emotional needs. Option A may overwhelm or confuse the patient with technical jargon. Option C dismisses her concerns without addressing them adequately. Option D might be premature without first understanding and addressing her immediate concerns.

Question 101: Correct Answer: C) Encourage him to express his feelings and fears.

Rationale: Encouraging Mr. Johnson to express his feelings and fears (Option C) is a core therapeutic communication technique that allows the patient to feel heard and supported. This approach helps build trust and provides an opportunity for the nurse to address specific concerns. Reassuring him that the pain will be minimal (Option A) might minimize his feelings, while sharing a personal story (Option B) shifts focus away from the patient. Distracting with unrelated conversation (Option D) ignores his anxiety altogether.

Question 102: Correct Answer: A) Wechsler Intelligence Scale for Children (WISC)

Rationale: The WISC is designed to assess various aspects of intelligence in children aged 6-16 years and includes subtests that evaluate memory and problem-solving skills. The Stanford-Binet also measures intelligence but is less commonly used in this age group compared to the WISC. KABC focuses on processing and achievement but may not provide as comprehensive an assessment of memory retention and problem-solving as the WISC. Bayley Scales are intended for infants and toddlers up to age 3 and are inappropriate for Emily's age group.

Question 103: Correct Answer: B) Using professional medical interpreters

Rationale: Professional medical interpreters ensure accurate communication, reducing misunderstandings and improving patient outcomes. Speaking slowly and loudly (A), providing English-only instructions (C), or relying on family members (D) can lead to miscommunication due to language barriers or lack of medical knowledge. Utilizing trained interpreters aligns with best practices for cultural competence, ensuring that discharge instructions are clearly understood by patients regardless of their language proficiency.

Question 104: Correct Answer: D) Trail Making Test Part B (TMT-B)

Rationale: The TMT-B is specifically designed to assess executive function, including task switching and working memory, which are crucial for diagnosing early-stage dementia. While the MMSE and MoCA are broader cognitive assessments, they do not focus solely on executive function. The CDT evaluates visuospatial and executive functions but lacks the complexity of TMT-B. Therefore, TMT-B is more accurate in assessing executive function deficits.

Question 105: Correct Answer: A) Oxygen saturation levels

Rationale: Hypoxia due to COPD can lead to significant cognitive impairment as low oxygen levels affect brain function. While blood glucose levels, medication review, and nutritional status are important considerations, they are secondary in this context. Hyperglycemia can cause confusion but is less directly linked to the immediate respiratory condition. Medication side effects and nutritional deficiencies can contribute to cognitive issues but are not as acutely impactful as hypoxia in this scenario.

Question 106: Correct Answer: A) Central venous catheter

Rationale: A central venous catheter allows for accurate measurement of central venous pressure (CVP), administration of vasoactive medications, and obtaining central venous oxygen saturation ($ScvO_2$), all critical components of early goal-directed therapy in sepsis management. Pulmonary artery catheters are more invasive, non-invasive cardiac output monitors do not measure CVP or allow medication administration, and peripheral IV lines are inadequate for these purposes. Thus, the central venous catheter is essential.

Question 107: Correct Answer: B) Listening actively to the patient's concerns
Rationale: Active listening is crucial for building trust, as it demonstrates empathy and understanding. Providing detailed explanations (Option A), offering reassurance (Option C), and maintaining professional boundaries (Option D) are important aspects of communication, but active listening directly fosters trust by making patients feel heard and valued.

Question 108: Correct Answer: C) Lung Cancer
Rationale: Lung cancer often presents with chronic cough, hemoptysis (coughing up blood), unintentional weight loss, and finger clubbing due to chronic hypoxia. COPD (A) includes chronic cough but lacks hemoptysis and significant weight loss typically seen in lung cancer. Tuberculosis (B) can cause hemoptysis but usually has night sweats as well. Pneumonia (D) causes acute symptoms like fever and productive cough without the chronicity or finger clubbing seen in lung cancer.

Question 109: Correct Answer: B) Sudden onset of severe headache
Rationale: A sudden onset of severe headache, often described as the "worst headache of my life," can be indicative of serious neurological conditions such as subarachnoid hemorrhage. Intermittent joint pain (Option A) typically relates to musculoskeletal issues, occasional dizziness when standing quickly (Option C) may be due to orthostatic hypotension, and chronic fatigue (Option D) can have numerous causes including psychological or systemic diseases. The critical point is the acute and severe nature of the headache in Option B that warrants immediate attention.

Question 110: Correct Answer: C) Allowing Mrs. Lee to practice injections under supervision
Rationale: Allowing Mrs. Lee to practice injections under supervision ensures she gains hands-on experience and immediate feedback, which builds confidence and competence in self-administration (C). Written instructions with diagrams (A), while helpful, do not provide practical experience. Demonstrating on an orange (B) is informative but does not involve patient participation. Instructional videos (D) are useful but insufficient alone for skill acquisition. Active learning through practice is supported by contemporary research as most effective for skill-based education.

Question 111: Correct Answer: C) Performing hand hygiene before and after patient contact
Rationale: Hand hygiene is the single most effective measure to prevent hospital-acquired infections, reducing pathogen transmission between patients and healthcare providers. Option A (private room and contact precautions) may be necessary but secondary to hand hygiene. Option B (early ambulation and deep breathing exercises) aids recovery but does not directly prevent infection transmission. Option D (incentive spirometer use) prevents respiratory complications but does not address overall infection control.

Question 112: Correct Answer: C) Pulmonary crackles
Rationale: Pulmonary crackles are most strongly associated with left-sided heart failure due to fluid accumulation in the lungs from impaired left ventricular function. JVD and peripheral edema are more indicative of right-sided heart failure or biventricular failure. Hepatomegaly also points towards right-sided heart failure due to systemic congestion. Therefore, pulmonary crackles are the key finding suggesting left-sided heart failure specifically.

Question 113: Correct Answer: A) Administer oxygen and notify the physician.
Rationale: Sudden shortness of breath and chest pain postoperatively may indicate a pulmonary embolism (PE), a life-threatening condition requiring immediate intervention. Administering oxygen helps stabilize the patient while notifying the physician ensures prompt medical evaluation and treatment. Performing a full respiratory assessment (Option B) is important but secondary to stabilizing the patient. Encouraging deep breathing exercises (Option C) is preventive but not an immediate response to acute symptoms. Checking for infection signs (Option D) does not address the acute respiratory distress.

Question 114: Correct Answer: B) Montreal Cognitive Assessment (MoCA)
Rationale: The MoCA is specifically designed to detect mild cognitive impairment and early Alzheimer's disease, making it highly suitable for evaluating Sarah's symptoms. The MMSE, while useful, is less sensitive to mild cognitive impairment. The Clock Drawing Test is a component of broader assessments but not comprehensive alone. The GDS assesses depression, which can mimic cognitive decline but does not directly evaluate cognitive function.

Question 115: Correct Answer: A) Review Mr. Lee's blood glucose logs and medication adherence history.
Rationale: Reviewing blood glucose logs and medication adherence history provides essential data that will inform the endocrinologist's assessment and recommendations during the consult, ensuring it is effective and targeted. Option B is premature without knowing what changes will be recommended by the endocrinologist. Option C could be necessary later but isn't immediately relevant to ensuring an effective initial consult. Option D may be helpful but is secondary to providing accurate clinical data to inform the consultation process effectively.

Question 116: Correct Answer: A) Breast MRI
Rationale: Breast MRI is highly sensitive and particularly useful in women with dense breast tissue or those at high risk for breast cancer. It provides detailed images that can detect abnormalities missed by mammography alone. Ultrasound (B), while helpful in evaluating dense breasts, is less sensitive than MRI. Digital Mammography (C), although beneficial for initial screening, may not provide sufficient detail in dense breasts. Clinical Breast Exam (D), while important, lacks the imaging capabilities needed for thorough evaluation in this context.

Question 117: Correct Answer: B) Engaging in art therapy
Rationale: Art therapy has been shown to significantly reduce anxiety and improve mood in patients with chronic pain by providing a creative outlet for expression and distraction from discomfort. Watching television (A) and reading books (C) can be passive activities that may not fully engage the patient, while listening to music (D), though beneficial, may not provide the same level of active engagement and emotional expression as art therapy.

Question 118: Correct Answer: B) Initiating anticoagulant therapy immediately
Rationale: The symptoms described are indicative of a pulmonary embolism (PE), a common postoperative complication. Immediate initiation of anticoagulant therapy is critical to prevent further clot propagation and reduce mortality. Administering IV fluids (A) may be supportive but does not address the underlying issue. A chest X-ray (C) can help rule out other conditions but is not an immediate priority. Supplemental oxygen (D) helps with hypoxia but does not treat the embolus itself.

Question 119: Correct Answer: A) Administering benzodiazepines
Rationale: Benzodiazepines are first-line treatment for acute agitation and paranoia due to methamphetamine intoxication as they provide rapid sedation and anxiolysis. Antipsychotic medication (B), while useful in psychosis, may not address acute agitation as quickly. A quiet environment with reassurance (C), though helpful, is insufficient alone for severe agitation. Methadone therapy (D) is used for opioid dependence, not stimulant intoxication.

Question 120: Correct Answer: B) Montreal Cognitive Assessment (MoCA)
Rationale: The MoCA is specifically designed to detect mild cognitive impairment and provides a comprehensive evaluation of various cognitive domains including memory,

attention, language, and executive functions. The MMSE is also used for cognitive assessment but is less sensitive in detecting mild cognitive impairment compared to the MoCA. The CDT evaluates visuospatial abilities and executive function but does not provide a comprehensive assessment. The CAM is primarily used for diagnosing delirium rather than general cognitive impairment.

Question 121: Correct Answer: D) Individualized teaching sessions

Rationale: Individualized teaching sessions are most effective because they tailor the information to the specific needs, preferences, and comprehension levels of each patient, thereby improving adherence. Lecture-based education (Option A) may not address individual patient concerns. Interactive workshops (Option B) are beneficial but may not provide the personalized attention required. Written handouts (Option C) alone lack the interactive component necessary for ensuring understanding and adherence. Hence, individualized teaching sessions are superior in addressing complex medication regimens effectively.

Question 122: Correct Answer: D) Ensuring proper hand hygiene before and after catheter manipulation

Rationale: Proper hand hygiene before and after catheter manipulation is the most effective strategy for preventing CAUTIs. While antimicrobial-coated catheters (A) can reduce infection rates, they are not as universally effective as strict hand hygiene practices. Implementing a closed drainage system (B) is important but secondary to hand hygiene. Regularly changing the catheter every 48 hours (C) is unnecessary and can increase infection risk due to frequent manipulation. Hand hygiene directly reduces the transmission of pathogens, making it a critical component of infection prevention.

Question 123: Correct Answer: A) Administer intravenous calcium gluconate.

Rationale: In cases of hyperkalemia with ECG changes, the first line of treatment is to stabilize the cardiac membrane using intravenous calcium gluconate (Option A). Sodium polystyrene sulfonate (Option B), while effective in reducing potassium levels, acts more slowly and is not the initial treatment in acute settings. Hemodialysis (Option C) is reserved for severe cases unresponsive to other treatments or in patients with renal failure but is not the first step. Loop diuretics (Option D) can help excrete potassium but are also not the immediate intervention for stabilizing cardiac function.

Question 124: Correct Answer: C) Glomerular filtration rate (GFR)

Rationale: GFR is the most accurate measure of kidney function and is crucial for assessing the severity of CKD. While urinalysis (A) can detect abnormalities in urine, it does not directly measure kidney function. Serum electrolytes (B) provide information about electrolyte balance but not overall kidney function. CBC (D) can indicate anemia related to CKD but does not assess kidney function itself. GFR provides a precise assessment of how well the kidneys are filtering waste from the blood, making it the most appropriate test in this scenario.

Question 125: Correct Answer: C) International Normalized Ratio (INR)

Rationale: Amiodarone can increase the effects of warfarin, leading to an elevated INR and increased risk of bleeding. Monitoring INR is crucial to adjust warfarin dosage appropriately. Blood glucose levels (A), serum potassium levels (B), and liver function tests (D) are important but not directly impacted by the interaction between warfarin and amiodarone. Therefore, while these parameters are relevant for other reasons, they do not address the specific interaction in question.

MEDSURG-BC Exam Practice Questions [SET 2]

Question 1: During the health history collection of Mrs. Smith, who presents with fatigue and shortness of breath, Nurse John needs to determine if her symptoms are related to her cardiac function. Which question is most appropriate for this purpose?
A) "Have you noticed any swelling in your legs or ankles?"
B) "Do you experience headaches frequently?"
C) "How many hours do you sleep at night?"
D) "Do you have any dietary restrictions?"

Question 2: A 65-year-old patient named Mr. Johnson is admitted for elective knee replacement surgery. As a medical-surgical nurse, you are responsible for preoperative education. Which of the following is the most effective method to ensure Mr. Johnson retains the preoperative instructions?
A) Provide written instructions and ask him to read them.
B) Explain the instructions verbally and ask him to repeat them back.
C) Show a video of the procedure and provide written instructions.
D) Use a combination of verbal explanation, written materials, and teach-back method.

Question 3: Sarah, a 55-year-old patient with a history of smoking and hypertension, comes for a routine check-up. As part of her screening, which tool would be most appropriate to assess her risk for cardiovascular disease?
A) Framingham Risk Score
B) ASCVD Risk Calculator
C) QRISK3
D) Reynolds Risk Score

Question 4: Which of the following drug combinations is most likely to result in serotonin syndrome?
A) Fluoxetine and Tramadol
B) Metoprolol and Furosemide
C) Warfarin and Ciprofloxacin
D) Digoxin and Verapamil

Question 5: John, a 60-year-old male with no significant past medical history, presents for his annual physical exam. Which screening tool would be most appropriate to evaluate his risk of developing colorectal cancer?
A) Fecal Immunochemical Test (FIT)
B) Colonoscopy
C) Cologuard Test
D) Digital Rectal Exam (DRE)

Question 6: Which of the following vaccines is recommended annually for adults, especially those with chronic health conditions such as diabetes or heart disease?
A) Influenza vaccine
B) Hepatitis B vaccine
C) Pneumococcal vaccine
D) Tetanus, diphtheria, and pertussis (Tdap) vaccine

Question 7: In Piaget's theory of cognitive development, which stage is characterized by abstract thinking and hypothetical reasoning?
A) Sensorimotor Stage
B) Preoperational Stage
C) Concrete Operational Stage
D) Formal Operational Stage

Question 8: Maria, a 60-year-old female with diabetes, reports feeling overwhelmed by her diagnosis and expresses anxiety about her ability to manage her condition. During the psychosocial assessment, which approach should the nurse prioritize?
A) Provide Maria with educational materials on diabetes management.
B) Explore Maria's coping mechanisms and support systems.
C) Encourage Maria to attend diabetes self-management classes.
D) Discuss potential lifestyle changes that could improve her condition.

Question 9: Mrs. Johnson, a 68-year-old patient with a history of chronic obstructive pulmonary disease (COPD), presents with increased shortness of breath, wheezing, and productive cough. During your assessment, you notice her oxygen saturation is 88% on room air. What is the most appropriate initial nursing intervention?
A) Administer a bronchodilator as prescribed
B) Increase oxygen flow rate to 4 L/min via nasal cannula
C) Position the patient in high Fowler's position
D) Perform chest physiotherapy

Question 10: In assessing a patient's blood pressure, which Korotkoff sound is associated with diastolic pressure?
A) Phase I
B) Phase II
C) Phase III
D) Phase V

Question 11: David, a 50-year-old male with chronic pain, expresses feelings of worthlessness and has hinted at life not being worth living anymore. He denies any current plans or means to harm himself but appears withdrawn and disengaged during the assessment. What should be the nurse's next step?
A) Educate David about coping mechanisms for chronic pain.
B) Assess David's access to means of suicide.
C) Refer David to cognitive-behavioral therapy (CBT).
D) Schedule an appointment with David's primary care physician.

Question 12: In the context of health history collection for a patient presenting with unexplained weight loss, which component should be prioritized?
A) Dietary habits
B) Recent travel history
C) Psychological state
D) Occupational exposure

Question 13: Tom, a 60-year-old patient who had abdominal surgery, presents with a distended abdomen and decreased urine output on postoperative day four. His hematocrit has dropped significantly since surgery. What should be the nurse's priority action?
A) Insert a nasogastric tube.
B) Increase oral fluid intake.
C) Assess for signs of hypovolemic shock.
D) Encourage ambulation.

Question 14: Mrs. Johnson, an 82-year-old woman with mild cognitive impairment, is struggling with her ADLs, particularly bathing and dressing. What is the most appropriate initial intervention?
A) Referral to an occupational therapist for adaptive equipment training.
B) Initiating home health aide services for personal care assistance.

C) Providing Mrs. Johnson with written instructions on bathing and dressing techniques.
D) Encouraging Mrs. Johnson to attend a group exercise class to improve mobility.

Question 15: Which evidence-based approach is recommended for assessing the effectiveness of an educational intervention in improving clinical skills among medical-surgical nurses?
A) Pre- and post-tests
B) Peer reviews
C) Patient feedback surveys
D) Simulation assessments

Question 16: In assessing a patient's functional status related to Activities of Daily Living (ADLs), which factor is least likely to directly impact their ability to perform these activities?
A) Visual acuity
B) Cognitive impairment
C) Social support network
D) Range of motion

Question 17: Which laboratory test is most specific for diagnosing acute pancreatitis?
A) Serum amylase
B) Serum lipase
C) Serum bilirubin
D) Serum alkaline phosphatase

Question 18: John, a 45-year-old male patient undergoing treatment for hypertension, expresses anxiety about his career progression and the impact of his health on his ability to mentor younger colleagues at work. According to Erikson's stages of development, which stage is John most likely navigating?
A) Generativity vs. Stagnation
B) Intimacy vs. Isolation
C) Integrity vs. Despair
D) Identity vs. Role Confusion

Question 19: Mrs. Thompson, a 68-year-old patient, is admitted for evaluation of her cognitive function due to recent memory loss and confusion. The nurse plans to use the Mini-Mental State Examination (MMSE) as part of the cognitive assessment. Which aspect of cognitive function is primarily assessed by the MMSE?
A) Executive function
B) Short-term memory
C) Visuospatial skills
D) Orientation

Question 20: Mr. Johnson, a 55-year-old patient recovering from abdominal surgery, is experiencing anxiety and moderate pain. Which non-pharmacologic intervention should be prioritized to address both his anxiety and pain?
A) Guided Imagery
B) Biofeedback
C) Music Therapy
D) Massage Therapy

Question 21: Nurse Jamie is coordinating care for Ms. Patel, who requires multiple interdisciplinary consults including cardiology, nephrology, and nutrition services. Which action best demonstrates effective interdisciplinary healthcare team collaboration?
A) Scheduling all consults on different days to avoid overwhelming Ms. Patel.
B) Facilitating a case conference with all consultants to discuss Ms. Patel's care plan.
C) Prioritizing consults based on Ms. Patel's immediate medical needs without consulting other team members.
D) Documenting each consultant's recommendations separately in Ms. Patel's medical record.

Question 22: Sarah, a 65-year-old patient, underwent a hip replacement surgery. On the third postoperative day, she develops a fever of 38.5°C, redness, and swelling around the surgical site. Which of the following is the most appropriate initial intervention to prevent further infection complications?
A) Start broad-spectrum antibiotics immediately.
B) Obtain wound cultures before starting antibiotics.
C) Increase the frequency of dressing changes.
D) Administer antipyretics to control fever.

Question 23: When assessing a patient's ability to perform Activities of Daily Living (ADLs), which of the following would be considered an instrumental activity of daily living (IADL)?
A) Bathing
B) Dressing
C) Managing medications
D) Eating

Question 24: A nurse is caring for a terminally ill patient who requests assistance in hastening death. What should be the nurse's ethical response?
A) Provide information on palliative care options.
B) Assist in hastening death as per patient's request.
C) Refer the patient to another healthcare provider willing to assist.
D) Avoid discussing end-of-life options with the patient.

Question 25: Mr. Thompson, a 58-year-old male, reports experiencing sudden visual disturbances and confusion. During your assessment, you note that he has difficulty recognizing familiar objects and faces despite having intact vision. Which condition might be causing these symptoms?
A) Agnosia
B) Apraxia
C) Dysarthria
D) Hemianopia

Question 26: Nurse Jamie is caring for Mr. Smith, a post-operative patient who has just undergone abdominal surgery. To prevent the risk of deep vein thrombosis (DVT), which patient safety measure should Nurse Jamie prioritize?
A) Encourage early ambulation
B) Administer prophylactic antibiotics
C) Ensure adequate hydration
D) Monitor blood glucose levels

Question 27: In preparing a patient for an MRI scan, which of the following actions is most important to prevent complications?
A) Asking about any history of claustrophobia
B) Ensuring all metallic objects are removed from the patient's body
C) Confirming if the patient has any allergies to contrast agents
D) Educating the patient about remaining still during the scan

Question 28: A 68-year-old patient named Mr. Thompson is admitted to the surgical ward following a hip replacement surgery. The nurse needs to ensure accurate monitoring of his vital signs using medical equipment. Which piece of equipment is most appropriate for continuous monitoring of Mr. Thompson's oxygen saturation?
A) Sphygmomanometer
B) Electrocardiogram (ECG) monitor
C) Pulse oximeter

D) Capnograph

Question 29: During her night shift, Nurse Emily finds that Mr. Lee, a confused elderly patient, has managed to loosen his wrist restraints several times despite proper application techniques being used. What is the most appropriate action Nurse Emily should take next?
A) Apply mittens instead of wrist restraints.
B) Double-check and tighten the wrist restraints.
C) Request an order for chemical restraints.
D) Reassess Mr. Lee's cognitive status and environment.

Question 30: John, a 45-year-old male, has been recently diagnosed with chronic heart failure. During a psychosocial assessment, he expresses feelings of hopelessness and mentions that he no longer enjoys activities he used to love. Which of the following is the most appropriate initial nursing intervention?
A) Encourage John to join a support group for individuals with chronic illnesses.
B) Refer John to a psychiatrist for evaluation of potential depression.
C) Educate John about the importance of adhering to his medication regimen.
D) Schedule regular follow-up appointments to monitor John's physical condition.

Question 31: Which of the following is the most effective initial step in creating a comprehensive care plan for a patient with multiple chronic conditions?
A) Conducting a thorough patient assessment
B) Reviewing the patient's medical history
C) Establishing patient-centered goals
D) Consulting with interdisciplinary team members

Question 32: Which assessment tool is most appropriate for evaluating a patient's ability to perform Activities of Daily Living (ADLs) independently in a medical-surgical setting?
A) Barthel Index
B) Mini-Mental State Examination (MMSE)
C) Braden Scale
D) Glasgow Coma Scale

Question 33: During a neurological assessment, which finding is most suggestive of an upper motor neuron lesion?
A) Flaccid paralysis
B) Hyperreflexia
C) Muscle atrophy
D) Fasciculations

Question 34: Mr. Smith, a diabetic patient on metformin therapy, is advised to take his medication with meals. Which dietary consideration should the nurse emphasize to Mr. Smith?
A) Avoid consuming dairy products with metformin as it decreases drug absorption.
B) Ensure meals are high in carbohydrates to enhance metformin's effectiveness.
C) Avoid excessive alcohol consumption as it increases the risk of lactic acidosis.
D) Increase protein intake during meals for better drug metabolism.

Question 35: Michael, a 40-year-old male with liver cirrhosis, presents with ascites and peripheral edema. His serum albumin level is significantly low. Which treatment option would be most effective in addressing his fluid imbalance?
A) Sodium restriction diet
B) Spironolactone administration
C) Intravenous albumin infusion
D) Fluid restriction

Question 36: Maria, a 45-year-old woman recovering from a hysterectomy, reports feeling dizzy and lightheaded on postoperative day three. Her blood pressure is 90/60 mmHg and her heart rate is 110 bpm. What is the most likely cause of her symptoms?
A) Dehydration
B) Postoperative hemorrhage
C) Pain medication side effects
D) Orthostatic hypotension

Question 37: What is the primary benefit of involving family members in patient teaching sessions for chronic disease management?
A) Ensuring someone else understands the care plan
B) Increasing emotional support for the patient
C) Enhancing adherence through shared responsibility
D) Allowing family members to make decisions on behalf of the patient

Question 38: Which of the following laboratory findings is most indicative of acute pancreatitis?
A) Elevated serum amylase
B) Elevated serum lipase
C) Elevated serum bilirubin
D) Elevated serum alkaline phosphatase

Question 39: Mrs. Smith, a 65-year-old female with chronic kidney disease, is found to have a potassium level of 6.5 mEq/L during routine blood work. Which nursing action should be prioritized?
A) Administer oral potassium supplements.
B) Initiate cardiac monitoring.
C) Encourage high-potassium foods.
D) Administer diuretics.

Question 40: Emily, a 45-year-old woman with no previous colorectal issues but a family history of colon cancer, seeks advice on colorectal cancer screening. What is the most appropriate initial screening test?
A) Fecal Immunochemical Test (FIT)
B) Colonoscopy
C) Flexible Sigmoidoscopy
D) CT Colonography

Question 41: Nurse Emily is caring for Mr. Chen, a 70-year-old Chinese immigrant who has been diagnosed with hypertension. Mr. Chen prefers using traditional Chinese medicine (TCM) along with his prescribed medications. How should Nurse Emily incorporate cultural competence in her care plan for Mr. Chen?
A) Advise Mr. Chen to stop using TCM and strictly follow the prescribed medications.
B) Collaborate with Mr. Chen to integrate TCM practices that do not interfere with his prescribed medications.
C) Ignore Mr. Chen's preference for TCM and focus solely on his prescribed medications.
D) Refer Mr. Chen to a TCM practitioner without considering his current medical regimen.

Question 42: When assessing a patient's ability to perform ADLs, which component is crucial in determining their level of independence?
A) Cognitive function
B) Muscle strength
C) Joint flexibility
D) Coordination

Question 43: Mrs. Thompson, a 78-year-old patient with hypertension, diabetes, and osteoarthritis, is on multiple medications. During a routine check-up, she complains of dizziness and fatigue. Which of the following actions

should the nurse prioritize to address potential polypharmacy issues?
A) Review her current medication list for possible drug interactions.
B) Increase her fluid intake to counteract dehydration.
C) Schedule an immediate appointment with a cardiologist.
D) Recommend over-the-counter supplements to boost energy.

Question 44: Michael, a 70-year-old male with COPD, is scheduled for elective surgery under general anesthesia. What preoperative preparation should be prioritized?
A) Performing pulmonary function tests (PFTs)
B) Withholding bronchodilators on the day of surgery
C) Initiating prophylactic antibiotics
D) Ensuring NPO status after midnight

Question 45: In the context of patient- and family-centered care, which strategy is most effective for involving family members in the care process?
A) Regularly scheduled family meetings
B) Providing educational materials
C) Open visitation policies
D) Family advisory councils

Question 46: In planning patient education for a diverse group of learners, which strategy best addresses varying learning preferences?
A) Using standardized written materials
B) Implementing a multimodal approach
C) Conducting group discussions only
D) Focusing solely on visual aids

Question 47: When planning an educational session for patients with chronic obstructive pulmonary disease (COPD), which topic should be prioritized to maximize patient outcomes?
A) Pathophysiology of COPD
B) Medication adherence strategies
C) Nutritional management
D) Breathing exercises

Question 48: Sarah, a 50-year-old female with chronic kidney disease (CKD), is scheduled for an MRI with contrast. What pre-procedure assessment is crucial in this case?
A) Checking serum potassium levels
B) Evaluating liver function tests
C) Assessing renal function through serum creatinine and GFR
D) Monitoring blood glucose levels

Question 49: A patient presents with hyperkalemia. Which of the following ECG changes is most indicative of this electrolyte imbalance?
A) Peaked T waves
B) Prolonged QT interval
C) ST segment depression
D) U waves

Question 50: David, a 60-year-old male smoker with chronic obstructive pulmonary disease (COPD), seeks advice on lifestyle modifications to improve his lung function and overall health. What is the most effective intervention he should prioritize?
A) Quitting smoking immediately
B) Using an air purifier at home
C) Practicing breathing exercises daily
D) Increasing omega-3 fatty acid intake

Question 51: Nurse Emily is preparing educational materials for a patient with newly diagnosed Type 2 Diabetes Mellitus. Which of the following supporting materials would be most effective in ensuring the patient comprehends and retains the information?
A) A detailed pamphlet with complex medical terminology
B) A video demonstrating glucose monitoring and insulin administration
C) A lengthy research article on the pathophysiology of diabetes
D) A PowerPoint presentation with bullet points and diagrams

Question 52: Which psychosocial factor is most important to assess when determining immediate suicide risk in hospitalized patients?
A) Recent loss or trauma
B) Employment status
C) Marital status
D) Educational level

Question 53: During a physical assessment, Nurse Emily observes that Mr. Johnson, a 68-year-old male with a history of chronic obstructive pulmonary disease (COPD), exhibits increased anteroposterior chest diameter. What is the most likely cause of this finding?
A) Pulmonary fibrosis
B) Kyphosis
C) Barrel chest
D) Pectus excavatum

Question 54: Which psychosocial assessment tool is most appropriate for evaluating the severity of depression in an adult patient?
A) Beck Depression Inventory (BDI)
B) Generalized Anxiety Disorder 7 (GAD-7)
C) Hamilton Anxiety Rating Scale (HAM-A)
D) Mini-Mental State Examination (MMSE)

Question 55: Which of the following is the most critical step in patient preparation for a colonoscopy to ensure accurate diagnostic results?
A) Administering a clear liquid diet 24 hours before the procedure
B) Ensuring the patient is NPO (nothing by mouth) for 8 hours before the procedure
C) Providing oral polyethylene glycol (PEG) solution for bowel cleansing
D) Administering a sedative to relax the patient during the procedure

Question 56: Which of the following strategies is most effective for ensuring patient adherence to a complex medication regimen post-discharge?
A) Providing written instructions and pamphlets
B) Utilizing teach-back methods to confirm understanding
C) Scheduling follow-up phone calls to remind patients
D) Recommending the use of a pill organizer

Question 57: Mr. Lee, a 48-year-old male with no significant past medical history, complains of frequent headaches and visual disturbances during his review of systems. He also reports occasional palpitations and sweating episodes. Which condition is most likely causing his symptoms?
A) Migraine
B) Hypertension
C) Pheochromocytoma
D) Hyperthyroidism

Question 58: Ms. Smith, a patient with chronic illness, expresses frustration about her condition during a routine check-up. What is the most appropriate therapeutic communication response from the nurse?
A) "I understand how you feel; my mother has the same

condition."
B) "Why don't you try focusing on the positives?"
C) "It sounds like you're feeling really overwhelmed right now."
D) "You should be grateful for the good days."

Question 59: In the context of chronic kidney disease (CKD), which electrolyte imbalance is most commonly observed?
A) Hyperkalemia
B) Hypokalemia
C) Hypercalcemia
D) Hypocalcemia

Question 60: What is the primary consideration for a nurse when evaluating the medication regimen of a patient with polypharmacy to prevent adverse effects?
A) Patient's age
B) Drug-drug interactions
C) Dosage frequency
D) Cost of medications

Question 61: When preparing a patient with diabetes mellitus for surgery, what is the primary consideration to prevent perioperative complications?
A) Monitoring blood glucose levels hourly during surgery
B) Administering insulin to maintain blood glucose below 100 mg/dL
C) Ensuring the patient has an early morning surgery slot
D) Adjusting insulin dosage based on preoperative blood glucose levels

Question 62: John, a 65-year-old male with a history of hypertension and diabetes, is scheduled for a colonoscopy. Which pre-procedure preparation is most critical to ensure accurate results and patient safety?
A) Administering a clear liquid diet for 24 hours before the procedure
B) Ensuring the patient stops taking antihypertensive medications 24 hours prior
C) Advising the patient to take their regular dose of insulin the morning of the procedure
D) Providing an enema the night before the procedure

Question 63: Which therapeutic communication technique is most effective in encouraging a patient to express their feelings about a recent diagnosis of chronic illness?
A) Providing reassurance
B) Using open-ended questions
C) Giving advice
D) Offering personal anecdotes

Question 64: Which principle best guides a medical-surgical nurse in maintaining patient confidentiality according to contemporary nursing ethics?
A) Beneficence
B) Nonmaleficence
C) Autonomy
D) Justice

Question 65: Which of the following actions best exemplifies the role of a medical-surgical nurse as an advocate for a patient experiencing difficulty in understanding their treatment options?
A) Recommending the patient to seek a second opinion from another physician.
B) Providing detailed explanations of the treatment options using layman's terms.
C) Encouraging the patient to research their condition independently.
D) Directing the patient to online forums for peer support.

Question 66: Sarah, a 45-year-old female, presents with fatigue, weight gain, and cold intolerance. Upon physical examination, you note dry skin and periorbital edema. Which of the following is the most likely diagnosis?
A) Hyperthyroidism
B) Hypothyroidism
C) Cushing's Syndrome
D) Addison's Disease

Question 67: Mr. Johnson, a 70-year-old patient with osteoarthritis, is having difficulty performing activities of daily living (ADLs). During your assessment, which intervention would most effectively help him maintain his independence?
A) Providing assistive devices such as grab bars and a raised toilet seat
B) Encouraging the use of pain medication before engaging in ADLs
C) Recommending complete bed rest to avoid joint strain
D) Suggesting physical therapy for muscle strengthening and joint flexibility

Question 68: For a postoperative patient experiencing severe pain unrelieved by standard analgesics, which advanced nursing intervention should be considered next?
A) Increasing the dose of current analgesic
B) Switching to a different class of analgesic
C) Implementing patient-controlled analgesia (PCA)
D) Utilizing non-pharmacological pain relief methods

Question 69: A patient with severe vomiting is likely to develop which of the following acid-base imbalances?
A) Metabolic alkalosis
B) Metabolic acidosis
C) Respiratory alkalosis
D) Respiratory acidosis

Question 70: In an interdisciplinary healthcare team, which strategy is most effective in ensuring that all team members contribute equally during patient care consultations?
A) Assigning roles based on seniority
B) Implementing structured communication tools like SBAR (Situation-Background-Assessment-Recommendation)
C) Conducting consultations via email to allow time for thoughtful responses
D) Rotating leadership roles among team members

Question 71: Which outcome measure is most appropriate for evaluating the effectiveness of a pain management plan in post-operative patients?
A) Reduction in patient-reported pain scores
B) Decrease in opioid usage
C) Improvement in patient mobility
D) Increase in patient satisfaction

Question 72: John, a 55-year-old male with a history of hypertension and obesity, is seeking advice on improving his overall health. As his medical-surgical nurse, which of the following interventions would be most effective in promoting John's health and wellness?
A) Encouraging him to reduce sodium intake to less than 2,300 mg per day.
B) Recommending he engage in at least 150 minutes of moderate-intensity aerobic activity per week.
C) Advising him to consume a diet rich in fruits and vegetables while limiting red meat intake.
D) Suggesting he monitor his blood pressure daily and keep a log for review during follow-up visits.

Question 73: John, a 55-year-old male with a history of chronic kidney disease (CKD), presents to the

emergency department with confusion, muscle weakness, and cardiac arrhythmias. His laboratory results show a serum potassium level of 6.5 mEq/L. What is the most appropriate initial treatment for his condition?
A) Administration of calcium gluconate
B) Administration of sodium bicarbonate
C) Administration of insulin and glucose
D) Administration of loop diuretics

Question 74: Which electrolyte imbalance is most likely to cause a prolonged QT interval on an electrocardiogram (ECG) in a patient with medical-surgical conditions?
A) Hypokalemia
B) Hypercalcemia
C) Hypocalcemia
D) Hypermagnesemia

Question 75: In preventing medication errors, which strategy is considered the most effective?
A) Double-checking medications with a second nurse
B) Utilizing barcode medication administration (BCMA)
C) Educating patients about their medications
D) Standardizing medication administration times

Question 76: Which screening tool is most appropriate for assessing the risk of falls in hospitalized adult patients?
A) Braden Scale
B) Morse Fall Scale
C) Mini-Mental State Examination (MMSE)
D) Norton Scale

Question 77: Nurse Alex is planning care for Mrs. Johnson, who has a high risk of falls due to her recent stroke. Which intervention should be implemented first to ensure her safety?
A) Place fall risk signs on her door and above her bed
B) Use bed alarms to alert staff if she tries to get up unassisted
C) Provide non-slip footwear and keep personal items within reach
D) Conduct hourly rounds to check on her status

Question 78: John, a 58-year-old male, underwent a total hip replacement surgery. On postoperative day two, he begins to exhibit signs of internal bleeding. Which of the following is the most appropriate initial nursing intervention?
A) Increase the IV fluid rate.
B) Administer an anticoagulant.
C) Apply direct pressure to the surgical site.
D) Notify the surgeon immediately.

Question 79: When assessing a patient for dehydration, which physical examination finding is most reliable?
A) Dry mucous membranes
B) Decreased skin turgor
C) Orthostatic hypotension
D) Elevated blood urea nitrogen (BUN)

Question 80: A 65-year-old patient named Mr. Johnson presents with confusion, muscle weakness, and a history of congestive heart failure. His lab results show serum sodium levels of 128 mEq/L. What is the most appropriate initial intervention to manage his condition?
A) Administer hypertonic saline solution.
B) Restrict water intake.
C) Administer isotonic saline solution.
D) Encourage increased oral fluid intake.

Question 81: John, a 60-year-old man with no significant medical history, asks about prostate cancer screening. Which screening method should be recommended based on current guidelines?
A) Digital Rectal Exam (DRE)
B) Prostate-Specific Antigen (PSA) test
C) Transrectal Ultrasound
D) MRI of the prostate

Question 82: John, a 55-year-old male with a history of hypertension and obesity, is seeking advice on healthy lifestyle modifications to manage his conditions. Which of the following interventions is most likely to provide significant long-term benefits?
A) Adopting a Mediterranean diet
B) Reducing sodium intake to less than 2,300 mg per day
C) Engaging in moderate-intensity aerobic exercise for at least 150 minutes per week
D) Increasing daily fiber intake to 25-30 grams

Question 83: Which diagnostic tool is most effective in identifying a deep vein thrombosis (DVT) in a post-operative patient?
A) D-dimer test
B) Doppler ultrasound
C) Venography
D) MRI

Question 84: Which approach is most effective in minimizing surgical site infections (SSIs)?
A) Administering prophylactic antibiotics within one hour before incision
B) Using chlorhexidine-alcohol for preoperative skin antisepsis
C) Ensuring proper hand hygiene among surgical staff
D) Maintaining normothermia during surgery

Question 85: In assessing cognitive impairment, which test is known to have high sensitivity for detecting mild cognitive impairment (MCI)?
A) Mini-Cog
B) Montreal Cognitive Assessment (MoCA)
C) Mini-Mental State Examination (MMSE)
D) Addenbrooke's Cognitive Examination III (ACE-III)

Question 86: Lisa, who is being treated for hyperlipidemia with atorvastatin, loves grapefruit juice. What advice should the nurse provide Lisa about her favorite beverage?
A) Drink grapefruit juice daily as it enhances atorvastatin absorption.
B) Limit grapefruit juice intake to avoid increased blood levels of atorvastatin.
C) Substitute grapefruit juice with orange juice for better drug efficacy.
D) Consume grapefruit juice only in the morning to prevent interactions.

Question 87: According to Lawrence Kohlberg, at which level of moral development do individuals make decisions based on societal rules and laws?
A) Preconventional Level
B) Conventional Level
C) Postconventional Level
D) Autonomous Level

Question 88: A medical-surgical nurse notices that a patient's pain management plan is ineffective. What is the most appropriate advocacy action for the nurse to take?
A) Informing the patient's family about the issue.
B) Contacting the physician to discuss alternative pain management strategies.
C) Documenting the patient's pain levels without further

action.
D) Suggesting over-the-counter medications to the patient.

Question 89: Maria, a 45-year-old female with prediabetes and a sedentary lifestyle, wants to prevent the progression to type 2 diabetes through lifestyle changes. Which intervention should be prioritized?
A) Following a low-carbohydrate diet
B) Participating in a structured weight loss program
C) Taking daily multivitamins
D) Drinking green tea regularly

Question 90: Mrs. Thompson, a 65-year-old female with a history of chronic obstructive pulmonary disease (COPD), is preparing for her annual physical examination. As part of her health and wellness promotion, which vaccination should be prioritized to reduce her risk of complications from respiratory infections?
A) Influenza vaccine
B) Hepatitis B vaccine
C) Meningococcal vaccine
D) Human papillomavirus (HPV) vaccine

Question 91: Mr. Garcia, a 50-year-old diabetic patient, visits the clinic for his routine check-up. Considering his age and chronic condition, which vaccination should be emphasized to prevent potential complications associated with his diabetes?
A) Tetanus-diphtheria-pertussis (Tdap) vaccine
B) Pneumococcal polysaccharide vaccine (PPSV23)
C) Varicella (chickenpox) vaccine
D) Measles-mumps-rubella (MMR) vaccine

Question 92: In a patient with suspected myocardial infarction (MI), which biomarker is considered the gold standard for diagnosis?
A) CK-MB
B) Myoglobin
C) Troponin I
D) LDH

Question 93: Nurse Taylor is assessing patient Lisa's learning about post-operative care following knee replacement surgery. Which strategy best evaluates Lisa's readiness for discharge?
A) Asking Lisa to list post-operative care instructions
B) Observing Lisa perform wound care and mobility exercises
C) Providing Lisa with a checklist to mark completed tasks
D) Having Lisa attend a group education session on post-operative care

Question 94: What is the most appropriate action if an irregular pulse is detected during vital signs assessment?
A) Immediately notify the physician
B) Reassess using a Doppler device
C) Count the pulse for a full minute
D) Document and continue with other assessments

Question 95: Which of the following best describes orthostatic hypotension?
A) A drop in systolic blood pressure of 10 mmHg upon standing
B) An increase in diastolic blood pressure of 10 mmHg upon standing
C) A drop in systolic blood pressure of 20 mmHg or more upon standing
D) An increase in heart rate by 10 beats per minute upon standing

Question 96: John, a 65-year-old male with a history of chronic kidney disease, presents with muscle weakness, confusion, and an irregular heartbeat. His lab results show a potassium level of 6.5 mEq/L. What is the most appropriate initial intervention?
A) Administer IV insulin and glucose
B) Administer oral potassium supplements
C) Administer IV calcium gluconate
D) Administer a loop diuretic

Question 97: Nurse Sarah is implementing an evidence-based practice protocol for preventing pressure ulcers in immobile patients like Mr. Garcia, who has limited mobility due to a stroke. Which intervention should she prioritize?
A) Repositioning the patient every two hours.
B) Using pressure-relieving mattresses.
C) Applying barrier creams to protect skin integrity.
D) Conducting daily skin assessments.

Question 98: What is the primary benefit of including a pharmacist in an interdisciplinary healthcare team managing complex medical-surgical patients?
A) Enhanced medication reconciliation accuracy
B) Improved nutritional support planning
C) Streamlined discharge processes
D) Increased patient satisfaction scores

Question 99: Which screening tool is most effective for identifying malnutrition in hospitalized surgical patients?
A) Malnutrition Universal Screening Tool (MUST)
B) Nutritional Risk Screening (NRS-2002)
C) Mini Nutritional Assessment (MNA)
D) Subjective Global Assessment (SGA)

Question 100: In surgical settings, which practice is most critical in preventing surgical site infections (SSIs)?
A) Administering prophylactic antibiotics within one hour before incision
B) Shaving surgical sites immediately prior to surgery
C) Using sterile gloves during all stages of surgery
D) Applying antiseptic solutions to surgical instruments

Question 101: Maria, a 30-year-old female, was recently diagnosed with major depressive disorder and has expressed passive suicidal ideation. She lives alone and has limited social support. During her follow-up visit, she reports feeling slightly better but still struggles with thoughts of self-harm. What should be the nurse's priority action?
A) Increase the frequency of follow-up visits.
B) Develop a safety plan with Maria.
C) Encourage Maria to join a support group.
D) Adjust Maria's medication dosage.

Question 102: In assessing a patient's functional status related to Activities of Daily Living (ADLs), which factor is least likely to directly impact their ability to perform these activities?
A) Visual acuity
B) Cognitive impairment
C) Social support network
D) Range of motion

Question 103: Sarah, a 55-year-old female with severe vomiting for three days, presents with dizziness and hypotension. Her lab results reveal a sodium level of 125 mEq/L. Which of the following treatments is most appropriate?
A) Administer isotonic saline solution
B) Restrict water intake
C) Administer hypertonic saline solution

D) Increase oral fluid intake

Question 104: During a health history interview with Mrs. Garcia, a 60-year-old diabetic patient who reports frequent episodes of hypoglycemia, what should the nurse prioritize in her assessment?
A) Mrs. Garcia's diet and meal patterns
B) Her medication adherence
C) Her physical activity level
D) Her emotional stress levels

Question 105: Ms. Smith, a 70-year-old female with chronic obstructive pulmonary disease (COPD), reports shortness of breath and increased sputum production. Her vital signs are: BP 130/80 mmHg, HR 88 bpm, RR 28 breaths/min, Temp 99°F, SpO2 88%. What should be the immediate nursing intervention?
A) Increase her oxygen flow rate.
B) Administer a bronchodilator via nebulizer.
C) Position her in high Fowler's position.
D) Start an antibiotic therapy.

Question 106: During a psychosocial assessment, what is the primary purpose of exploring a patient's cultural background?
A) To identify potential language barriers
B) To understand the patient's health beliefs and practices
C) To assess socioeconomic status
D) To determine educational level

Question 107: Mrs. Smith, a 55-year-old patient recovering from abdominal surgery, has the following vital signs: BP 120/80 mmHg, HR 90 bpm, RR 28 breaths/min, and SpO2 93%. She reports feeling short of breath. Which vital sign is most concerning in this context?
A) Blood Pressure
B) Heart Rate
C) Respiratory Rate
D) Oxygen Saturation

Question 108: Mr. Lee, a 55-year-old male post-operative patient following abdominal surgery, has vital signs as follows: BP 140/90 mmHg, HR 58 bpm, RR 16 breaths/min, Temp 100.4°F. He complains of feeling cold and shivering. What should be the nurse's initial action?
A) Apply warm blankets and monitor temperature.
B) Administer antipyretic medication for fever control.
C) Assess for signs of infection at the surgical site.
D) Notify the surgeon immediately about bradycardia.

Question 109: When considering medication administration in a patient with renal impairment, which pharmacokinetic parameter is most crucial to monitor?
A) Absorption
B) Distribution
C) Metabolism
D) Excretion

Question 110: Which of the following medication combinations is most likely to result in serotonin syndrome?
A) Fluoxetine and Tramadol
B) Metoprolol and Simvastatin
C) Lisinopril and Hydrochlorothiazide
D) Atorvastatin and Amlodipine

Question 111: In a situation where a patient refuses a life-saving treatment due to personal beliefs, what is the nurse's primary ethical responsibility?
A) Persuade the patient to accept treatment.
B) Respect the patient's autonomy and document their decision.
C) Seek a court order to override the patient's decision.
D) Inform the patient's family and encourage them to intervene.

Question 112: Maria, a 30-year-old patient, presents with recurrent urinary tract infections (UTIs). During a private conversation, she confides that her partner forces sexual intercourse even when she refuses due to pain from UTIs. What should be the nurse's initial response?
A) Advise Maria on safe sexual practices.
B) Provide information about local shelters and support services.
C) Conduct a thorough physical examination for additional injuries.
D) Encourage Maria to talk to her partner about consent.

Question 113: Which of the following components is most critical when collecting a patient's health history to ensure accurate diagnosis and treatment planning?
A) Family medical history
B) Current medications
C) Chief complaint
D) Social history

Question 114: Nurse Jamie is planning an educational session for a group of post-operative patients about wound care management. Which educational strategy is most effective in ensuring that patients understand and retain the information provided?
A) Providing written instructions only
B) Demonstrating the wound care procedure
C) Using a combination of verbal instructions, demonstrations, and written materials
D) Conducting a one-time lecture on wound care

Question 115: In the context of planning and implementing patient education, which barrier is most likely to affect adherence to post-operative care instructions?
A) Patient's cognitive impairment
B) Cultural beliefs about health
C) Complexity of medical terminology
D) Patient's socioeconomic status

Question 116: In enhancing patient education for chronic disease management, which skill should nurses develop to improve patient adherence to treatment plans?
A) Simplifying medical terminology
B) Using visual aids during explanations
C) Establishing mutual goals with the patient
D) Providing written instructions only

Question 117: Sarah, a 68-year-old patient with congestive heart failure (CHF), is admitted to the hospital with worsening dyspnea and edema. As part of the nursing care plan, which of the following interventions should be prioritized to address her fluid overload?
A) Administering prescribed diuretics and monitoring electrolyte levels
B) Encouraging increased fluid intake to promote renal perfusion
C) Providing high-sodium diet to maintain electrolyte balance
D) Restricting physical activity to reduce cardiac workload

Question 118: Michael, a 70-year-old patient with coronary artery disease, is on clopidogrel therapy. He has been recently prescribed omeprazole for gastroesophageal reflux disease (GERD). What potential drug-drug interaction should concern the nurse?
A) Increased risk of thrombosis
B) Decreased efficacy of clopidogrel

C) Increased gastrointestinal bleeding
D) Elevated blood pressure

Question 119: During discharge planning for a patient named Mrs. Smith who had a myocardial infarction (MI), which educational strategy would best ensure she understands her new medication regimen?
A) Provide detailed pamphlets about each medication.
B) Schedule a follow-up appointment with her primary care provider.
C) Review each medication with her verbally and use the teach-back method.
D) Encourage her to attend a cardiac rehabilitation program.

Question 120: When evaluating supporting materials for evidence-based practice, which criterion is most critical to assess their validity?
A) Publication date
B) Author credentials
C) Sample size of study
D) Methodology used

Question 121: John, a 60-year-old diabetic patient, is started on metformin therapy. Which laboratory test should be prioritized before initiating this medication?
A) Liver function tests
B) Serum creatinine level
C) Complete blood count (CBC)
D) Electrolyte panel

Question 122: At what developmental stage, according to Piaget, do children begin to develop logical thinking but still struggle with abstract concepts?
A) Sensorimotor Stage
B) Preoperational Stage
C) Concrete Operational Stage
D) Formal Operational Stage

Question 123: Michael, a 70-year-old male with heart failure, presents with shortness of breath and swelling in his legs. His lab results show a serum osmolality of 260 mOsm/kg and low urine sodium levels. What is the most likely diagnosis?
A) Syndrome of Inappropriate Antidiuretic Hormone Secretion (SIADH)
B) Dehydration
C) Hypervolemic hyponatremia
D) Diabetes Insipidus

Question 124: While performing a gastrointestinal review of systems, which symptom would most likely suggest an upper gastrointestinal bleed?
A) Hematochezia
B) Melena
C) Steatorrhea
D) Jaundice

Question 125: Emily, a 35-year-old female with a history of Crohn's disease, presents with severe abdominal pain and dehydration. Her lab results indicate hypomagnesemia. Which symptom is most likely associated with her condition?
A) Hyperreflexia
B) Hypotension
C) Bradycardia
D) Hypercalcemia

ANSWER WITH DETAILED EXPLANATION SET [2]

Question 1: Correct Answer: A) "Have you noticed any swelling in your legs or ankles?"
Rationale: Edema in the legs or ankles can be indicative of heart failure, making Option A the most pertinent question for assessing potential cardiac issues. While B), C), and D) provide useful information for overall health assessment, they do not directly address symptoms that could be related to cardiac function as effectively as A).
Question 2: Correct Answer: D) Use a combination of verbal explanation, written materials, and teach-back method.
Rationale: The combination of verbal explanation, written materials, and the teach-back method ensures comprehensive understanding and retention. Verbal explanations clarify doubts immediately, written materials serve as references, and the teach-back method confirms understanding by having Mr. Johnson repeat information in his own words. Option A relies solely on reading, which may not address all learning styles or confirm comprehension. Option B lacks supplementary material for reference. Option C combines visual aids with written instructions but does not confirm understanding through active engagement like the teach-back method.
Question 3: Correct Answer: B) ASCVD Risk Calculator
Rationale: The ASCVD Risk Calculator is specifically designed to estimate the 10-year risk for atherosclerotic cardiovascular disease, considering factors such as age, smoking status, blood pressure, and cholesterol levels. While the Framingham Risk Score (A) and QRISK3 (C) are also used for cardiovascular risk assessment, they are less specific to the U.S. population compared to the ASCVD calculator. The Reynolds Risk Score (D) includes additional biomarkers like hs-CRP but is not as widely recommended for general use as the ASCVD calculator.
Question 4: Correct Answer: A) Fluoxetine and Tramadol
Rationale: Serotonin syndrome can occur when medications that increase serotonin levels are combined. Fluoxetine (an SSRI) and Tramadol (a weak SNRI) both increase serotonin, posing a high risk for serotonin syndrome. Metoprolol and Furosemide do not affect serotonin levels. Warfarin and Ciprofloxacin interact by increasing bleeding risk, not serotonin syndrome. Digoxin and Verapamil interaction can cause bradycardia, but not serotonin syndrome.
Question 5: Correct Answer: B) Colonoscopy
Rationale: Colonoscopy is considered the gold standard for colorectal cancer screening due to its ability to visualize the entire colon and remove polyps during the procedure. The Fecal Immunochemical Test (FIT) (A) is less invasive but not as comprehensive. The Cologuard Test (C), while effective in detecting DNA mutations associated with cancer, is not as definitive as colonoscopy. Digital Rectal Exam (DRE) (D), though useful for prostate evaluation, is inadequate for comprehensive colorectal cancer screening.
Question 6: Correct Answer: A) Influenza vaccine
Rationale: The influenza vaccine is recommended annually for all adults, particularly those with chronic health conditions like diabetes or heart disease, due to their increased risk of complications from the flu. The Hepatitis B vaccine (B) is typically given in a series and not annually. The Pneumococcal vaccine (C) is generally administered once or twice in a lifetime, depending on age and health status. The Tdap vaccine (D) is recommended every ten years. Annual vaccination against influenza is crucial because the virus strains change frequently, necessitating yearly updates to the vaccine.
Question 7: Correct Answer: D) Formal Operational Stage
Rationale: Piaget's Formal Operational Stage (beginning around age 12) involves abstract thinking and hypothetical reasoning. The Sensorimotor Stage (birth-2 years) focuses on sensory experiences and motor actions, the Preoperational Stage (2-7 years) involves symbolic thinking but lacks logical operations, and the Concrete Operational Stage (7-11 years) includes logical thinking about concrete events but not abstract concepts. The correct answer emphasizes advanced cognitive abilities unique to adolescents and adults.
Question 8: Correct Answer: B) Explore Maria's coping mechanisms and support systems.
Rationale: Prioritizing the exploration of coping mechanisms and support systems (B) is essential in understanding Maria's psychosocial needs and providing holistic care. Providing educational materials (A), encouraging self-management classes (C), and discussing lifestyle changes (D), while beneficial, do not address her immediate emotional distress. Understanding her current coping strategies allows for tailored interventions that can reduce anxiety and improve overall management.
Question 9: Correct Answer: C) Position the patient in high Fowler's position
Rationale: Positioning the patient in high Fowler's position helps to maximize lung expansion and improve oxygenation, which is critical for a COPD patient experiencing increased shortness of breath. Administering a bronchodilator (Option A) is also important but should follow proper positioning. Increasing oxygen flow rate (Option B) can be helpful but must be done cautiously to avoid CO_2 retention in COPD patients. Chest physiotherapy (Option D) may assist with secretion clearance but is not the immediate priority.
Question 10: Correct Answer: D) Phase V
Rationale: Diastolic pressure is identified at Korotkoff sound Phase V, where sounds disappear completely. This phase indicates the point at which blood flow through the artery returns to normal, uninterrupted flow. Phase I (A) marks the systolic pressure with the first appearance of faint tapping sounds. Phases II (B) and III (C) represent intermediate sounds that occur between systolic and diastolic pressures but do not indicate diastolic pressure themselves. Understanding these phases is crucial for accurate blood pressure measurement.
Question 11: Correct Answer: B) Assess David's access to means of suicide.
Rationale: Assessing David's access to means of suicide (B) is critical in evaluating his immediate risk level. This step helps determine if he has the capability to act on suicidal thoughts. Educating about coping mechanisms (A), referring to CBT (C), and scheduling an appointment with his primary care physician (D), while important for long-term management, do not address the immediate risk assessment needed in this scenario.
Question 12: Correct Answer: A) Dietary habits
Rationale: Dietary habits (A) should be prioritized when collecting health history for unexplained weight loss because they provide direct insight into potential causes such as malnutrition or eating disorders. Although recent travel history (B), psychological state (C), and occupational exposure (D) can contribute valuable information, they are less likely to be primary factors in unexplained weight loss compared to dietary habits. Understanding what and how much the patient eats can help identify nutritional deficiencies or other dietary issues contributing to weight loss.
Question 13: Correct Answer: C) Assess for signs of hypovolemic shock.
Rationale: The significant drop in hematocrit along with abdominal distension and decreased urine output indicates potential intra-abdominal bleeding leading to hypovolemic shock, requiring immediate assessment and intervention. Inserting a nasogastric tube (Option A), increasing oral fluid intake (Option B), or encouraging ambulation (Option D) are not immediate priorities and could delay critical care needed for hypovolemic shock management.

Question 14: Correct Answer: A) Referral to an occupational therapist for adaptive equipment training.
Rationale: An occupational therapist can assess Mrs. Johnson's specific needs and train her in using adaptive equipment, which promotes independence in ADLs like bathing and dressing. Home health aide services (B) offer support but do not foster independence initially. Written instructions (C) may be ineffective due to her cognitive impairment.
Question 15: Correct Answer: D) Simulation assessments
Rationale: Simulation assessments (D) are recommended as they provide a realistic and controlled environment to evaluate clinical skills effectively. Pre- and post-tests (A), while useful, may not fully capture practical competencies. Peer reviews (B) can be subjective, and patient feedback surveys (C), though valuable, do not directly measure clinical skills. Research highlights simulation as a robust method for assessing practical abilities and identifying areas needing improvement in clinical practice.
Question 16: Correct Answer: C) Social support network
Rationale: While social support networks play a critical role in overall well-being and recovery, they do not directly impact the physical or cognitive ability to perform ADLs. Visual acuity, cognitive impairment, and range of motion are direct factors influencing one's capability to complete ADLs independently. Understanding these distinctions helps prioritize assessment areas.
Question 17: Correct Answer: B) Serum lipase
Rationale: Serum lipase is the most specific test for diagnosing acute pancreatitis due to its higher specificity compared to serum amylase. While serum amylase can be elevated in various conditions such as mumps and renal failure, serum lipase levels are more specifically elevated in pancreatic inflammation. Serum bilirubin and alkaline phosphatase are related to liver function and biliary tract disorders, not specifically pancreatitis.
Question 18: Correct Answer: A) Generativity vs. Stagnation
Rationale: In Erikson's theory, individuals aged 40-65 are in the "Generativity vs. Stagnation" stage, where they focus on contributing to society and guiding the next generation through career and mentorship roles. John's anxiety about career progression and mentoring aligns with this stage's emphasis on productivity and societal contribution. "Intimacy vs. Isolation" applies to young adulthood (20-40 years), focusing on forming close relationships. "Integrity vs. Despair" pertains to late adulthood (65+ years), involving reflection on life's achievements or regrets. "Identity vs. Role Confusion" is relevant during adolescence (12-18 years), centering on personal identity formation.
Question 19: Correct Answer: D) Orientation
Rationale: The MMSE primarily assesses orientation, including awareness of time and place, which is crucial for diagnosing cognitive impairments like dementia. While it also evaluates other cognitive domains such as short-term memory (B), visuospatial skills (C), and executive function (A), these are secondary components. Orientation questions in the MMSE help determine if the patient is aware of their surroundings, an essential aspect in early detection of cognitive decline. Incorrect options are closely related but do not represent the primary focus of the MMSE.
Question 20: Correct Answer: C) Music Therapy
Rationale: Music therapy has been demonstrated to effectively reduce both anxiety and pain in postoperative patients by providing a distraction, promoting relaxation, and decreasing stress hormones. Guided imagery (A) also reduces anxiety but may not be as effective for pain management. Biofeedback (B), while useful for chronic conditions involving muscle tension, is less immediate in its effects on acute postoperative states. Massage therapy (D), although beneficial for pain relief, primarily addresses physical discomfort rather than psychological symptoms like anxiety.
Question 21: Correct Answer: B) Facilitating a case conference with all consultants to discuss Ms. Patel's care plan.
Rationale: Facilitating a case conference demonstrates effective interdisciplinary healthcare team collaboration by ensuring all consultants can discuss and align their recommendations for a cohesive care plan. Option A might be considerate but does not promote collaboration among consultants. Option C ignores the collaborative aspect necessary for comprehensive care planning. Option D, while important for documentation, does not actively engage in collaboration or coordination among team members.
Question 22: Correct Answer: B) Obtain wound cultures before starting antibiotics.
Rationale: Obtaining wound cultures before starting antibiotics is crucial for identifying the causative organism and selecting the appropriate antibiotic therapy. Starting broad-spectrum antibiotics (Option A) without culture results may lead to resistance and inappropriate treatment. Increasing dressing changes (Option C) is supportive but not diagnostic or therapeutic in this scenario. Administering antipyretics (Option D) addresses symptoms but not the underlying infection. Cultures ensure targeted therapy, preventing complications.
Question 23: Correct Answer: C) Managing medications
Rationale: Managing medications is classified as an Instrumental Activity of Daily Living (IADL), which requires more complex cognitive and physical skills compared to basic ADLs like bathing, dressing, and eating. IADLs are crucial for independent living but are not considered basic self-care tasks. This distinction helps clinicians develop comprehensive care plans.
Question 24: Correct Answer: A) Provide information on palliative care options.
Rationale: Providing information on palliative care aligns with ethical principles of beneficence, offering comfort without compromising legal or professional standards. Assisting in hastening death (Option B) violates legal and ethical norms in many jurisdictions. Referring (Option C) could imply endorsement of illegal actions. Avoiding discussion (Option D) neglects duty of care, leaving patients unsupported in distressing times. Palliative care respects dignity and provides holistic support within ethical boundaries.
Question 25: Correct Answer: A) Agnosia
Rationale: Agnosia refers to the inability to recognize familiar objects or faces despite having intact sensory function, often due to damage in the occipital or temporal lobes. Mr. Thompson's intact vision rules out hemianopia (D), which involves loss of vision in half the visual field. Apraxia (B) affects motor planning for movements despite normal muscle function and coordination; dysarthria (C) involves impaired articulation due to muscle weakness affecting speech production but does not impact object recognition.
Question 26: Correct Answer: A) Encourage early ambulation
Rationale: Early ambulation is a key preventive measure for DVT in post-operative patients, promoting blood circulation and reducing clot formation. Administering prophylactic antibiotics (Option B) prevents infection but does not address DVT. Ensuring adequate hydration (Option C) aids in overall recovery but is less directly impactful on DVT prevention than ambulation. Monitoring blood glucose levels (Option D) is crucial for diabetic patients but not specifically related to DVT prevention.
Question 27: Correct Answer: B) Ensuring all metallic objects are removed from the patient's body
Rationale: Removing all metallic objects from the patient's body is critical to prevent serious complications such as burns or injury due to magnetic field interactions during an MRI scan. While assessing claustrophobia (Option A), checking allergies to contrast agents (Option C), and educating about stillness (Option D) are important, they do

not address immediate safety concerns posed by metal objects in an MRI environment. Proper removal of metal items ensures patient safety and prevents adverse events related to strong magnetic fields.

Question 28: Correct Answer: C) Pulse oximeter

Rationale: A pulse oximeter is specifically designed for continuous monitoring of oxygen saturation (SpO2) and pulse rate, making it the most appropriate choice for Mr. Thompson post-surgery. While a sphygmomanometer measures blood pressure, an ECG monitor tracks heart rhythms, and a capnograph measures carbon dioxide levels in exhaled air, none of these provide direct continuous monitoring of oxygen saturation like a pulse oximeter does.

Question 29: Correct Answer: D) Reassess Mr. Lee's cognitive status and environment.

Rationale: Reassessing Mr. Lee's cognitive status and environment (Option D) helps identify factors contributing to his agitation or confusion, potentially resolving issues without increasing restraint use. Applying mittens (Option A), tightening wrist restraints (Option B), or requesting chemical restraints (Option C) are reactive measures that do not address underlying causes or ensure long-term safety and comfort based on contemporary best practices in nursing care focused on least restrictive measures first.

Question 30: Correct Answer: B) Refer John to a psychiatrist for evaluation of potential depression.

Rationale: While all options are important in managing chronic illness, referring John to a psychiatrist is critical due to his expressed feelings of hopelessness and anhedonia, which are key indicators of depression. Encouraging support group participation (A) and educating about medication adherence (C) are supportive measures but secondary. Regular follow-ups (D) focus on physical rather than mental health. Early psychiatric intervention can provide necessary treatment and prevent worsening of depressive symptoms.

Question 31: Correct Answer: A) Conducting a thorough patient assessment

Rationale: Conducting a thorough patient assessment is crucial as it provides a comprehensive understanding of the patient's current health status, needs, and priorities. This step ensures that subsequent planning, goal-setting, and interventions are based on accurate and detailed information. While reviewing medical history (B), establishing goals (C), and consulting with team members (D) are important, they rely on the data gathered during the initial assessment to be effective. Without a detailed assessment, other steps may be misguided or incomplete.

Question 32: Correct Answer: A) Barthel Index

Rationale: The Barthel Index is specifically designed to measure a patient's ability to perform ADLs independently, such as feeding, bathing, dressing, and toileting. The MMSE assesses cognitive function, the Braden Scale evaluates pressure ulcer risk, and the Glasgow Coma Scale measures consciousness levels. The Barthel Index focuses directly on ADLs, making it the most appropriate tool in this context.

Question 33: Correct Answer: B) Hyperreflexia

Rationale: Hyperreflexia is indicative of an upper motor neuron lesion due to loss of inhibitory control from higher brain centers. Flaccid paralysis (A), muscle atrophy (C), and fasciculations (D) are more characteristic of lower motor neuron lesions. Upper motor neuron lesions typically present with spasticity and exaggerated reflexes due to disrupted descending pathways that normally inhibit spinal reflexes.

Question 34: Correct Answer: C) Avoid excessive alcohol consumption as it increases the risk of lactic acidosis.

Rationale: Excessive alcohol consumption can increase the risk of lactic acidosis, a serious side effect of metformin. Dairy products (Option A), carbohydrate-rich meals (Option B), and protein intake (Option D) do not have significant impacts on metformin's primary concern, which is lactic acidosis.

Question 35: Correct Answer: C) Intravenous albumin infusion

Rationale: Intravenous albumin infusion helps restore colloid osmotic pressure in patients with hypoalbuminemia due to liver cirrhosis, thereby reducing ascites and edema more effectively than other treatments. Sodium restriction diet (A) can help manage fluid retention but does not address the underlying hypoalbuminemia. Spironolactone (B), an aldosterone antagonist, helps reduce fluid retention but may not be sufficient alone without addressing low albumin levels. Fluid restriction (D), while helpful in preventing further fluid overload, does not correct the underlying cause related to low serum albumin levels.

Question 36: Correct Answer: B) Postoperative hemorrhage

Rationale: The combination of dizziness, low blood pressure, and tachycardia strongly suggests postoperative hemorrhage. Dehydration (Option A) could cause similar symptoms but less acutely severe changes in vital signs. Pain medication side effects (Option C) are less likely to present with such hemodynamic instability. Orthostatic hypotension (Option D) would typically present with symptoms upon standing rather than at rest.

Question 37: Correct Answer: C) Enhancing adherence through shared responsibility

Rationale: Involving family members enhances adherence by distributing responsibility and providing additional support, making it easier for patients to follow care plans. Option A ensures understanding but doesn't directly affect adherence. Option B increases emotional support but doesn't necessarily improve adherence. Option D may undermine patient autonomy if not handled appropriately.

Question 38: Correct Answer: B) Elevated serum lipase

Rationale: Elevated serum lipase is the most specific and sensitive marker for acute pancreatitis, often rising within hours of onset and remaining elevated longer than amylase. While elevated serum amylase (Option A) is also indicative, it can be elevated in other conditions such as mumps or renal failure. Elevated serum bilirubin (Option C) and alkaline phosphatase (Option D) are more indicative of biliary obstruction or liver pathology rather than acute pancreatitis.

Question 39: Correct Answer: B) Initiate cardiac monitoring.

Rationale: Hyperkalemia (potassium >5.0 mEq/L) can lead to life-threatening cardiac arrhythmias; thus, initiating cardiac monitoring is crucial to detect early changes in heart rhythm. Administering oral potassium supplements (A) or encouraging high-potassium foods (C) would exacerbate hyperkalemia. Diuretics (D), particularly those that are potassium-sparing, may not be immediately effective in reducing potassium levels and are secondary measures after ensuring patient safety via monitoring.

Question 40: Correct Answer: B) Colonoscopy

Rationale: Colonoscopy is the most appropriate initial screening test for Emily due to her family history of colon cancer. It allows direct visualization and biopsy/removal of polyps. FIT (A), while non-invasive, is less comprehensive than colonoscopy. Flexible sigmoidoscopy (C), though useful, examines only part of the colon. CT colonography (D), while effective, requires follow-up colonoscopy if abnormalities are found. Colonoscopy's comprehensive nature makes it superior in this scenario.

Question 41: Correct Answer: B) Collaborate with Mr. Chen to integrate TCM practices that do not interfere with his prescribed medications.

Rationale: Integrating culturally competent care involves respecting and incorporating patients' cultural preferences into their treatment plans when safe and appropriate. Option B allows Nurse Emily to respect Mr. Chen's cultural beliefs while ensuring his safety by monitoring for potential interactions between TCM and prescribed medications. Option A disregards Mr. Chen's cultural preferences, potentially reducing adherence to the treatment plan. Option C ignores the importance of cultural competence altogether, and Option D could lead to unsafe practices without proper coordination of care.

Question 42: Correct Answer: A) Cognitive function

Rationale: Cognitive function is crucial in determining a patient's ability to perform ADLs because it encompasses memory, attention, and problem-solving skills necessary for executing daily tasks safely and efficiently. Muscle strength, joint flexibility, and coordination are also important but secondary factors. Without adequate cognitive function, even patients with good physical health may struggle with planning and executing ADLs. Thus, assessing cognitive function is paramount in evaluating overall independence.

Question 43: Correct Answer: A) Review her current medication list for possible drug interactions.

Rationale: Reviewing the medication list is crucial in identifying potential drug interactions that could cause dizziness and fatigue. Increasing fluid intake (B) might help if dehydration were the issue but does not address polypharmacy. Scheduling an appointment with a cardiologist (C) could be necessary but isn't the first step in addressing polypharmacy. Recommending supplements (D) without reviewing medications could exacerbate interactions.

Question 44: Correct Answer: A) Performing pulmonary function tests (PFTs)

Rationale: Performing pulmonary function tests (PFTs) helps assess respiratory status and guide anesthesia management in COPD patients. Withholding bronchodilators (B) can exacerbate respiratory issues. Prophylactic antibiotics (C) are not routinely indicated unless there's an infection risk. NPO status after midnight (D) is standard but does not address specific respiratory concerns in COPD patients like PFTs do.

Question 45: Correct Answer: C) Open visitation policies

Rationale: Open visitation policies are the most effective strategy for involving family members as they allow continuous access to the patient, fostering real-time involvement in care decisions. Regularly scheduled family meetings (A) provide structured engagement but lack immediacy. Educational materials (B) enhance understanding but do not ensure active involvement. Family advisory councils (D) offer strategic input but are less impactful on day-to-day care. Open visitation policies promote immediate support, real-time communication, and collaborative decision-making.

Question 46: Correct Answer: B) Implementing a multimodal approach

Rationale: A multimodal approach caters to various learning preferences by incorporating visual, auditory, kinesthetic, and reading/writing methods. Standardized written materials (A) may not address all preferences. Group discussions (C), while beneficial, predominantly support auditory learners. Solely focusing on visual aids (D) neglects other preferences. By combining different strategies, educators can ensure comprehensive understanding and retention across diverse learners.

Question 47: Correct Answer: D) Breathing exercises

Rationale: Breathing exercises should be prioritized as they directly improve respiratory function and quality of life in COPD patients. Understanding pathophysiology (Option A), while important, does not immediately impact daily management. Medication adherence strategies (Option B), though crucial, may not be as immediately beneficial as techniques that improve breathing efficiency. Nutritional management (Option C), although supportive, does not address the primary symptom of breathlessness as effectively as breathing exercises do. Thus, focusing on breathing exercises maximizes immediate patient outcomes in COPD management.

Question 48: Correct Answer: C) Assessing renal function through serum creatinine and GFR

Rationale: Assessing renal function through serum creatinine and GFR is crucial before administering contrast in patients with CKD to prevent contrast-induced nephropathy. Serum potassium levels (A) are important but not specific to contrast administration. Liver function tests (B) are less relevant unless hepatotoxicity is suspected. Blood glucose levels (D) are necessary in diabetic patients but not directly related to contrast use.

Question 49: Correct Answer: A) Peaked T waves

Rationale: Hyperkalemia is characterized by elevated potassium levels in the blood, which affects cardiac conduction and can lead to peaked T waves on an ECG. Prolonged QT interval (B) is more commonly associated with hypocalcemia or hypokalemia. ST segment depression (C) is typically seen in myocardial ischemia. U waves (D) are indicative of hypokalemia, not hyperkalemia. Recognizing these specific ECG changes helps in the prompt diagnosis and treatment of electrolyte imbalances.

Question 50: Correct Answer: A) Quitting smoking immediately

Rationale: Quitting smoking immediately is the most effective intervention for improving lung function and overall health in patients with COPD. Smoking cessation halts further damage to lung tissue and can significantly slow disease progression. While using an air purifier (B), practicing breathing exercises (C), and increasing omega-3 fatty acid intake (D) can provide additional benefits, they do not address the primary cause of lung damage—smoking. Smoking cessation leads to substantial improvements in respiratory symptoms, reduces exacerbations, and enhances quality of life more effectively than any other single intervention.

Question 51: Correct Answer: B) A video demonstrating glucose monitoring and insulin administration

Rationale: Videos are effective because they engage multiple senses, making it easier for patients to understand and remember procedures. Unlike pamphlets or articles that can be overwhelming due to complex terminology, videos provide visual and auditory learning cues. PowerPoint presentations are useful but may not be as engaging as videos. Therefore, a video demonstrating practical skills like glucose monitoring and insulin administration is most effective.

Question 52: Correct Answer: A) Recent loss or trauma

Rationale: Recent loss or trauma is a critical psychosocial factor that can precipitate suicidal ideation and behavior. It often leads to intense emotional distress and feelings of hopelessness. Employment status, marital status, and educational level are important contextual factors but do not have the immediate impact on emotional state that recent traumatic events do. Employment status might affect long-term stability; marital status could influence support systems; educational level may affect access to resources. However, recent trauma directly correlates with acute emotional responses that heighten immediate suicide risk.

Question 53: Correct Answer: C) Barrel chest

Rationale: The increased anteroposterior chest diameter observed in Mr. Johnson is indicative of a barrel chest, commonly seen in patients with COPD due to chronic overinflation of the lungs. Pulmonary fibrosis (Option A) leads to stiffening and scarring of lung tissue but does not typically cause barrel chest. Kyphosis (Option B) involves spinal curvature affecting posture but not necessarily the anteroposterior diameter. Pectus excavatum (Option D) is a congenital deformity resulting in a sunken chest appearance, unlike the outward expansion seen in barrel chest.

Question 54: Correct Answer: A) Beck Depression Inventory (BDI)

Rationale: The Beck Depression Inventory (BDI) is specifically designed to assess the severity of depression symptoms. The GAD-7 and HAM-A are focused on anxiety, not depression, while the MMSE evaluates cognitive function rather than mood disorders. The BDI's focus on depressive symptoms makes it the most suitable tool for this assessment.

Question 55: Correct Answer: C) Providing oral polyethylene glycol (PEG) solution for bowel cleansing

Rationale: The administration of oral polyethylene glycol (PEG) solution is crucial for effective bowel cleansing, which is essential for clear visualization during a colonoscopy. While a clear liquid diet (Option A) and NPO status (Option B) are important, they do not ensure complete bowel preparation. Sedatives (Option D), although helpful for patient comfort, do not contribute to bowel cleanliness. PEG solution effectively clears the bowel, reducing the risk of missed lesions or inaccurate diagnoses.

Question 56: Correct Answer: B) Utilizing teach-back methods to confirm understanding

Rationale: Teach-back methods ensure that the patient comprehends the instructions by having them repeat the information in their own words. This technique is superior because it actively engages the patient and verifies understanding, reducing errors. Option A, while helpful, does not confirm comprehension. Option C provides reminders but does not ensure initial understanding. Option D helps with organization but doesn't address understanding of the regimen.

Question 57: Correct Answer: C) Pheochromocytoma

Rationale: Pheochromocytoma should be considered due to its classic triad of headaches, palpitations, and sweating episodes resulting from catecholamine-secreting tumors. These symptoms align closely with Mr. Lee's presentation. While migraines (A) can cause headaches and visual disturbances, they do not typically include palpitations or sweating episodes. Hypertension (B), although common in pheochromocytoma patients, does not explain all symptoms comprehensively without considering an underlying cause like pheochromocytoma itself. Hyperthyroidism (D) might present with palpitations and sweating but is less likely to cause severe headaches or visual disturbances without other systemic signs.

Question 58: Correct Answer: C) "It sounds like you're feeling really overwhelmed right now."

Rationale: Reflecting Ms. Smith's feelings by acknowledging her sense of being overwhelmed (Option C) validates her emotions and demonstrates empathy, which are key components of therapeutic communication. Sharing personal anecdotes (Option A), suggesting she focus on positives (Option B), or telling her to be grateful (Option D) can come across as dismissive or minimizing her experience, rather than providing support.

Question 59: Correct Answer: A) Hyperkalemia

Rationale: Hyperkalemia is a common electrolyte imbalance in CKD due to decreased renal excretion of potassium. Hypokalemia (Option B) is less common as the kidneys lose their ability to excrete potassium. Hypercalcemia (Option C) can occur but is less frequent compared to hypocalcemia (Option D), which results from decreased activation of vitamin D and impaired calcium absorption. Thus, hyperkalemia is the most prevalent and clinically significant electrolyte imbalance in CKD.

Question 60: Correct Answer: B) Drug-drug interactions

Rationale: The primary consideration is drug-drug interactions because they are a common cause of adverse effects in patients with polypharmacy. While patient's age (Option A), dosage frequency (Option C), and cost (Option D) are important, they do not directly address the immediate risk posed by potential interactions between multiple drugs. Identifying and managing these interactions can prevent significant harm.

Question 61: Correct Answer: D) Adjusting insulin dosage based on preoperative blood glucose levels

Rationale: Adjusting insulin dosage based on preoperative blood glucose levels is essential to maintain glycemic control and prevent perioperative complications such as hyperglycemia or hypoglycemia. Monitoring blood glucose hourly (Option A) is important but secondary to initial dose adjustment. Maintaining blood glucose below 100 mg/dL (Option B) can risk hypoglycemia. Early morning surgery slots (Option C), while beneficial, do not directly manage glycemic control. Proper insulin adjustment ensures stable blood glucose levels throughout the perioperative period.

Question 62: Correct Answer: A) Administering a clear liquid diet for 24 hours before the procedure

Rationale: Administering a clear liquid diet for 24 hours before a colonoscopy is essential to ensure that the bowel is adequately cleansed, allowing for accurate visualization. Stopping antihypertensive medications can lead to uncontrolled blood pressure (B), which is unsafe. Taking regular insulin without adjusting for fasting can cause hypoglycemia (C). While enemas (D) might be used, they are not as effective alone as a clear liquid diet combined with bowel prep.

Question 63: Correct Answer: B) Using open-ended questions

Rationale: Open-ended questions facilitate a deeper conversation and allow patients to express their feelings and concerns, which is essential for understanding their emotional state. Providing reassurance (A) may minimize their feelings, giving advice (C) can be perceived as directive rather than supportive, and offering personal anecdotes (D) shifts the focus away from the patient. Thus, using open-ended questions is the most effective technique.

Question 64: Correct Answer: C) Autonomy

Rationale: Autonomy refers to respecting the patient's right to make their own decisions, including the right to privacy and confidentiality. Beneficence (A) involves actions that benefit the patient, while Nonmaleficence (B) means avoiding harm. Justice (D) pertains to fairness and equality in care. Although these principles are integral to nursing ethics, Autonomy specifically addresses confidentiality by emphasizing respect for the patient's personal rights and informed consent.

Question 65: Correct Answer: B) Providing detailed explanations of the treatment options using layman's terms.

Rationale: Providing detailed explanations of treatment options in layman's terms ensures that patients can make informed decisions about their care, which is a fundamental aspect of advocacy. Recommending a second opinion (A) or encouraging independent research (C) are supportive but do not directly address immediate understanding. Directing to online forums (D) might help with peer support but does not substitute for professional guidance. Ensuring comprehension through clear communication aligns with ethical principles and supports patient autonomy.

Question 66: Correct Answer: B) Hypothyroidism

Rationale: Hypothyroidism is characterized by symptoms such as fatigue, weight gain, cold intolerance, dry skin, and periorbital edema due to decreased thyroid hormone production. Hyperthyroidism (A) presents with weight loss and heat intolerance. Cushing's Syndrome (C) involves weight gain but with features like moon face and central obesity. Addison's Disease (D) includes symptoms like hyperpigmentation and hypotension. The combination of Sarah's symptoms aligns best with hypothyroidism.

Question 67: Correct Answer: A) Providing assistive devices such as grab bars and a raised toilet seat

Rationale: Providing assistive devices like grab bars and a raised toilet seat can significantly enhance Mr. Johnson's ability to perform ADLs independently by reducing strain on his joints. While pain medication (Option B) can help manage symptoms, it does not directly address functional independence. Complete bed rest (Option C) may lead to muscle atrophy and decreased mobility. Physical therapy (Option D) is beneficial but may not provide immediate assistance for daily tasks. Thus, Option A is the most effective intervention.

Question 68: Correct Answer: C) Implementing patient-controlled analgesia (PCA)

Rationale: Patient-controlled analgesia (PCA) allows patients to manage their pain more effectively by self-administering predetermined doses of pain medication, often leading to better pain control and satisfaction. Increasing the dose of the current analgesic (A) may not be effective if tolerance has developed. Switching to a different class of analgesic (B) could help but lacks the immediate control PCA offers. Non-pharmacological methods (D), while supportive, are insufficient alone for severe postoperative pain.

Question 69: Correct Answer: A) Metabolic alkalosis

Rationale: Severe vomiting leads to a loss of gastric acid (HCl), resulting in a decrease in hydrogen ion concentration and subsequent metabolic alkalosis. Metabolic acidosis (B) would occur with conditions that increase acid or decrease bicarbonate, such as renal failure. Respiratory alkalosis (C) results from hyperventilation, causing CO2 loss. Respiratory acidosis (D) occurs with hypoventilation, leading to CO2 retention. Understanding these mechanisms helps nurses identify and manage acid-base imbalances effectively.

Question 70: Correct Answer: B) Implementing structured communication tools like SBAR (Situation-Background-Assessment-Recommendation)

Rationale: Implementing structured communication tools like SBAR ensures that each team member can contribute effectively and equally by providing a clear framework for sharing information. Assigning roles based on seniority (A) may limit contributions from less experienced members, while conducting consultations via email (C) lacks immediacy and dynamic interaction. Rotating leadership roles (D), although beneficial, does not inherently ensure balanced contributions. SBAR promotes organized and concise communication, facilitating comprehensive input from all disciplines involved.

Question 71: Correct Answer: A) Reduction in patient-reported pain scores

Rationale: Reduction in patient-reported pain scores directly measures the primary goal of pain management. While B (Decrease in opioid usage), C (Improvement in patient mobility), and D (Increase in patient satisfaction) are important, they are indirect indicators. Pain scores provide a direct, quantifiable measure of pain relief effectiveness, aligning closely with contemporary research emphasizing patient-centered outcomes.

Question 72: Correct Answer: B) Recommending he engage in at least 150 minutes of moderate-intensity aerobic activity per week.

Rationale: Engaging in regular physical activity is crucial for managing both hypertension and obesity. The American Heart Association recommends at least 150 minutes of moderate-intensity aerobic activity weekly to improve cardiovascular health and aid in weight management. While reducing sodium intake (Option A), consuming a healthy diet (Option C), and monitoring blood pressure (Option D) are beneficial, they are supplementary strategies. Physical activity has the most significant impact on overall health improvement for John's specific conditions.

Question 73: Correct Answer: A) Administration of calcium gluconate

Rationale: Calcium gluconate is the most appropriate initial treatment for hyperkalemia because it stabilizes the cardiac membrane, reducing the risk of life-threatening arrhythmias. While insulin and glucose (C) help shift potassium into cells, they do not act as quickly as calcium gluconate in stabilizing cardiac activity. Sodium bicarbonate (B) can also shift potassium into cells but is less effective for immediate cardiac protection. Loop diuretics (D) promote renal excretion of potassium but are not suitable for immediate intervention in severe hyperkalemia.

Question 74: Correct Answer: C) Hypocalcemia

Rationale: Hypocalcemia is most likely to cause a prolonged QT interval on an ECG due to delayed ventricular repolarization. Hypokalemia can also affect the ECG but typically causes U waves and flattened T waves. Hypercalcemia shortens the QT interval, while hypermagnesemia can lead to prolonged PR intervals and widened QRS complexes. Understanding these differences is crucial for accurate diagnosis and treatment.

Question 75: Correct Answer: B) Utilizing barcode medication administration (BCMA)

Rationale: Barcode medication administration (BCMA) is the most effective strategy for preventing medication errors as it ensures accurate patient identification and correct medication dispensing through technology. Double-checking with a second nurse (Option A), while important, is prone to human error. Educating patients (Option C) enhances awareness but doesn't prevent errors during administration. Standardizing times (Option D) improves workflow but doesn't directly address verification accuracy. BCMA integrates multiple safety checks and has been shown to significantly reduce errors.

Question 76: Correct Answer: B) Morse Fall Scale

Rationale: The Morse Fall Scale is specifically designed to assess the risk of falls in hospitalized adult patients by evaluating factors such as history of falling, secondary diagnosis, ambulatory aids, intravenous therapy, gait, and mental status. The Braden Scale and Norton Scale are used for pressure ulcer risk assessment, while the MMSE assesses cognitive impairment. Thus, although the other tools are valuable in clinical settings, they do not directly address fall risk assessment.

Question 77: Correct Answer: B) Use bed alarms to alert staff if she tries to get up unassisted

Rationale: Bed alarms provide immediate alerts when a high-risk patient attempts to move unassisted, allowing quick intervention and preventing falls. Fall risk signs (Option A) increase awareness but do not provide real-time alerts. Non-slip footwear and accessible personal items (Option C) are helpful but less immediate in preventing falls than alarms. Hourly rounds (Option D) are important but may miss critical moments between checks.

Question 78: Correct Answer: D) Notify the surgeon immediately.

Rationale: The immediate notification of the surgeon is critical in managing postoperative internal bleeding to enable prompt diagnostic and therapeutic interventions. Increasing IV fluid rate (Option A) could exacerbate bleeding. Administering an anticoagulant (Option B) is contraindicated as it may worsen the bleeding. Applying direct pressure (Option C) is ineffective for internal bleeding and may delay necessary surgical intervention.

Question 79: Correct Answer: C) Orthostatic hypotension

Rationale: Orthostatic hypotension is a reliable indicator of dehydration as it reflects intravascular volume depletion leading to decreased blood pressure upon standing. While dry mucous membranes (A), decreased skin turgor (B), and elevated BUN (D) can be signs of dehydration, they can also be influenced by other factors such as age and renal function. Orthostatic hypotension directly measures the body's response to fluid status changes, making it a more specific indicator.

Question 80: Correct Answer: B) Restrict water intake.

Rationale: The most appropriate initial intervention for hyponatremia, particularly in a patient with congestive heart failure, is to restrict water intake to prevent further dilution of serum sodium levels. Administering hypertonic saline (Option A) is typically reserved for severe or symptomatic hyponatremia. Isotonic saline (Option C) may not be effective in correcting the underlying issue and could exacerbate fluid overload in heart failure. Encouraging increased oral fluid intake (Option D) would worsen the hyponatremia by further diluting serum sodium.

Question 81: Correct Answer: B) Prostate-Specific Antigen (PSA) test

Rationale: The PSA test is currently recommended for prostate cancer screening in men aged 55-69 after discussing potential benefits and harms. The DRE (A), while used in conjunction with PSA, is less sensitive alone. Transrectal ultrasound (C) and MRI of the prostate (D) are more diagnostic than screening tools. PSA testing provides a balance between sensitivity and specificity, making it the preferred initial screening method.

Question 82: Correct Answer: C) Engaging in moderate-intensity aerobic exercise for at least 150 minutes per week
Rationale: Engaging in regular moderate-intensity aerobic exercise has been shown to significantly improve cardiovascular health, reduce blood pressure, and aid in weight management. While adopting a Mediterranean diet (A), reducing sodium intake (B), and increasing fiber intake (D) are all beneficial, consistent physical activity provides the most comprehensive long-term benefits. Exercise improves endothelial function, enhances insulin sensitivity, and promotes overall well-being. The other options support cardiovascular health but do not offer the same broad spectrum of benefits as regular aerobic exercise.
Question 83: Correct Answer: B) Doppler ultrasound
Rationale: Doppler ultrasound is the most effective and non-invasive diagnostic tool for identifying DVT, as it visualizes blood flow and detects abnormalities. The D-dimer test, while useful, can produce false positives and is less specific. Venography, though accurate, is invasive and less commonly used. MRI can detect DVT but is more expensive and not typically the first-line diagnostic tool. Doppler ultrasound combines accuracy with non-invasiveness, making it the preferred choice.
Question 84: Correct Answer: A) Administering prophylactic antibiotics within one hour before incision
Rationale: Administering prophylactic antibiotics within one hour before incision is the most effective approach to minimize SSIs as it ensures optimal antibiotic levels at the surgical site when contamination risk is highest. Chlorhexidine-alcohol antisepsis (Option B), while effective, works best in conjunction with antibiotics. Proper hand hygiene (Option C), though critical, primarily prevents cross-contamination rather than direct site infection. Maintaining normothermia (Option D) reduces complications but isn't as directly impactful on SSIs as timely antibiotic administration according to guidelines and research findings.
Question 85: Correct Answer: B) Montreal Cognitive Assessment (MoCA)
Rationale: The MoCA has been validated to have high sensitivity for detecting MCI, outperforming the MMSE in this regard. While the Mini-Cog is useful for quick screening and the ACE-III provides a comprehensive assessment, neither matches the MoCA's sensitivity for MCI. The MMSE is less sensitive to subtle cognitive changes seen in MCI compared to MoCA.
Question 86: Correct Answer: B) Limit grapefruit juice intake to avoid increased blood levels of atorvastatin.
Rationale: Grapefruit juice can inhibit CYP3A4 enzymes, leading to higher blood levels of atorvastatin and increasing the risk of adverse effects like myopathy. Drinking it daily (Option A), substituting with orange juice (Option C), or timing consumption (Option D) do not adequately address this interaction's risks. Limiting intake is essential for safety.
Question 87: Correct Answer: B) Conventional Level
Rationale: At the Conventional Level, individuals conform to societal rules and laws to maintain social order. The Preconventional Level is characterized by self-interest and obedience to avoid punishment, while the Postconventional Level involves principles of justice and individual rights beyond societal laws. The Autonomous Level is not a recognized stage in Kohlberg's theory. The distinguishing factor is adherence to societal norms at the Conventional Level.
Question 88: Correct Answer: B) Contacting the physician to discuss alternative pain management strategies.
Rationale: Advocacy involves taking proactive steps to ensure optimal patient care. Contacting the physician to discuss alternative strategies (B) directly addresses and aims to resolve the issue. Informing family (A) may provide support but does not directly change care plans. Simply documenting pain levels (C) without action does not fulfill advocacy responsibilities. Suggesting over-the-counter medications (D), while potentially helpful, bypasses proper medical channels and could be unsafe without physician approval. Therefore, engaging with the physician reflects appropriate advocacy and interprofessional collaboration.
Question 89: Correct Answer: B) Participating in a structured weight loss program
Rationale: Participating in a structured weight loss program is crucial for preventing the progression of prediabetes to type 2 diabetes. Weight loss has been shown to improve insulin sensitivity and glucose metabolism. While following a low-carbohydrate diet (A) can help manage blood sugar levels, it may not be sustainable long-term without professional guidance. Taking daily multivitamins (C) and drinking green tea (D) have limited evidence supporting their effectiveness in preventing diabetes progression compared to structured weight loss programs that focus on comprehensive dietary and physical activity modifications.
Question 90: Correct Answer: A) Influenza vaccine
Rationale: The influenza vaccine is critical for Mrs. Thompson due to her age and underlying COPD, which increases her risk of severe complications from the flu. The Hepatitis B vaccine is important but not immediately relevant to her respiratory condition. The Meningococcal vaccine is typically prioritized for younger individuals or those in specific risk groups. The HPV vaccine is recommended for younger adults to prevent cervical and other cancers. Therefore, the influenza vaccine is the most pertinent for reducing respiratory infection risks in this scenario.
Question 91: Correct Answer: B) Pneumococcal polysaccharide vaccine (PPSV23)
Rationale: Diabetic patients are at increased risk for pneumococcal infections, making the PPSV23 vaccination crucial in preventing severe pneumococcal diseases. While Tdap is important for preventing tetanus, diphtheria, and pertussis, it does not specifically address the increased risk posed by diabetes. The Varicella and MMR vaccines are essential but generally administered earlier in life or based on specific exposure risks. Therefore, PPSV23 is the most relevant for Mr. Garcia's health maintenance.
Question 92: Correct Answer: C) Troponin I
Rationale: Troponin I is the gold standard biomarker for diagnosing myocardial infarction due to its high sensitivity and specificity for cardiac muscle injury. CK-MB can be elevated in other muscle injuries, myoglobin rises quickly but lacks specificity, and LDH is less specific and has a slower rise time. Therefore, Troponin I provides the most accurate diagnostic information for MI.
Question 93: Correct Answer: B) Observing Lisa perform wound care and mobility exercises
Rationale: Observing Lisa perform wound care and mobility exercises directly assesses her practical readiness for discharge. Listing instructions (A), using checklists (C), or attending group sessions (D) do not confirm her ability to perform necessary tasks independently. Direct observation ensures she can manage her care effectively at home, reducing risks of complications.
Question 94: Correct Answer: C) Count the pulse for a full minute
Rationale: Counting the pulse for a full minute is crucial when an irregular pulse is detected to accurately determine its rate and rhythm. Immediate notification of a physician (Option A) should follow if there are significant findings, but accurate assessment must come first. Using a Doppler device (Option B) may help detect pulses but won't provide rhythm information. Documenting and continuing assessments (Option D) without thorough evaluation could overlook critical details, thus delaying necessary interventions.
Question 95: Correct Answer: C) A drop in systolic blood pressure of 20 mmHg or more upon standing
Rationale: Orthostatic hypotension is characterized by a drop in systolic blood pressure of 20 mmHg or more upon standing, indicating inadequate physiological response to postural changes. Option A describes an insufficient drop to

qualify as orthostatic hypotension. Option B incorrectly suggests an increase in diastolic pressure, which isn't characteristic of this condition. Option D focuses on heart rate changes rather than blood pressure criteria, although increased heart rate often accompanies orthostatic hypotension but isn't diagnostic on its own.

Question 96: Correct Answer: C) Administer IV calcium gluconate

Rationale: The most appropriate initial intervention for hyperkalemia (potassium level of 6.5 mEq/L) is to stabilize the cardiac membrane by administering IV calcium gluconate. This does not lower potassium levels but prevents life-threatening arrhythmias. Insulin and glucose (Option A) shift potassium into cells but are not the first step. Oral potassium supplements (Option B) would worsen hyperkalemia. Loop diuretics (Option D) help excrete potassium but are not immediate.

Question 97: Correct Answer: A) Repositioning the patient every two hours.

Rationale: Repositioning every two hours is a fundamental intervention in preventing pressure ulcers by alleviating pressure on vulnerable areas. While using pressure-relieving mattresses (Option B), applying barrier creams (Option C), and conducting daily skin assessments (Option D) are all essential components of a comprehensive prevention plan, repositioning directly addresses the primary cause of pressure ulcers—sustained pressure on bony prominences. This frequent repositioning ensures that no single area bears weight for too long, thereby reducing ulcer risk effectively.

Question 98: Correct Answer: A) Enhanced medication reconciliation accuracy

Rationale: Including a pharmacist enhances medication reconciliation accuracy (A), which is crucial for preventing medication errors and adverse drug interactions in complex cases. While pharmacists can contribute to nutritional support planning (B), it is not their primary role compared to dietitians. Streamlined discharge processes (C) benefit from multidisciplinary input but hinge more on case management roles. Increased patient satisfaction scores (D), though important, are an indirect benefit rather than the primary role of pharmacists. Studies show that accurate medication reconciliation significantly reduces readmission rates and improves overall patient safety.

Question 99: Correct Answer: B) Nutritional Risk Screening (NRS-2002)

Rationale: The NRS-2002 is specifically validated for identifying malnutrition in hospitalized surgical patients by considering nutritional status and disease severity. While MUST and MNA are also used for malnutrition screening, they are more general and not tailored to the surgical population. SGA involves a comprehensive assessment but is more subjective compared to the NRS-2002. Hence, NRS-2002 is the most suitable tool for this specific patient group.

Question 100: Correct Answer: A) Administering prophylactic antibiotics within one hour before incision

Rationale: Administering prophylactic antibiotics within one hour before incision is crucial for preventing SSIs by ensuring adequate tissue levels during surgery. Shaving surgical sites immediately prior to surgery (B) can increase infection risk due to micro-abrasions. Using sterile gloves (C) is essential but not as impactful alone without timely antibiotic administration. Applying antiseptic solutions to instruments (D) is necessary but secondary; preoperative antibiotics target potential pathogens directly within tissues, significantly reducing SSI risk.

Question 101: Correct Answer: B) Develop a safety plan with Maria.

Rationale: Developing a safety plan (B) is crucial as it provides Maria with specific strategies and resources she can use during crises, thereby directly addressing her immediate risk of self-harm. Increasing follow-up visits (A), joining support groups (C), and adjusting medication (D) are supportive actions but do not provide an immediate framework for managing acute suicidal thoughts.

Question 102: Correct Answer: C) Social support network

Rationale: While social support networks play a critical role in overall well-being and recovery, they do not directly impact the physical or cognitive ability to perform ADLs. Visual acuity, cognitive impairment, and range of motion are direct factors influencing one's capability to complete ADLs independently. Understanding these distinctions helps prioritize assessment areas.

Question 103: Correct Answer: C) Administer hypertonic saline solution

Rationale: Severe hyponatremia (sodium level of 125 mEq/L), especially with symptoms like dizziness and hypotension, requires careful correction with hypertonic saline solution to avoid cerebral edema. Isotonic saline (Option A) may be insufficient for severe cases. Water restriction (Option B) helps in chronic hyponatremia but not in acute severe cases. Increasing oral fluids (Option D) could worsen hyponatremia.

Question 104: Correct Answer: A) Mrs. Garcia's diet and meal patterns

Rationale: Prioritizing Mrs. Garcia's diet and meal patterns (Option A) is essential because dietary intake directly influences blood glucose levels in diabetic patients, particularly concerning hypoglycemia. Medication adherence (Option B), physical activity level (Option C), and emotional stress levels (Option D) are also important factors but secondary to understanding her nutritional intake, which has an immediate impact on glucose control.

Question 105: Correct Answer: B) Administer a bronchodilator via nebulizer.

Rationale: The immediate nursing intervention should be administering a bronchodilator via nebulizer (Option B), which helps open airways and improve breathing in COPD patients experiencing exacerbation. Increasing oxygen flow rate (Option A) may be necessary but should follow bronchodilator administration for maximum effectiveness. Positioning her in high Fowler's position (Option C) aids breathing but is secondary to bronchodilator therapy. Starting antibiotic therapy (Option D) may be needed if an infection is suspected but is not the immediate priority for acute symptom relief.

Question 106: Correct Answer: B) To understand the patient's health beliefs and practices

Rationale: Understanding a patient's cultural background helps healthcare providers comprehend their health beliefs and practices, which can significantly impact care delivery and patient outcomes. While language barriers, socioeconomic status, and educational level are important factors, they do not provide as comprehensive an understanding of health beliefs and practices as cultural background does.

Question 107: Correct Answer: C) Respiratory Rate

Rationale: Mrs. Smith's respiratory rate (RR) of 28 breaths/min indicates tachypnea and suggests respiratory distress or potential complications such as pulmonary embolism or infection. Her blood pressure (BP), heart rate (HR), and oxygen saturation (SpO2) are within acceptable limits for her condition; however, the elevated RR requires immediate assessment and intervention to determine the underlying cause.

Question 108: Correct Answer: A) Apply warm blankets and monitor temperature.

Rationale: The initial action should be applying warm blankets and monitoring temperature (Option A). Shivering can increase metabolic demand and discomfort post-operatively; warming measures help alleviate these symptoms while monitoring ensures prompt identification of changes. Administering antipyretics (Option B) may be needed if fever persists but isn't the first step without assessing non-pharmacologic measures first. Assessing for infection (Option C) is important but secondary to addressing immediate comfort needs. Notifying the surgeon about bradycardia (Option D), though necessary if persistent or symptomatic bradycardia occurs, isn't immediately required here given other stable vitals and context.

Question 109: Correct Answer: D) Excretion

Rationale: In patients with renal impairment, excretion is the most crucial pharmacokinetic parameter to monitor because the kidneys are primarily responsible for eliminating many medications and their metabolites. Impaired renal function can lead to drug accumulation and toxicity. While absorption, distribution, and metabolism are also important, they do not directly address the elimination of drugs from the body. For instance, metabolism (C) primarily involves the liver, not the kidneys. Monitoring excretion helps in adjusting dosages to prevent adverse effects.

Question 110: Correct Answer: A) Fluoxetine and Tramadol

Rationale: Serotonin syndrome is a potentially life-threatening condition caused by excessive serotonin. Fluoxetine, a selective serotonin reuptake inhibitor (SSRI), and Tramadol, an opioid analgesic with serotonin reuptake inhibition properties, can significantly increase serotonin levels when used together. Metoprolol and Simvastatin, Lisinopril and Hydrochlorothiazide, and Atorvastatin and Amlodipine do not significantly impact serotonin levels. Thus, combining Fluoxetine with Tramadol poses the highest risk for serotonin syndrome.

Question 111: Correct Answer: B) Respect the patient's autonomy and document their decision.

Rationale: Respecting patient autonomy is fundamental in nursing ethics, acknowledging their right to make informed decisions about their care. Option A undermines autonomy by pressuring acceptance. Option C disregards personal beliefs and legal rights without exploring all avenues of consent. Option D involves family but may violate confidentiality and autonomy principles. Documenting ensures clarity and legal compliance while honoring patient choice.

Question 112: Correct Answer: B) Provide information about local shelters and support services.

Rationale: The nurse's initial response should be providing information about local shelters and support services (Option B). This empowers Maria by offering immediate resources for escaping an abusive environment. Advising on safe sexual practices (Option A), conducting a physical examination (Option C), or encouraging dialogue about consent (Option D), while important, do not directly address her need for safety and support in an abusive relationship. Ensuring Maria knows where to find help can significantly impact her ability to leave the abusive situation safely.

Question 113: Correct Answer: C) Chief complaint

Rationale: The chief complaint is the most critical component as it directs the focus of the clinical assessment and subsequent diagnostic process. While family medical history, current medications, and social history provide essential background information, they are secondary to understanding the primary issue prompting the patient's visit. The chief complaint allows for targeted questioning and examination, which is crucial for accurate diagnosis and effective treatment planning. Family medical history (A), current medications (B), and social history (D) are important but do not provide the immediate focal point needed for diagnostic accuracy.

Question 114: Correct Answer: C) Using a combination of verbal instructions, demonstrations, and written materials

Rationale: Research shows that using multimodal teaching strategies enhances patient understanding and retention. Combining verbal instructions, demonstrations, and written materials caters to different learning styles and reinforces information through repetition. Option A lacks engagement; Option B is effective but limited without reinforcement; Option D does not accommodate varied learning preferences or provide ongoing support.

Question 115: Correct Answer: A) Patient's cognitive impairment

Rationale: Cognitive impairment significantly affects a patient's ability to understand and adhere to post-operative care instructions. Cultural beliefs (Option B), while important, can often be navigated with culturally sensitive education. Complexity of medical terminology (Option C) can be simplified by using layman's terms. Socioeconomic status (Option D) impacts access to resources but not directly comprehension of instructions. Cognitive impairment directly influences the patient's capacity to process and retain critical health information, making it a primary barrier.

Question 116: Correct Answer: C) Establishing mutual goals with the patient

Rationale: Establishing mutual goals with the patient enhances adherence by involving them in their care plan, fostering ownership and motivation. Simplifying terminology (Option A), using visual aids (Option B), and providing written instructions (Option D) are helpful but insufficient alone. Mutual goal setting ensures that education is personalized and relevant, making other educational tools more effective by aligning them with the patient's understanding and preferences.

Question 117: Correct Answer: A) Administering prescribed diuretics and monitoring electrolyte levels

Rationale: Administering diuretics helps reduce fluid overload by promoting urine output, which is crucial for managing CHF. Monitoring electrolytes ensures safe diuretic use. Option B is incorrect as increased fluid intake can worsen fluid overload. Option C is incorrect because a high-sodium diet can exacerbate edema. Option D, while reducing cardiac workload, does not directly address fluid overload.

Question 118: Correct Answer: B) Decreased efficacy of clopidogrel

Rationale: Omeprazole can inhibit CYP2C19, an enzyme crucial for converting clopidogrel into its active form, thereby reducing its antiplatelet effect and increasing the risk of cardiovascular events. Increased risk of thrombosis (A) is a consequence of decreased efficacy but not a direct interaction mechanism. Increased gastrointestinal bleeding (C) and elevated blood pressure (D) are not primary concerns related to this interaction. Hence, understanding enzyme inhibition helps manage medication efficacy in polypharmacy scenarios effectively.

Question 119: Correct Answer: C) Review each medication with her verbally and use the teach-back method.

Rationale: Reviewing each medication verbally and using the teach-back method ensures Mrs. Smith understands her regimen by having her explain it back in her own words, confirming comprehension. Option A provides information but does not verify understanding or allow for immediate clarification of questions. Option B is important for ongoing care but does not address immediate understanding of medications. Option D supports overall recovery but does not directly focus on ensuring she understands her medications at discharge.

Question 120: Correct Answer: D) Methodology used

Rationale: The methodology used in a study is critical for assessing its validity because it determines how the research was conducted and whether the results are reliable and reproducible. While publication date ensures currency, author credentials indicate expertise, and sample size affects generalizability, none of these alone can confirm the robustness of a study like a well-designed methodology can. A sound methodology includes proper design, data collection, and analysis techniques that ensure accurate and unbiased results.

Question 121: Correct Answer: B) Serum creatinine level

Rationale: Metformin is contraindicated in patients with impaired renal function due to the risk of lactic acidosis. Serum creatinine provides an estimate of kidney function and helps determine if metformin can be safely administered. Liver function tests (A) are secondary since metformin is primarily renally excreted. CBC (C) and electrolyte panel (D) are important but less critical than assessing kidney function before starting metformin.

Question 122: Correct Answer: C) Concrete Operational Stage

Rationale: In the Concrete Operational Stage (ages 7-11), children develop logical thinking about concrete events but struggle with abstract concepts. The Sensorimotor Stage involves sensory and motor interactions (birth-2 years), the Preoperational Stage (ages 2-7) involves symbolic play and egocentrism, and the Formal Operational Stage (ages 12 and up) involves abstract reasoning. The critical distinction is that logical thinking about concrete events emerges in the Concrete Operational Stage.

Question 123: Correct Answer: C) Hypervolemic hyponatremia

Rationale: Michael's symptoms and lab results suggest hypervolemic hyponatremia due to heart failure. Serum osmolality below normal (260 mOsm/kg), low urine sodium, and signs of fluid overload indicate this condition. SIADH (Option A) typically shows high urine sodium levels despite low serum osmolality. Dehydration (Option B) would present with high serum osmolality. Diabetes Insipidus (Option D) involves high serum osmolality due to water loss, not fluid overload.

Question 124: Correct Answer: B) Melena

Rationale: Melena, or black tarry stools, suggests an upper gastrointestinal bleed due to the digestion of blood as it passes through the GI tract. Hematochezia (bright red blood per rectum) typically indicates lower GI bleeding. Steatorrhea (fatty stools) relates to malabsorption syndromes and not bleeding. Jaundice indicates liver dysfunction or bile duct obstruction rather than GI bleeding. The presence of melena specifically points to bleeding above the ligament of Treitz in the GI tract.

Question 125: Correct Answer: A) Hyperreflexia

Rationale: Hypomagnesemia often leads to neuromuscular excitability, manifesting as hyperreflexia due to magnesium's role in stabilizing nerve function. Hypotension (B), while possible, is less directly associated with hypomagnesemia compared to neuromuscular symptoms. Bradycardia (C) is typically linked to hypermagnesemia rather than hypomagnesemia. Hypercalcemia (D) is unrelated to low magnesium levels; instead, hypocalcemia can occur concurrently due to impaired parathyroid hormone secretion.

MEDSURG-BC Exam Practice Questions [SET 3]

Question 1: Which method is most effective for evaluating a patient's understanding of self-care instructions after surgery?
A) Written test
B) Verbal questioning
C) Demonstration/return demonstration
D) Patient self-report

Question 2: Jane, a 45-year-old patient, has just been diagnosed with Type 2 Diabetes. During your initial consultation, she expresses feelings of anxiety and confusion about managing her condition. Which therapeutic communication skill is most appropriate to help Jane understand and manage her diagnosis?
A) Providing detailed medical information about diabetes management
B) Encouraging Jane to express her feelings and concerns
C) Referring Jane to a diabetes support group
D) Scheduling frequent follow-up appointments

Question 3: Which developmental theory emphasizes the importance of resolving conflicts at different stages to achieve healthy psychological development in adults?
A) Jean Piaget's Cognitive Development Theory
B) Erik Erikson's Psychosocial Development Theory
C) Sigmund Freud's Psychosexual Development Theory
D) Lawrence Kohlberg's Moral Development Theory

Question 4: Which approach is most appropriate for evaluating long-term retention of patient education about medication adherence?
A) Immediate post-instruction testing
B) Scheduled follow-up phone calls
C) Periodic in-person assessments
D) Reviewing refill records over several months

Question 5: In the context of evidence-based practice, which source of knowledge is considered most reliable for guiding clinical decision-making?
A) Expert opinion
B) Randomized controlled trials
C) Case studies
D) Clinical experience

Question 6: What is the primary rationale for administering fresh frozen plasma (FFP) in a postoperative patient with active bleeding?
A) To increase hemoglobin levels rapidly
B) To provide clotting factors and correct coagulopathies
C) To expand intravascular volume quickly
D) To supply platelets for clot formation

Question 7: Mr. Lee, a 72-year-old male with a history of heart failure, reports sudden weight gain and swelling in his legs. During your assessment, which finding would most likely indicate worsening heart failure?
A) Elevated jugular venous pressure (JVP)
B) Clear lung sounds
C) Bradycardia
D) Decreased urinary output

Question 8: Mrs. Patel, a 75-year-old woman with mild cognitive impairment, undergoes a clock-drawing test as part of her cognitive assessment. What specific type of impairment is best identified by this test?
A) Language deficits
B) Executive dysfunction
C) Short-term memory loss
D) Visuospatial disorientation

Question 9: For a patient with chronic obstructive pulmonary disease (COPD), which intervention is most effective in slowing disease progression?
A) Long-term oxygen therapy
B) Smoking cessation
C) Pulmonary rehabilitation
D) Inhaled corticosteroids

Question 10: Mrs. Johnson is taking warfarin for atrial fibrillation and has been prescribed ciprofloxacin for a urinary tract infection. What adverse effect should the nurse be most concerned about?
A) Increased risk of bleeding
B) Decreased efficacy of warfarin
C) Increased risk of thrombosis
D) Decreased efficacy of ciprofloxacin

Question 11: In assessing a patient with chronic heart failure, which laboratory test result would most likely indicate worsening condition?
A) Elevated serum creatinine
B) Increased B-type natriuretic peptide (BNP)
C) Low hemoglobin level
D) Elevated liver enzymes

Question 12: Which diagnostic test is most appropriate for evaluating a patient's acid-base balance in the context of suspected metabolic acidosis?
A) Serum lactate level
B) Arterial blood gas (ABG)
C) Serum bicarbonate level
D) Urine pH

Question 13: A patient named Ms. Garcia complains of persistent cough, night sweats, and unintentional weight loss over the past two months. Which condition should the nurse consider as a priority during the review of systems?
A) Tuberculosis
B) Asthma
C) Chronic obstructive pulmonary disease (COPD)
D) Gastroesophageal reflux disease (GERD)

Question 14: Nurse Alex needs to delegate wound care for Ms. Johnson, a patient with a complex surgical wound that requires sterile dressing changes. Which team member is most appropriate for this delegation?
A) A certified nursing assistant (CNA)
B) A licensed practical nurse (LPN)
C) Another registered nurse (RN)
D) A student nurse under direct supervision

Question 15: When performing a neurological assessment, which skill is paramount in determining the level of consciousness in a patient?
A) Checking pupil response to light
B) Assessing motor response to stimuli
C) Evaluating verbal response to questions
D) Monitoring vital signs

Question 16: A patient's arterial blood gas (ABG) results show pH 7.30, $PaCO_2$ 50 mm Hg, and HCO_3^- 24 mEq/L. What is the most appropriate nursing intervention for this patient?
A) Encourage deep breathing exercises
B) Prepare for intubation and mechanical ventilation
C) Administer sodium bicarbonate intravenously
D) Increase oxygen flow rate via nasal cannula

Question 17: During a physical assessment, which of the following findings is most indicative of early-stage left-sided heart failure?
A) Bilateral pitting edema in the lower extremities
B) Crackles heard at the lung bases during auscultation
C) Jugular venous distention
D) Hepatomegaly

Question 18: John, a 55-year-old patient post-abdominal surgery, reports severe pain at the surgical site. Which nursing intervention should be included in his care plan to effectively manage his pain?
A) Encouraging deep breathing exercises and early ambulation
B) Administering prescribed analgesics as per pain assessment
C) Applying ice packs intermittently to the surgical site
D) Educating on non-pharmacological pain relief methods like meditation

Question 19: Which complementary and alternative medicine (CAM) practice is most supported by contemporary research for reducing anxiety in preoperative patients?
A) Aromatherapy
B) Reiki
C) Acupuncture
D) Yoga

Question 20: Mr. Lee, a 55-year-old patient recovering from coronary artery bypass graft surgery, needs education on lifestyle modifications to prevent further cardiac events. Which teaching strategy should the nurse use to effectively communicate this information?
A) Give Mr. Lee written instructions on dietary changes.
B) Demonstrate and practice physical exercises with him.
C) Discuss stress management techniques during his visit.
D) Use multimedia tools to explain lifestyle modifications.

Question 21: Which of the following interventions is most effective in reducing the risk of falls in hospitalized elderly patients?
A) Hourly rounding by nursing staff
B) Use of bed alarms
C) Application of non-slip socks
D) Implementation of a fall risk assessment tool

Question 22: A patient with heart failure presents with hyponatremia. Which of the following is the most appropriate initial treatment to correct this electrolyte imbalance?
A) Administration of hypertonic saline
B) Fluid restriction
C) Administration of loop diuretics
D) Sodium supplementation

Question 23: In advocating for a patient's right to informed consent, what should be a medical-surgical nurse's primary focus?
A) Ensuring that all consent forms are signed by the patient.
B) Verifying that all information provided is understandable and comprehensive.
C) Encouraging patients to agree with recommended treatments.
D) Confirming that family members are aware of treatment plans.

Question 24: Which adverse effect is most likely to occur with long-term use of proton pump inhibitors (PPIs)?
A) Renal failure
B) Osteoporosis-related fractures
C) Hepatic encephalopathy
D) Myocardial infarction

Question 25: In patients with hyponatremia due to SIADH (Syndrome of Inappropriate Antidiuretic Hormone), which treatment option is most appropriate?
A) Fluid restriction
B) Administration of isotonic saline
C) Administration of hypotonic saline
D) Increased oral salt intake

Question 26: Mrs. Johnson, a 70-year-old patient with a history of hypertension, presents with sudden onset of right-sided weakness and facial droop. Upon assessment, she has difficulty with speech articulation but can comprehend language well. Which type of aphasia is she most likely experiencing?
A) Global aphasia
B) Broca's aphasia
C) Wernicke's aphasia
D) Anomic aphasia

Question 27: Mr. Smith, a 70-year-old patient with a history of osteoarthritis, is being assessed for his ability to perform activities of daily living (ADLs). Which of the following assessments would provide the most accurate indication of his functional status?
A) Observing Mr. Smith as he performs a simulated meal preparation.
B) Asking Mr. Smith to fill out a self-report questionnaire on his ADLs.
C) Reviewing Mr. Smith's medical records for previous ADL assessments.
D) Conducting an interview with Mr. Smith's family members about his ADLs.

Question 28: Which of the following foods should be avoided by a patient taking warfarin due to its potential to decrease the drug's anticoagulant effect?
A) Spinach
B) Grapefruit
C) Bananas
D) Apples

Question 29: John, a 45-year-old male recovering from a traumatic brain injury, shows signs of impaired executive function. Which developmental age-related cognitive assessment would best evaluate his executive functioning skills?
A) Trail Making Test Part B
B) Stroop Test
C) Wechsler Adult Intelligence Scale (WAIS)
D) Mini-Cog

Question 30: Which assessment finding is most indicative of early hypovolemic shock in a postoperative patient?
A) Blood pressure of 90/60 mmHg
B) Heart rate of 120 beats per minute
C) Respiratory rate of 22 breaths per minute
D) Urine output of 25 mL/hour

Question 31: Which theory emphasizes the importance of matching instructional methods with individual learning styles in medical-surgical nursing education?
A) Behaviorist Theory
B) Cognitive Load Theory
C) Gardner's Multiple Intelligences Theory
D) VARK Model

Question 32: John, a 72-year-old patient with diabetes mellitus, is recovering from abdominal surgery. On postoperative day five, he presents with increased pain at the incision site, purulent drainage, and an elevated

white blood cell count. What is the most important nursing action to prevent sepsis?
A) Administer prescribed analgesics for pain relief.
B) Notify the healthcare provider immediately.
C) Apply a warm compress to the incision site.
D) Encourage ambulation to improve circulation.

Question 33: Sarah, a 70-year-old patient with chronic heart failure, frequently misses her follow-up appointments and struggles with self-care instructions. She lives alone and has limited social interactions. What is the primary barrier affecting Sarah's self-care?
A) Cognitive impairment
B) Social isolation
C) Financial constraints
D) Transportation issues

Question 34: Which screening tool is recommended for early detection of delirium in critically ill patients?
A) Confusion Assessment Method for the ICU (CAM-ICU)
B) Richmond Agitation-Sedation Scale (RASS)
C) Glasgow Coma Scale (GCS)
D) Mini-Cog

Question 35: Nurse Alex is working with Mrs. Smith, who has been diagnosed with diabetes mellitus type 2. Mrs. Smith expresses anxiety about managing her condition at home. What is the most effective strategy Nurse Alex can use to empower Mrs. Smith in managing her diabetes?
A) Encourage her to join a diabetes support group.
B) Provide extensive written instructions on diabetes management.
C) Demonstrate how to use her glucometer and insulin pen.
D) Discuss the benefits of regular exercise and diet control.

Question 36: Which intervention is most critical in the initial management of acute myocardial infarction (AMI) to improve patient outcomes?
A) Administering oxygen
B) Initiating IV nitroglycerin
C) Providing aspirin
D) Performing early coronary angiography

Question 37: During a physical assessment of Mr. Johnson, a 68-year-old male with a history of chronic obstructive pulmonary disease (COPD), the nurse notes an increased anteroposterior diameter of the chest. What is the most likely underlying cause of this finding?
A) Pulmonary fibrosis
B) Chronic bronchitis
C) Emphysema
D) Pneumonia

Question 38: Which laboratory test is most appropriate for assessing therapeutic levels of a medication with a narrow therapeutic index?
A) Complete Blood Count (CBC)
B) Serum Creatinine
C) Therapeutic Drug Monitoring (TDM)
D) Liver Function Tests (LFTs)

Question 39: Which of the following interventions is most effective in preventing postoperative pulmonary complications in a high-risk patient?
A) Incentive spirometry
B) Early ambulation
C) Deep breathing exercises
D) Prophylactic antibiotics

Question 40: Ms. Lee, a 45-year-old patient with hypertension, has been advised to adopt lifestyle changes to better manage her condition. Which self-management strategy should be prioritized to achieve optimal blood pressure control?
A) Following the DASH diet
B) Engaging in weekly yoga sessions
C) Limiting alcohol intake to weekends
D) Taking prescribed antihypertensive medications

Question 41: John, a 60-year-old male with chronic kidney disease, is receiving a transfusion of fresh frozen plasma (FFP). What is the primary reason for administering FFP in this patient?
A) To increase red blood cell count
B) To correct coagulopathy
C) To provide platelets
D) To treat hypovolemia

Question 42: Mrs. Smith, a 55-year-old female with a history of hypertension, presents with sudden onset of severe headache and blurred vision. During the physical assessment, which finding would most strongly indicate a hypertensive crisis?
A) Blood pressure of 150/90 mmHg
B) Retinal hemorrhages on fundoscopic examination
C) Mild ankle edema
D) Heart rate of 100 beats per minute

Question 43: Mrs. Smith, a 58-year-old female with diabetes mellitus, presents with a non-healing ulcer on her right foot. Which assessment finding would most strongly suggest the presence of peripheral arterial disease (PAD)?
A) Warm skin around the ulcer
B) Bounding pedal pulses
C) Delayed capillary refill time
D) Increased hair growth on lower extremities

Question 44: A nurse discovers that a colleague has been documenting care that was not provided. What is the most ethical course of action for the nurse to take?
A) Discuss the issue directly with the colleague.
B) Report the incident to the nursing supervisor.
C) Document the discrepancy in the patient's medical record.
D) Ignore the incident to maintain team harmony.

Question 45: What is the primary reason for using compression stockings in postoperative patients to prevent emboli?
A) Increase arterial blood flow
B) Reduce venous stasis
C) Enhance lymphatic drainage
D) Prevent superficial thrombophlebitis

Question 46: During a multidisciplinary team meeting, Nurse Sarah advocates for Mr. Thompson's discharge plan but encounters resistance from other team members who believe he needs more inpatient care despite his expressed wish to go home. What is Sarah's most appropriate advocacy action in this situation?
A) Agreeing with the team to avoid conflict.
B) Presenting evidence of Mr. Thompson's readiness for discharge.
C) Encouraging Mr. Thompson to demand discharge against medical advice.
D) Suggesting an extended stay without further discussion.

Question 47: In managing chronic heart failure, which pharmacological agent is primarily used to reduce mortality and morbidity by blocking neurohormonal activation?
A) Furosemide
B) Digoxin
C) Carvedilol
D) Spironolactone

Question 48: Patient David, a 70-year-old male with diabetes mellitus, presents with lethargy and abdominal pain. His lab results indicate serum calcium of 11.5 mg/dL. What is the most appropriate initial management?
A) Administer intravenous bisphosphonates
B) Increase oral calcium intake
C) Administer intravenous normal saline
D) Restrict dietary calcium

Question 49: In a patient with heart failure, which dietary modification is most effective in managing fluid retention?
A) Increase potassium intake.
B) Reduce sodium intake.
C) Limit protein consumption.
D) Increase calcium intake.

Question 50: Mrs. Johnson, a 65-year-old patient recovering from hip replacement surgery, is experiencing anxiety and restlessness during her hospital stay. Which diversional activity is most appropriate to help alleviate her symptoms?
A) Encouraging her to watch television
B) Providing her with a puzzle book
C) Engaging her in a guided imagery session
D) Offering her a selection of magazines

Question 51: Nurse Alex is assessing a post-operative patient, Mr. Johnson, who has undergone abdominal surgery. He complains of severe pain and exhibits signs of distress. Which skill should Nurse Alex prioritize to assess the patient's pain effectively?
A) Use a numerical pain scale
B) Perform a physical examination of the surgical site
C) Administer prescribed analgesics immediately
D) Evaluate vital signs for abnormalities

Question 52: A 65-year-old patient named Mr. Smith is admitted with a suspected stroke. During the neurological assessment, you notice that he has difficulty understanding spoken language, although his speech is fluent but nonsensical. Which area of the brain is most likely affected?
A) Broca's area
B) Wernicke's area
C) Occipital lobe
D) Cerebellum

Question 53: Mr. Johnson, a 68-year-old patient with chronic osteoarthritis, is experiencing severe pain despite being on a stable regimen of NSAIDs and acetaminophen. The healthcare team decides to introduce an opioid for better pain control. Which of the following considerations is most important when initiating opioid therapy in this patient?
A) Start with a high dose to quickly achieve pain relief.
B) Consider the patient's renal function before selecting an opioid.
C) Combine opioids with NSAIDs to enhance analgesic effect.
D) Monitor for gastrointestinal side effects as the primary concern.

Question 54: During a review of systems, a nurse assesses a patient for cardiovascular abnormalities. Which symptom is most indicative of left-sided heart failure?
A) Peripheral edema
B) Jugular vein distention
C) Orthopnea
D) Hepatomegaly

Question 55: Which developmental stage according to Havighurst's developmental tasks theory involves achieving emotional independence from parents and preparing for marriage and family life?
A) Infancy and Early Childhood
B) Middle Childhood
C) Adolescence
D) Early Adulthood

Question 56: During a routine check-up, Mr. Lee, a 45-year-old male with no significant medical history, has the following vital signs: BP 130/85 mmHg, HR 58 bpm, RR 16 breaths/min, and SpO2 98%. He mentions feeling dizzy occasionally but denies any chest pain or shortness of breath. Which vital sign should be further evaluated?
A) Blood Pressure
B) Heart Rate
C) Respiratory Rate
D) Oxygen Saturation

Question 57: Nurse Emily is planning a teaching session for Mr. Johnson, a 65-year-old patient recently diagnosed with diabetes. To ensure the teaching is effective, she assesses his learning preferences. Mr. Johnson mentions he enjoys reading and often takes notes to remember important information. Based on this information, which learning preference does Mr. Johnson most likely have?
A) Visual
B) Auditory
C) Kinesthetic
D) Read/Write

Question 58: Mr. Lee is recovering from surgery and expresses fear about potential complications he read about online. Which response by the nurse exemplifies effective therapeutic communication?
A) "Don't worry; those complications are very rare."
B) "Tell me more about what you read and how it makes you feel."
C) "You shouldn't believe everything you read online."
D) "Let's focus on your recovery instead of worrying."

Question 59: In managing a patient with diabetic ketoacidosis (DKA), which intervention should be prioritized to stabilize the patient?
A) Administering subcutaneous insulin
B) Initiating intravenous fluid replacement
C) Providing oral glucose
D) Monitoring blood glucose every hour

Question 60: For a patient experiencing acute blood loss from trauma, which blood product should be prioritized to improve oxygen-carrying capacity?
A) Packed Red Blood Cells (PRBCs)
B) Fresh Frozen Plasma (FFP)
C) Whole Blood
D) Platelets

Question 61: In the context of a neurological review of systems, which finding would be most concerning for a nurse assessing a patient with suspected increased intracranial pressure (ICP)?
A) Bradycardia
B) Hyperreflexia
C) Hypotension
D) Mydriasis

Question 62: Which cranial nerve assessment finding would be most concerning for a nurse evaluating a patient with suspected increased intracranial pressure?

A) Unilateral pupil dilation
B) Bilateral pupil constriction
C) Impaired upward gaze
D) Loss of corneal reflex

Question 63: Which ethical theory primarily focuses on the outcomes or consequences of actions when making a decision in medical-surgical nursing?
A) Deontology
B) Virtue ethics
C) Utilitarianism
D) Principlism

Question 64: What is the primary reason for administering prophylactic anticoagulants to a postoperative patient?
A) To prevent deep vein thrombosis (DVT)
B) To reduce postoperative pain
C) To enhance wound healing
D) To decrease infection risk

Question 65: What is the primary concern when combining Warfarin with Amiodarone?
A) Increased risk of bleeding
B) Decreased effectiveness of Warfarin
C) Increased risk of QT prolongation
D) Reduced heart rate variability

Question 66: During a post-operative teaching session, Nurse Sarah notices that Mrs. Thompson prefers to watch videos and look at diagrams to understand her recovery exercises better. Which learning preference should Nurse Sarah consider when planning further education for Mrs. Thompson?
A) Visual
B) Auditory
C) Kinesthetic
D) Read/Write

Question 67: Mr. Smith, a 70-year-old patient with congestive heart failure (CHF), needs education on dietary modifications to manage his condition better. Which educational method should the nurse employ to maximize Mr. Smith's adherence to dietary changes?
A) Providing a list of foods to avoid
B) Conducting a one-on-one dietary counseling session
C) Referring him to a nutritionist for meal planning
D) Using interactive tools like food diaries and apps

Question 68: Which of the following is the most accurate method for measuring core body temperature in a critically ill patient?
A) Oral thermometer
B) Axillary thermometer
C) Tympanic thermometer
D) Rectal thermometer

Question 69: John, a 60-year-old patient recovering from surgery, expresses frustration about his slow recovery progress. Despite following his prescribed physical therapy exercises, he feels demotivated due to pain and limited mobility. Which barrier is most likely hindering John's recovery?
A) Pain management issues
B) Lack of motivation
C) Insufficient physical therapy sessions
D) Nutritional deficiencies

Question 70: Which cognitive assessment tool is most effective for detecting early-stage impairment in older adults?
A) Mini-Mental State Examination (MMSE)
B) Montreal Cognitive Assessment (MoCA)
C) Clock Drawing Test
D) Geriatric Depression Scale

Question 71: In assessing the effectiveness of a patient education program on diabetes management, which evaluation method provides the most comprehensive assessment?
A) Pre-test and post-test comparisons
B) Patient satisfaction surveys
C) Monitoring blood glucose levels over time
D) Follow-up appointments for direct observation

Question 72: In the context of therapeutic communication, which approach should a nurse take when dealing with a patient from a different cultural background who is reluctant to express pain?
A) Accept the patient's reluctance without further inquiry
B) Use culturally sensitive pain assessment tools
C) Encourage the patient to express pain using familiar medical terminology
D) Rely on non-verbal cues alone for pain assessment

Question 73: Maria, a 40-year-old female with no significant medical history, wants to adopt a healthier lifestyle to prevent chronic diseases. Which primary prevention strategy should be prioritized?
A) Initiating annual mammograms starting at age 40.
B) Encouraging her to receive an annual influenza vaccination.
C) Advising her to follow a balanced diet low in saturated fats and high in fiber.
D) Recommending she undergo regular blood glucose screening.

Question 74: Emily, a 35-year-old patient with a history of peptic ulcer disease, is prescribed NSAIDs for chronic pain management. What should be the primary consideration to minimize adverse effects?
A) Prescribing a proton pump inhibitor concurrently
B) Monitoring blood pressure regularly
C) Advising increased fluid intake
D) Scheduling regular liver function tests

Question 75: When initiating a consult for a patient with complex medical needs, which is the most critical first step to ensure effective interdisciplinary collaboration?
A) Identifying the primary care physician
B) Reviewing the patient's complete medical history
C) Clarifying the specific question or need for the consult
D) Scheduling a multidisciplinary team meeting

Question 76: In creating a nursing care plan for a patient with chronic heart failure, which intervention should be prioritized to prevent hospital readmissions?
A) Educating the patient on medication adherence
B) Scheduling regular follow-up appointments
C) Implementing dietary modifications
D) Encouraging daily physical activity

Question 77: Which screening tool is most appropriate for identifying alcohol use disorder in a medical-surgical patient?
A) CAGE Questionnaire
B) AUDIT-C
C) CIWA-Ar
D) T-ACE

Question 78: Which screening method is recommended for lung cancer detection in a high-risk population, such as long-term smokers aged 55-80?
A) Chest X-ray annually
B) Low-dose computed tomography (LDCT) annually
C) Sputum cytology annually

D) MRI of the chest annually

Question 79: When conducting a psychosocial assessment, which factor is most critical in understanding a patient's coping mechanisms?
A) Social support network
B) Financial status
C) Physical health
D) Employment history

Question 80: In a patient with congestive heart failure, which nursing diagnosis should be prioritized to ensure optimal patient outcomes?
A) Activity Intolerance
B) Fluid Volume Excess
C) Impaired Gas Exchange
D) Decreased Cardiac Output

Question 81: During discharge planning for Ms. Garcia, who underwent hip replacement surgery, her family expresses concerns about her mobility at home. How should you address their concerns to ensure patient- and family-centered care?
A) Reassure them that she will adapt over time.
B) Provide them with contact information for physical therapy services.
C) Discuss potential home modifications and safety measures.
D) Suggest hiring a private caregiver temporarily.

Question 82: During a review of systems, which symptom is most indicative of a potential cardiovascular issue?
A) Persistent cough
B) Chest pain on exertion
C) Frequent headaches
D) Unexplained weight loss

Question 83: During the evaluation phase of patient teaching in medical-surgical nursing, which barrier most commonly hinders accurate assessment of patient understanding?
A) Nurse's time constraints
B) Patient's fear or anxiety
C) Use of medical jargon by the nurse
D) Patient's literacy level

Question 84: Mrs. Smith, a 65-year-old patient with chronic heart failure (CHF), is being discharged from the hospital. The nurse is developing a self-management plan to prevent readmission. Which component of the plan is most critical for Mrs. Smith's successful self-management at home?
A) Daily weight monitoring
B) Weekly telehealth check-ins
C) Monthly medication reviews
D) Quarterly cardiac rehabilitation sessions

Question 85: In assessing a patient's cognitive status, which test is most appropriate for evaluating executive function?
A) Mini-Mental State Examination (MMSE)
B) Glasgow Coma Scale (GCS)
C) Trail Making Test Part B
D) Rancho Los Amigos Scale

Question 86: Nurse Sarah is conducting a physical assessment on Mrs. Lee, a 55-year-old female presenting with generalized weakness and fatigue. Upon auscultation, she notes a systolic murmur best heard at the second right intercostal space. What is the most likely diagnosis?
A) Mitral valve prolapse
B) Aortic stenosis
C) Tricuspid regurgitation
D) Pulmonary hypertension

Question 87: When delegating tasks to unlicensed assistive personnel (UAP), which principle must the medical-surgical nurse prioritize?
A) Ensuring the UAP has completed similar tasks before
B) Confirming that the task is within the UAP's job description
C) Assessing the complexity of the patient's condition
D) Verifying that the UAP has received recent training

Question 88: Maria, a 45-year-old patient recovering from abdominal surgery, has a nursing care plan focused on preventing postoperative complications. Which outcome demonstrates effective prevention?
A) Maria will ambulate in the hallway twice daily.
B) Maria's incision site will show no signs of infection within one week.
C) Maria will perform deep breathing exercises hourly.
D) Maria's pain level will be managed at or below a score of 4 out of 10.

Question 89: During psychosocial assessment of a patient with suspected opioid use disorder, which factor should be prioritized to determine the risk of overdose?
A) Duration of opioid use
B) Frequency of opioid use
C) History of previous overdose
D) Concurrent use of benzodiazepines

Question 90: According to recognized theories, which approach is most likely to foster sustained self-management behaviors in patients?
A) Educating patients about their condition and treatment options
B) Involving family members in the care plan
C) Setting specific, achievable goals with the patient
D) Providing continuous professional monitoring

Question 91: Ms. Davis, a 45-year-old female, presents with jaundice and abdominal pain. Her liver function tests reveal elevated bilirubin levels and abnormal liver enzymes. Which imaging study should be conducted next to evaluate her condition?
A) Abdominal ultrasound
B) Magnetic resonance imaging (MRI)
C) Computed tomography (CT) scan
D) Hepatobiliary iminodiacetic acid (HIDA) scan

Question 92: In assessing a patient with suspected acute pancreatitis, which laboratory test is most indicative of this condition?
A) Serum amylase
B) Serum lipase
C) Liver function tests (LFTs)
D) Complete blood count (CBC)

Question 93: Which diagnostic test is considered the gold standard for confirming a diagnosis of pulmonary embolism?
A) Chest X-ray
B) D-dimer test
C) Ventilation-perfusion (V/Q) scan
D) Computed Tomography Pulmonary Angiography (CTPA)

Question 94: Maria, a nurse, is educating a newly diagnosed hypertensive patient, David, about lifestyle modifications. Which teaching strategy best demonstrates the use of effective communication skills?
A) Providing David with pamphlets on hypertension management

B) Using teach-back method to confirm David's understanding
C) Giving David a list of dietary restrictions
D) Scheduling a follow-up appointment in one month

Question 95: In a patient presenting with confusion, muscle weakness, and an ECG showing a prolonged QT interval, which electrolyte imbalance should be suspected?
A) Hypokalemia
B) Hypocalcemia
C) Hypermagnesemia
D) Hyperphosphatemia

Question 96: Mrs. Smith, an 82-year-old woman with mild cognitive impairment, is struggling with bathing independently. What is the best approach to ensure her safety while promoting her autonomy?
A) Supervising her closely during the entire bathing process
B) Installing a walk-in shower and providing a shower chair
C) Bathing her entirely yourself to prevent any accidents
D) Limiting her baths to once a week to reduce risk

Question 97: Nurse James is preparing an educational plan for Mr. Lee, who has expressed difficulty in understanding medical concepts through reading alone but finds it easier when he can discuss them in person or hear explanations from others. What is Mr. Lee's primary learning preference?
A) Visual
B) Auditory
C) Kinesthetic
D) Read/Write

Question 98: Which of the following interventions is most effective in reducing the risk of postoperative surgical site infections (SSIs) in patients undergoing abdominal surgery?
A) Administering prophylactic antibiotics within 60 minutes before incision
B) Maintaining normothermia during the perioperative period
C) Using chlorhexidine-alcohol for preoperative skin antisepsis
D) Ensuring tight glucose control in diabetic patients

Question 99: During the night shift, Nurse Lee notices that Mr. Thompson, who is on high doses of opioids for pain management, appears overly sedated and has shallow breathing. What should be Nurse Lee's immediate action?
A) Call the physician immediately
B) Administer naloxone as per protocol
C) Decrease the opioid dosage
D) Increase monitoring frequency

Question 100: In the evaluation phase of nursing care planning, which skill is essential for assessing patient outcomes accurately?
A) Critical thinking
B) Documentation accuracy
C) Patient interviewing techniques
D) Clinical judgment

Question 101: Which of the following is most critical to assess during the initial health history collection for a patient with a chronic illness?
A) Family medical history
B) Current medications
C) Past surgical history
D) Social history

Question 102: Jane, a 65-year-old patient with hypertension, has been prescribed warfarin. She enjoys eating green leafy vegetables daily. What should the nurse advise Jane regarding her diet?
A) Increase the intake of green leafy vegetables to enhance the effectiveness of warfarin.
B) Maintain a consistent intake of green leafy vegetables to avoid fluctuations in INR levels.
C) Completely eliminate green leafy vegetables from her diet to prevent any interaction with warfarin.
D) Consume green leafy vegetables only occasionally to minimize the risk of interaction with warfarin.

Question 103: For a patient with chronic obstructive pulmonary disease (COPD), which nursing diagnosis should be prioritized to prevent complications?
A) Ineffective Breathing Pattern
B) Risk for Infection
C) Activity Intolerance
D) Imbalanced Nutrition: Less than Body Requirements

Question 104: Ms. Lee, a 60-year-old female with chronic obstructive pulmonary disease (COPD), has been hospitalized due to an acute exacerbation. Upon discharge, what should be prioritized in her discharge education?
A) Instruction on proper inhaler technique.
B) Information on smoking cessation programs.
C) Education on recognizing early signs of exacerbation.
D) Guidance on physical activity limitations.

Question 105: A 65-year-old patient named Mr. Johnson presents with acute abdominal pain and a history of diverticulitis. During the physical assessment, you note guarding and rebound tenderness in the lower left quadrant. Which diagnostic skill is most critical to further evaluate his condition?
A) Percussion
B) Auscultation
C) Palpation
D) Inspection

Question 106: Which of the following strategies is most effective for enhancing self-management in patients with chronic illnesses according to contemporary research?
A) Providing detailed written instructions
B) Regular follow-up phone calls by healthcare providers
C) Utilizing digital health interventions like mobile apps
D) Encouraging peer support group participation

Question 107: During a multidisciplinary team meeting, Nurse Jane is advocating for her patient, Mr. Smith, who has complex medical needs. The team is considering a new treatment plan. Which of the following actions best demonstrates Nurse Jane's professional role in this scenario?
A) Presenting evidence-based research to support the proposed treatment plan.
B) Agreeing with the physician's recommendation without questioning it.
C) Delegating the decision-making process to another nurse.
D) Focusing solely on Mr. Smith's emotional well-being during the discussion.

Question 108: Sarah, a 55-year-old patient with hypertension, has been prescribed lisinopril. She also takes ibuprofen regularly for chronic back pain. What adverse effect should the nurse be most concerned about due to this drug-drug interaction?
A) Hyperkalemia
B) Hypotension
C) Renal impairment
D) Gastrointestinal bleeding

Question 109: Mr. Lewis, a 72-year-old man with a

history of hypertension and diabetes, presents with difficulty in performing daily tasks and frequent forgetfulness. The nurse decides to use the Montreal Cognitive Assessment (MoCA). What specific cognitive domain does the MoCA test that is not covered by the MMSE?
A) Language
B) Attention
C) Executive function
D) Memory recall

Question 110: Which electrolyte imbalance is commonly associated with prolonged nasogastric suctioning?
A) Hyperkalemia
B) Hypocalcemia
C) Hypokalemia
D) Hypernatremia

Question 111: In assessing potential drug interactions, which enzyme system is most commonly involved in metabolizing medications?
A) Cytochrome P450
B) Renin-Angiotensin System
C) Sodium-Potassium Pump
D) Glutathione S-transferase

Question 112: Nurse Sarah discovers that her colleague, Nurse Mike, has been documenting patient care inaccurately to cover up medication errors. What is Nurse Sarah's most ethical course of action?
A) Confront Nurse Mike privately about the inaccuracies.
B) Report Nurse Mike's behavior to the nursing supervisor immediately.
C) Correct the documentation errors herself without informing anyone.
D) Ignore the situation as it is not her responsibility.

Question 113: Which diagnostic test is most appropriate for confirming a suspected pulmonary embolism in a patient with sudden onset dyspnea and chest pain?
A) Chest X-ray
B) Electrocardiogram (ECG)
C) D-dimer assay
D) CT pulmonary angiography

Question 114: Maria, a 58-year-old patient who recently underwent colorectal surgery, reports new-onset diarrhea and abdominal cramping on postoperative day seven. She has been on broad-spectrum antibiotics since her surgery. What should be the nurse's priority action?
A) Discontinue all antibiotics immediately.
B) Collect a stool sample for Clostridium difficile testing.
C) Increase fluid intake to prevent dehydration.
D) Administer antidiarrheal medication as prescribed.

Question 115: In the context of postoperative care, which skill is essential for early detection of complications such as hemorrhage or infection?
A) Monitoring blood pressure trends
B) Inspecting surgical site for signs of infection
C) Measuring body temperature regularly
D) Assessing pain levels frequently

Question 116: In evidence-based practice, which type of research study provides the highest level of evidence for determining best practices?
A) Randomized controlled trials (RCTs)
B) Cohort studies
C) Case-control studies
D) Expert opinion

Question 117: Ms. Lee, a 45-year-old immunocompromised patient, is undergoing chemotherapy. Which strategy should be prioritized to minimize her risk of infection during her hospital stay?
A) Regularly disinfecting all surfaces in her room
B) Restricting visitors to immediate family members only
C) Implementing strict neutropenic precautions
D) Providing her with a high-protein diet

Question 118: Mrs. Lee, an elderly patient with chronic heart failure, has her son as her primary caregiver. He feels overwhelmed and uncertain about managing her medications. What should be your priority action as a nurse to support them?
A) Provide detailed written instructions on medication administration.
B) Arrange for a home health nurse to visit regularly.
C) Offer to demonstrate proper medication administration techniques.
D) Encourage him to attend a caregiver support group.

Question 119: Which principle is most crucial in ensuring effective patient- and family-centered care in a medical-surgical setting?
A) Respect and dignity
B) Information sharing
C) Collaboration
D) Participation

Question 120: A patient's laboratory results reveal a serum calcium level of 7.8 mg/dL. Which clinical sign should the nurse assess first?
A) Chvostek's sign
B) Trousseau's sign
C) Deep tendon reflexes
D) Babinski's reflex

Question 121: Which model is widely used for integrating evidence-based practice into nursing care and involves steps such as assessing the need for change, linking problems with interventions, synthesizing best evidence, designing practice changes, implementing changes, and evaluating outcomes?
A) The Iowa Model of Evidence-Based Practice
B) The Stetler Model of Research Utilization
C) The Johns Hopkins Nursing Evidence-Based Practice Model
D) The ACE Star Model of Knowledge Transformation

Question 122: A medical-surgical unit is implementing a new electronic health record (EHR) system. Jane, a nurse on this unit, notices that some team members are struggling with using the new system efficiently. What should Jane do to promote successful interdisciplinary collaboration during this transition?
A) Offer individual training sessions for those struggling.
B) Organize regular team meetings to discuss challenges and share tips.
C) Report inefficiencies to hospital administration for further action.
D) Assign tech-savvy staff members to assist those having difficulties.

Question 123: Which approach is considered most comprehensive in promoting smoking cessation among adults?
A) Nicotine replacement therapy (NRT)
B) Behavioral counseling
C) Pharmacotherapy combined with behavioral counseling
D) Public health campaigns

Question 124: Nurse Emily is caring for a post-operative patient, Mr. Johnson, who has undergone abdominal surgery. She needs to implement a pain management

plan that minimizes opioid use due to the patient's history of substance abuse. Which intervention should she prioritize?

A) Administering scheduled acetaminophen and NSAIDs.
B) Utilizing patient-controlled analgesia (PCA) with low-dose opioids.
C) Incorporating non-pharmacological methods such as guided imagery and relaxation techniques.
D) Prescribing a combination of acetaminophen and low-dose opioids as needed.

Question 125: When educating diabetic patients about foot care, which recommendation is most critical to prevent complications?

A) Soaking feet daily in warm water
B) Walking barefoot at home
C) Inspecting feet daily for injuries
D) Using over-the-counter corn removers

ANSWER WITH DETAILED EXPLANATION SET [3]

Question 1: Correct Answer: C) Demonstration/return demonstration

Rationale: Demonstration/return demonstration is the most effective method for evaluating a patient's understanding of self-care instructions. It allows the nurse to directly observe the patient performing the task, ensuring they have comprehended and can apply the instructions correctly. While verbal questioning (B) and written tests (A) can assess knowledge, they do not confirm practical application. Patient self-report (D) relies on subjective feedback, which may not be accurate. Thus, return demonstration provides concrete evidence of learning.

Question 2: Correct Answer: B) Encouraging Jane to express her feelings and concerns

Rationale: Encouraging Jane to express her feelings and concerns (Option B) aligns with the principles of therapeutic communication by fostering an open environment where she feels heard and supported. This approach helps build trust and allows for a deeper understanding of her emotional state. While providing detailed medical information (Option A), referring to a support group (Option C), and scheduling follow-ups (Option D) are important, they do not directly address her immediate emotional needs, which are crucial for effective communication and patient-centered care.

Question 3: Correct Answer: B) Erik Erikson's Psychosocial Development Theory

Rationale: Erikson's theory focuses on resolving conflicts at various stages, such as trust vs. mistrust and identity vs. role confusion, to foster healthy psychological development. Piaget's theory centers on cognitive development stages, Freud's theory addresses psychosexual stages, and Kohlberg's theory involves moral reasoning stages. The key difference is that Erikson emphasizes psychosocial conflict resolution as crucial for adult psychological health.

Question 4: Correct Answer: D) Reviewing refill records over several months

Rationale: Reviewing refill records over several months is most appropriate for evaluating long-term retention of medication adherence education. This method provides objective data on whether patients continue to adhere to their medication regimen over time. Immediate post-instruction testing (A) only assesses short-term recall. Scheduled follow-up phone calls (B) rely on self-reported adherence, which may be inaccurate. Periodic in-person assessments (C), while useful, may not capture ongoing adherence as effectively as refill records do over an extended period.

Question 5: Correct Answer: B) Randomized controlled trials

Rationale: Randomized controlled trials (RCTs) are considered the gold standard in evidence-based practice due to their rigorous methodology that minimizes bias and establishes causality. Expert opinion (A), while valuable, lacks empirical testing. Case studies (C), though detailed, often lack generalizability. Clinical experience (D), although important, is subjective and less reliable than RCTs. RCTs provide high-quality evidence that supports clinical decision-making with robust data.

Question 6: Correct Answer: B) To provide clotting factors and correct coagulopathies

Rationale: Fresh frozen plasma (FFP) is administered to provide essential clotting factors and correct coagulopathies in patients with active bleeding. Increasing hemoglobin levels rapidly (Option A) is achieved through red blood cell transfusions, not FFP. Expanding intravascular volume quickly (Option C) can be managed with crystalloids or colloids. Supplying platelets for clot formation (Option D) requires platelet transfusions specifically. Thus, FFP's primary purpose is to address deficiencies in clotting factors, making Option B correct.

Question 7: Correct Answer: A) Elevated jugular venous pressure (JVP)

Rationale: Elevated JVP is a direct indicator of increased central venous pressure and fluid overload in heart failure. Clear lung sounds (B), while normal, do not indicate worsening heart failure as they do not reflect fluid status in this context. Bradycardia (C), although it can occur in advanced heart failure, is less indicative than JVP elevation. Decreased urinary output (D), while relevant, is less specific compared to JVP for immediate assessment of worsening heart failure.

Question 8: Correct Answer: D) Visuospatial disorientation

Rationale: The clock-drawing test effectively identifies visuospatial disorientation by requiring patients to accurately represent numbers and hands on a clock face. This task assesses spatial planning and visual perception abilities. While executive dysfunction (B) can influence performance due to planning requirements, visuospatial disorientation is more directly evaluated by this test. Language deficits (A) and short-term memory loss (C) are less relevant in this context since they do not directly affect clock-drawing ability.

Question 9: Correct Answer: B) Smoking cessation

Rationale: Smoking cessation is the most effective intervention for slowing COPD progression, as it directly addresses the primary cause of the disease. Long-term oxygen therapy (A), while beneficial for hypoxemic patients, does not alter disease progression. Pulmonary rehabilitation (C) improves quality of life and exercise capacity but does not slow progression. Inhaled corticosteroids (D), though helpful in reducing exacerbations, do not impact the underlying decline in lung function caused by ongoing smoking. Contemporary research strongly supports smoking cessation as the cornerstone of COPD management.

Question 10: Correct Answer: A) Increased risk of bleeding

Rationale: Ciprofloxacin can inhibit the metabolism of warfarin, leading to increased levels of warfarin and a higher risk of bleeding. Decreased efficacy of warfarin (Option B) would occur if an inducer was used instead. Increased risk of thrombosis (Option C) would result from decreased warfarin levels, not increased levels. Ciprofloxacin's efficacy (Option D) is not significantly affected by warfarin.

Question 11: Correct Answer: B) Increased B-type natriuretic peptide (BNP)

Rationale: BNP levels increase with ventricular stretch and volume overload, directly correlating with heart failure severity and worsening condition. Elevated serum creatinine indicates renal impairment but isn't specific to heart failure progression. Low hemoglobin can contribute to symptoms but doesn't directly indicate heart failure status. Elevated liver enzymes may suggest hepatic congestion secondary to heart failure but are less specific than BNP levels for assessing cardiac function deterioration. Thus, BNP is the most reliable marker among these options for worsening heart failure.

Question 12: Correct Answer: B) Arterial blood gas (ABG)

Rationale: ABG analysis is the gold standard for evaluating acid-base balance as it provides direct measurements of pH, PaCO2, and HCO3-. Serum lactate levels can indicate lactic acidosis but do not provide a complete acid-base picture. Serum bicarbonate levels are part of ABG analysis but are insufficient alone. Urine pH reflects renal compensation but does not diagnose systemic acid-base disorders comprehensively.

Question 13: Correct Answer: A) Tuberculosis

Rationale: Tuberculosis (TB) should be considered due to its hallmark symptoms of persistent cough, night sweats, and unintentional weight loss. Asthma (B), while causing cough, does not typically present with night sweats or significant weight loss. COPD (C), although chronic and causing cough, usually involves sputum production and dyspnea rather than night sweats or weight loss. GERD (D), primarily affecting the gastrointestinal tract, may cause cough due to aspiration but lacks systemic symptoms like night sweats or significant weight loss seen in TB cases. Prioritizing TB ensures timely diagnosis and treatment of this infectious disease.

Question 14: Correct Answer: B) A licensed practical nurse (LPN)

Rationale: LPNs have the training and licensure required to perform sterile dressing changes independently, making them suitable for this delegation. CNAs do not have the necessary training for complex wound care involving sterile techniques. While an RN could perform the task, it would be more efficient to delegate it to an LPN so that the RN can focus on more critical aspects of patient care. Student nurses under direct supervision are not ideal as they are still learning and may not yet be proficient in sterile techniques.

Question 15: Correct Answer: C) Evaluating verbal response to questions

Rationale: Evaluating verbal response to questions is key in determining the level of consciousness, as it directly assesses cognitive function and awareness. Checking pupil response to light (Option A), assessing motor response to stimuli (Option B), and monitoring vital signs (Option D) are important but do not provide as comprehensive an assessment of consciousness as verbal responses.

Question 16: Correct Answer: A) Encourage deep breathing exercises

Rationale: The ABG results indicate respiratory acidosis, likely due to hypoventilation. Encouraging deep breathing increases alveolar ventilation, helping to expel CO2 and correct acidosis. Intubation (B) is considered if less invasive measures fail. Sodium bicarbonate (C) is used in metabolic acidosis, not respiratory acidosis. Increasing oxygen flow rate (D) does not address CO2 retention, the primary issue here.

Question 17: Correct Answer: B) Crackles heard at the lung bases during auscultation

Rationale: Crackles at the lung bases are a hallmark sign of pulmonary congestion due to left-sided heart failure. This occurs as fluid backs up into the lungs. Bilateral pitting edema (A) and hepatomegaly (D) are more commonly associated with right-sided heart failure. Jugular venous distention (C) is also indicative of right-sided heart failure or severe biventricular failure. Therefore, crackles are more specific to early left-sided heart failure.

Question 18: Correct Answer: B) Administering prescribed analgesics as per pain assessment

Rationale: Administering analgesics based on pain assessment ensures effective pain management tailored to the patient's needs. Option A aids in recovery but does not directly address severe pain. Option C might provide some relief but is not sufficient for severe pain. Option D is beneficial but should complement pharmacological interventions rather than replace them.

Question 19: Correct Answer: C) Acupuncture

Rationale: Contemporary research supports acupuncture as an effective CAM practice for reducing anxiety in preoperative patients. Studies have shown that acupuncture can modulate the autonomic nervous system, reducing stress and anxiety levels. Aromatherapy (A), while beneficial, lacks consistent evidence for significant anxiety reduction. Reiki (B) has limited empirical support for preoperative anxiety. Yoga (D), though effective for chronic anxiety, may not be practical in a preoperative setting. Therefore, acupuncture is the most evidence-based option among those listed.

Question 20: Correct Answer: D) Use multimedia tools to explain lifestyle modifications.

Rationale: Using multimedia tools can enhance understanding by providing visual and auditory learning aids, making complex information more accessible and engaging for Mr. Lee. While A provides necessary information, it may not be as engaging or comprehensive. B is useful but focuses only on one aspect (exercise). C addresses stress but not other critical lifestyle changes like diet or exercise comprehensively. Therefore, D offers a holistic approach that can cater to various learning styles and improve retention of information.

Question 21: Correct Answer: A) Hourly rounding by nursing staff

Rationale: Hourly rounding by nursing staff is the most effective intervention as it proactively addresses patient needs, reduces anxiety, and allows for timely assistance, thus significantly reducing fall risk. While bed alarms (Option B) and non-slip socks (Option C) are useful, they are reactive rather than proactive measures. The fall risk assessment tool (Option D) helps identify high-risk patients but does not directly prevent falls. Research supports that consistent hourly rounding leads to better patient outcomes and safety.

Question 22: Correct Answer: B) Fluid restriction

Rationale: Fluid restriction is the most appropriate initial treatment for hyponatremia in a patient with heart failure, as it helps to reduce fluid overload and improve sodium concentration. Hypertonic saline (A) is typically reserved for severe symptomatic cases. Loop diuretics (C) may exacerbate hyponatremia by increasing water loss more than sodium loss. Sodium supplementation (D) is not effective in dilutional hyponatremia caused by fluid overload.

Question 23: Correct Answer: B) Verifying that all information provided is understandable and comprehensive.

Rationale: Advocacy for informed consent centers on ensuring that patients fully understand their treatment options, risks, and benefits, enabling them to make informed decisions (B). Simply obtaining signed forms (A), while necessary, does not ensure comprehension. Encouraging agreement with treatments (C) undermines autonomy. Keeping family members informed (D), though important, is secondary to ensuring patient understanding. Comprehensive and understandable information respects ethical principles and empowers patients in their healthcare decisions, embodying true advocacy.

Question 24: Correct Answer: B) Osteoporosis-related fractures

Rationale: Long-term use of proton pump inhibitors (PPIs) can lead to decreased calcium absorption, increasing the risk of osteoporosis-related fractures. While renal failure, hepatic encephalopathy, and myocardial infarction are serious conditions that may be linked to various medications or underlying diseases, they are not commonly associated with long-term PPI use. The risk of osteoporosis-related fractures is well-documented in patients on prolonged PPI therapy due to impaired calcium absorption.

Question 25: Correct Answer: A) Fluid restriction

Rationale: SIADH causes water retention and dilutional hyponatremia; thus, fluid restriction is the primary treatment to prevent further dilution of sodium. Administration of isotonic saline (B) or hypotonic saline (C) could worsen hyponatremia by increasing fluid volume without correcting the underlying issue. Increased oral salt intake (D), while theoretically increasing sodium levels, does not address the water retention problem and can be less effective than fluid restriction. Understanding these treatment strategies ensures proper management of electrolyte imbalances in SIADH patients.

Question 26: Correct Answer: B) Broca's aphasia

Rationale: Broca's aphasia results from damage to Broca's area in the frontal lobe, affecting speech production while preserving comprehension. Mrs. Johnson's symptoms of right-sided weakness and facial droop suggest a stroke affecting the left hemisphere where Broca's area is located. Global aphasia (A) involves severe impairment in both comprehension and production. Wernicke's aphasia (C) affects comprehension with fluent but nonsensical speech. Anomic aphasia (D) involves difficulty finding words but not articulation or comprehension.

Question 27: Correct Answer: A) Observing Mr. Smith as he performs a simulated meal preparation.
Rationale: Observing Mr. Smith performing a simulated meal preparation provides direct and objective evidence of his functional abilities, particularly fine motor skills and coordination. Self-report questionnaires (B) can be subjective and may not accurately reflect current abilities. Reviewing medical records (C) gives historical data but may not represent current status. Family interviews (D) provide valuable insights but are second-hand and can be biased or inaccurate.
Question 28: Correct Answer: A) Spinach
Rationale: Spinach is high in vitamin K, which can counteract the anticoagulant effects of warfarin, making it less effective. Grapefruit is known to interact with other medications but not specifically with warfarin. Bananas and apples do not have significant interactions with warfarin. The key difference lies in the vitamin K content, which directly impacts warfarin's efficacy.
Question 29: Correct Answer: A) Trail Making Test Part B
Rationale: The Trail Making Test Part B specifically assesses executive function, including task switching and attention, which are often affected in traumatic brain injury. The Stroop Test also evaluates executive function but focuses more on inhibitory control rather than task switching. WAIS measures overall intelligence and includes some executive function components but is broader in scope. Mini-Cog screens for dementia rather than specific executive function deficits.
Question 30: Correct Answer: B) Heart rate of 120 beats per minute
Rationale: Tachycardia (heart rate of 120 bpm) is an early compensatory mechanism in hypovolemic shock, as the body attempts to maintain cardiac output. Blood pressure (90/60 mmHg) may remain normal initially due to compensatory vasoconstriction. Respiratory rate (22 breaths per minute) can be elevated for various reasons and is less specific. Reduced urine output (25 mL/hour) indicates decreased renal perfusion but occurs later in the progression of shock. Therefore, tachycardia is the earliest indicator among the options provided.
Question 31: Correct Answer: D) VARK Model
Rationale: The VARK Model emphasizes tailoring instructional methods to individual learning styles—Visual, Auditory, Reading/Writing, and Kinesthetic—ensuring that educational interventions are more effective. Behaviorist Theory (A) focuses on observable behaviors rather than internal processes like learning preferences. Cognitive Load Theory (B), while relevant in managing cognitive resources during learning, does not specifically address individual styles. Gardner's Multiple Intelligences Theory (C), though recognizing diverse intelligences, does not provide a specific framework for matching instructional methods to these intelligences as directly as the VARK Model does.
Question 32: Correct Answer: B) Notify the healthcare provider immediately.
Rationale: Immediate notification of the healthcare provider is essential for prompt evaluation and intervention to prevent sepsis. Administering analgesics (Option A) addresses pain but not infection control. Warm compresses (Option C) could worsen an infection by increasing local blood flow and spreading bacteria. Encouraging ambulation (Option D) improves circulation but does not address infection directly. Timely medical intervention can prevent systemic infection progression.
Question 33: Correct Answer: B) Social isolation
Rationale: Social isolation is a primary barrier for elderly patients like Sarah in managing chronic conditions. It impacts their ability to adhere to self-care instructions and attend follow-up appointments due to lack of support and encouragement. Cognitive impairment could be a factor but would need assessment; financial constraints and transportation issues are secondary concerns that may result from or be exacerbated by social isolation.
Question 34: Correct Answer: A) Confusion Assessment Method for the ICU (CAM-ICU)
Rationale: CAM-ICU is designed specifically to detect delirium in critically ill patients by assessing acute onset or fluctuating course, inattention, disorganized thinking, and altered level of consciousness. RASS measures sedation and agitation levels but does not diagnose delirium. GCS evaluates overall consciousness but lacks specificity for delirium. Mini-Cog screens for cognitive impairment but is less suited for acute settings like ICUs. Therefore, CAM-ICU remains the gold standard for early delirium detection in critically ill patients.
Question 35: Correct Answer: C) Demonstrate how to use her glucometer and insulin pen.
Rationale: Demonstrating the use of essential tools like a glucometer and insulin pen provides practical, hands-on learning that directly addresses Mrs. Smith's immediate needs, reducing anxiety through competence building. While joining a support group (A), receiving written instructions (B), or discussing lifestyle changes (D) are beneficial, they do not immediately equip her with the skills necessary for daily self-management as effectively as direct demonstration does.
Question 36: Correct Answer: D) Performing early coronary angiography
Rationale: Early coronary angiography is essential as it allows for immediate visualization and treatment of the occluded artery, significantly improving outcomes by restoring perfusion. While administering oxygen (A), initiating IV nitroglycerin (B), and providing aspirin (C) are important supportive measures, they do not directly address the occlusion. Early reperfusion through angiography has been shown in contemporary research to reduce mortality and preserve myocardial function more effectively than these other interventions.
Question 37: Correct Answer: C) Emphysema
Rationale: The increased anteroposterior diameter, often referred to as "barrel chest," is most commonly associated with emphysema, a form of COPD. Emphysema leads to hyperinflation of the lungs and loss of lung elasticity, causing the chest to expand. Pulmonary fibrosis (A) typically results in restrictive lung patterns and does not cause barrel chest. Chronic bronchitis (B), another form of COPD, primarily affects the airways rather than causing significant changes in chest shape. Pneumonia (D) is an acute infection and does not lead to chronic changes like barrel chest.
Question 38: Correct Answer: C) Therapeutic Drug Monitoring (TDM)
Rationale: Therapeutic Drug Monitoring (TDM) is specifically designed to measure drug concentrations in the blood to ensure they are within the therapeutic range, especially for medications with a narrow therapeutic index. This helps in preventing toxicity while ensuring efficacy. While CBC (A), Serum Creatinine (B), and LFTs (D) provide valuable information about overall health and organ function, they do not directly measure drug levels or ensure that they remain within the safe and effective range.
Question 39: Correct Answer: B) Early ambulation
Rationale: Early ambulation is the most effective intervention to prevent postoperative pulmonary complications, such as atelectasis and pneumonia. It promotes lung expansion, increases circulation, and enhances overall recovery. While incentive spirometry (A) and deep breathing exercises (C) are beneficial for lung expansion, they are less effective without the increased circulation provided by ambulation. Prophylactic antibiotics (D) do not address pulmonary complications directly but rather prevent infections. Therefore, early ambulation is the most comprehensive approach.
Question 40: Correct Answer: A) Following the DASH diet
Rationale: The DASH diet is specifically designed to lower blood pressure through dietary changes rich in fruits, vegetables, whole grains, and low-fat dairy products while

reducing sodium intake. This comprehensive approach addresses multiple dietary factors influencing hypertension. Weekly yoga sessions (B), while beneficial for stress reduction, do not directly impact dietary sodium or nutrient intake as effectively as the DASH diet. Limiting alcohol intake to weekends (C), although helpful, does not provide the same broad-spectrum dietary benefits. Taking prescribed medications (D) is essential but should be complemented by dietary changes like those promoted by the DASH diet for optimal control.

Question 41: Correct Answer: B) To correct coagulopathy

Rationale: Fresh frozen plasma (FFP) is primarily used to correct coagulopathy by supplying deficient clotting factors. Increasing red blood cell count (A), providing platelets (C), and treating hypovolemia (D) are not primary functions of FFP. FFP contains clotting factors necessary for proper coagulation, making it essential for patients like John with coagulopathy due to chronic kidney disease.

Question 42: Correct Answer: B) Retinal hemorrhages on fundoscopic examination

Rationale: Retinal hemorrhages observed during fundoscopic examination are indicative of target organ damage due to severe hypertension and suggest a hypertensive crisis. A blood pressure reading of 150/90 mmHg (A), while elevated, is not high enough to indicate a crisis without additional symptoms or findings. Mild ankle edema (C) can be associated with various conditions and is not specific to hypertensive crisis. A heart rate of 100 beats per minute (D), though elevated, does not specifically indicate hypertensive crisis without other critical signs.

Question 43: Correct Answer: C) Delayed capillary refill time

Rationale: Delayed capillary refill time indicates poor perfusion, strongly suggesting PAD. Warm skin around the ulcer (A) is more indicative of infection or inflammation rather than PAD. Bounding pedal pulses (B) are inconsistent with PAD, which typically presents with weak or absent pulses. Increased hair growth on lower extremities (D) is not associated with PAD; rather, hair loss is more common due to poor circulation.

Question 44: Correct Answer: B) Report the incident to the nursing supervisor.

Rationale: Reporting to a nursing supervisor aligns with ethical principles of accountability and patient safety, ensuring proper investigation and corrective action. Option A, while promoting direct communication, may not resolve systemic issues. Option C focuses on documentation but does not address broader ethical concerns. Option D compromises ethical standards by prioritizing team harmony over patient safety and integrity. Reporting ensures transparency and adherence to professional standards.

Question 45: Correct Answer: B) Reduce venous stasis

Rationale: Compression stockings primarily reduce venous stasis by applying pressure to the legs, promoting blood flow back to the heart and preventing clot formation. Increasing arterial blood flow (A) is not their main function. Enhancing lymphatic drainage (C) is a secondary benefit but not the primary purpose. Preventing superficial thrombophlebitis (D), while possible, is not their main objective; they are primarily used to prevent deep vein thrombosis and subsequent emboli.

Question 46: Correct Answer: B) Presenting evidence of Mr. Thompson's readiness for discharge.

Rationale: Effective advocacy requires using evidence-based practice to support patient preferences while ensuring safety and quality care (Option B). Agreeing without presenting evidence (Option A), encouraging against medical advice discharge (Option C), or suggesting an extended stay without discussion (Option D) do not adequately support or respect Mr. Thompson's wishes or clinical readiness based on objective data and collaborative decision-making principles in nursing ethics and professional roles.

Question 47: Correct Answer: C) Carvedilol

Rationale: Carvedilol, a beta-blocker, reduces mortality and morbidity in chronic heart failure by blocking neurohormonal activation, particularly sympathetic nervous system activity. Furosemide (A) is a diuretic used for symptom control but does not impact long-term survival. Digoxin (B) improves symptoms but does not significantly affect mortality. Spironolactone (D), while beneficial in reducing morbidity and mortality due to its aldosterone antagonism, does not have as broad an effect on neurohormonal pathways as carvedilol.

Question 48: Correct Answer: C) Administer intravenous normal saline

Rationale: The initial management for hypercalcemia often involves administering intravenous normal saline (C), which helps promote calcium excretion through the kidneys by increasing urine output. Intravenous bisphosphonates (A) are used but not as an initial step; they take longer to act. Increasing oral calcium intake (B) and restricting dietary calcium (D) do not address the acute need to lower serum calcium levels quickly.

Question 49: Correct Answer: B) Reduce sodium intake.

Rationale: Reducing sodium intake is essential in managing fluid retention because sodium promotes water retention, exacerbating heart failure symptoms. Increasing potassium intake (A) can be beneficial but must be monitored due to potential hyperkalemia. Limiting protein consumption (C) is not directly related to fluid management. Increasing calcium intake (D) does not influence fluid balance and is more relevant to bone health.

Question 50: Correct Answer: C) Engaging her in a guided imagery session

Rationale: Guided imagery is an evidence-based non-pharmacologic intervention that helps reduce anxiety and promote relaxation by encouraging patients to visualize calming scenes. Unlike watching television (A), which can be passive and less engaging, guided imagery (C) actively involves the patient's mental focus. A puzzle book (B) may be too mentally demanding for someone experiencing restlessness, and magazines (D) might not capture sufficient attention or provide the same level of relaxation as guided imagery.

Question 51: Correct Answer: A) Use a numerical pain scale

Rationale: Using a numerical pain scale is essential for quantifying the patient's subjective pain experience, allowing for accurate assessment and appropriate intervention. While performing a physical examination (Option B) and evaluating vital signs (Option D) are important, they do not directly quantify pain. Administering analgesics immediately (Option C) without proper assessment could lead to inappropriate dosing or masking underlying issues.

Question 52: Correct Answer: B) Wernicke's area

Rationale: Wernicke's area, located in the left temporal lobe, is responsible for language comprehension. Damage to this area results in Wernicke's aphasia, characterized by fluent but nonsensical speech and difficulty understanding spoken language. Broca's area (A) affects speech production, leading to non-fluent aphasia. The occipital lobe (C) is primarily involved in visual processing, and the cerebellum (D) coordinates voluntary movements and balance, not language comprehension.

Question 53: Correct Answer: B) Consider the patient's renal function before selecting an opioid.

Rationale: Renal function is crucial when initiating opioid therapy, especially in elderly patients, as impaired renal function can lead to accumulation of the drug or its metabolites, increasing the risk of toxicity. Starting with a high dose (A) can cause overdose and adverse effects. Combining opioids with NSAIDs (C) may enhance analgesia but doesn't address safety concerns specific to opioids. While monitoring for gastrointestinal side effects (D) is important, it is not the primary concern when starting opioids; renal function takes precedence due to its impact on drug clearance.

Question 54: Correct Answer: C) Orthopnea

Rationale: Orthopnea, or difficulty breathing when lying flat, is most indicative of left-sided heart failure due to pulmonary congestion. Peripheral edema and jugular vein distention are more commonly associated with right-sided heart failure. Hepatomegaly can occur in both types but is more prominent in right-sided heart failure. The key difference is that orthopnea directly results from fluid accumulation in the lungs, which is characteristic of left-sided heart failure.

Question 55: Correct Answer: C) Adolescence

Rationale: Havighurst identifies adolescence as the period where individuals achieve emotional independence from parents and prepare for marriage and family life. Infancy and Early Childhood focus on basic physical skills, Middle Childhood emphasizes developing friendships and academic skills, while Early Adulthood involves establishing a career and starting a family. The correct answer highlights key developmental tasks specific to adolescence, differentiating it from other stages with distinct priorities.

Question 56: Correct Answer: B) Heart Rate

Rationale: Mr. Lee's heart rate (HR) of 58 bpm indicates bradycardia, which could be benign in well-conditioned individuals but warrants further evaluation due to his reported dizziness. His blood pressure (BP), respiratory rate (RR), and oxygen saturation (SpO2) are within normal ranges. The occasional dizziness combined with bradycardia necessitates further investigation to rule out any underlying cardiac issues or other causes.

Question 57: Correct Answer: D) Read/Write

Rationale: Mr. Johnson's preference for reading and taking notes aligns with the read/write learning style, which emphasizes textual information and note-taking as key methods for understanding and retaining information. While visual learners prefer images and diagrams (A), auditory learners benefit from listening (B), and kinesthetic learners engage through hands-on activities (C), none of these align as closely with Mr. Johnson's stated preferences as read/write (D).

Question 58: Correct Answer: B) "Tell me more about what you read and how it makes you feel."

Rationale: Asking Mr. Lee to elaborate on what he read and how it makes him feel (Option B) opens up dialogue, allowing the nurse to address specific concerns and provide accurate information, fostering trust. Simply reassuring him that complications are rare (Option A), dismissing online information (Option C), or shifting focus away from his worries (Option D), does not address his underlying fears effectively or promote open communication.

Question 59: Correct Answer: B) Initiating intravenous fluid replacement

Rationale: The primary intervention for DKA is initiating intravenous fluid replacement to correct dehydration, electrolyte imbalance, and acidosis. Subcutaneous insulin (A) is less effective than intravenous insulin in acute management. Oral glucose (C) is contraindicated as it can exacerbate hyperglycemia. While monitoring blood glucose every hour (D) is essential, it does not directly stabilize the patient without concurrent fluid and insulin therapy.

Question 60: Correct Answer: A) Packed Red Blood Cells (PRBCs)

Rationale: Packed Red Blood Cells (PRBCs) are prioritized to improve oxygen-carrying capacity in acute blood loss situations due to their high concentration of hemoglobin. FFP is primarily used for coagulation factor replacement, whole blood provides both volume and red cells but is less commonly used due to risks of volume overload and transfusion reactions. Platelets are necessary for clotting but do not significantly impact oxygen-carrying capacity. Thus, PRBCs are the optimal choice for improving oxygen transport in acute blood loss.

Question 61: Correct Answer: A) Bradycardia

Rationale: Bradycardia is a component of Cushing's triad (along with hypertension and irregular respirations), indicating increased ICP. Hyperreflexia can be seen in various neurological conditions but is not specific to increased ICP. Hypotension typically does not accompany increased ICP; rather, hypertension does. Mydriasis (pupil dilation) can indicate brain herniation but is less specific than bradycardia when considering Cushing's triad.

Question 62: Correct Answer: A) Unilateral pupil dilation

Rationale: Unilateral pupil dilation (anisocoria), particularly if it is non-reactive to light, can indicate increased intracranial pressure affecting cranial nerve III (oculomotor nerve). This condition can result from brain herniation. Bilateral pupil constriction (B), while abnormal, is less specific for increased ICP and could result from opioid use or pontine hemorrhage. Impaired upward gaze (C) may indicate midbrain lesions but is less immediately concerning than anisocoria for ICP. Loss of corneal reflex (D), involving cranial nerves V and VII, suggests brainstem involvement but does not specifically point to increased ICP like unilateral pupil dilation does.

Question 63: Correct Answer: C) Utilitarianism

Rationale: Utilitarianism emphasizes the outcomes or consequences of actions, aiming for the greatest good for the greatest number. Deontology (A), on the other hand, focuses on duties and rules regardless of outcomes. Virtue ethics (B) centers on moral character rather than specific actions or consequences. Principlism (D) incorporates multiple ethical principles but does not focus solely on outcomes. Utilitarianism is distinct in its consequentialist approach, making it particularly relevant for decisions impacting patient populations.

Question 64: Correct Answer: A) To prevent deep vein thrombosis (DVT)

Rationale: The primary reason for administering prophylactic anticoagulants postoperatively is to prevent deep vein thrombosis (DVT), a common and serious complication. DVT can lead to pulmonary embolism if left untreated. Reducing postoperative pain (B), enhancing wound healing (C), and decreasing infection risk (D) are important but are not directly achieved through anticoagulants. Anticoagulants specifically target thrombus formation by inhibiting clotting factors, thereby preventing DVT effectively.

Question 65: Correct Answer: A) Increased risk of bleeding

Rationale: Amiodarone inhibits the metabolism of Warfarin, significantly increasing its anticoagulant effect and raising the risk of bleeding. Decreased effectiveness would be seen with inducers like Rifampin, not Amiodarone. QT prolongation is a concern with Amiodarone alone or combined with other QT-prolonging drugs, not Warfarin. Reduced heart rate variability is more related to beta-blockers or calcium channel blockers than Warfarin-Amiodarone interaction.

Question 66: Correct Answer: A) Visual

Rationale: Mrs. Thompson's preference for watching videos and looking at diagrams indicates a visual learning style, which involves using visual aids like charts, graphs, and videos to enhance comprehension. Auditory learners (B) benefit from listening to explanations, kinesthetic learners (C) need physical engagement, and read/write learners (D) prefer textual information. Therefore, visual (A) is the most appropriate choice given her preferences.

Question 67: Correct Answer: B) Conducting a one-on-one dietary counseling session

Rationale: Conducting a one-on-one dietary counseling session allows personalized education tailored to Mr. Smith's specific needs, preferences, and lifestyle, thus promoting adherence (B). A list of foods to avoid (A) lacks personalization and engagement. Referring him to a nutritionist (C), while beneficial, may not provide immediate support or tailored advice from the nurse's perspective. Interactive tools like food diaries and apps (D), though helpful for tracking progress, do not replace personalized initial education sessions that build foundational knowledge essential for long-term adherence.

Question 68: Correct Answer: D) Rectal thermometer
Rationale: The rectal thermometer is considered the gold standard for measuring core body temperature, especially in critically ill patients. This method provides a more accurate reflection of internal body temperature compared to oral (A), axillary (B), and tympanic (C) methods, which can be influenced by external factors such as ambient temperature and patient movement. Oral thermometers can be affected by recent intake of hot or cold substances, axillary readings are less reliable due to peripheral vasoconstriction, and tympanic measurements may be inaccurate due to earwax or improper positioning.

Question 69: Correct Answer: A) Pain management issues
Rationale: Pain management issues are a critical barrier in post-surgical recovery. Effective pain control can significantly improve mobility and motivation for physical therapy. While lack of motivation and insufficient therapy sessions are relevant barriers, they often stem from inadequate pain management. Nutritional deficiencies can impact recovery but are not as immediately influential as pain control.

Question 70: Correct Answer: B) Montreal Cognitive Assessment (MoCA)
Rationale: The MoCA is more sensitive than the MMSE in detecting mild cognitive impairment, particularly in early stages. The Clock Drawing Test is useful but less comprehensive, and the Geriatric Depression Scale assesses mood rather than cognition. The MoCA evaluates multiple cognitive domains, providing a thorough assessment that can detect subtle impairments.

Question 71: Correct Answer: A) Pre-test and post-test comparisons
Rationale: Pre-test and post-test comparisons provide a comprehensive assessment by measuring knowledge gained from the education program. They offer quantitative data on what patients knew before and after the intervention. While monitoring blood glucose levels (C) can indicate management effectiveness, it doesn't directly measure learning. Patient satisfaction surveys (B) gauge perception but not knowledge or skills. Follow-up appointments (D) allow for observation but may miss broader educational impacts. Therefore, pre- and post-tests best evaluate learning outcomes.

Question 72: Correct Answer: B) Use culturally sensitive pain assessment tools
Rationale: Using culturally sensitive pain assessment tools helps bridge communication gaps and ensures accurate pain evaluation by considering the patient's cultural context. Accepting reluctance (A), encouraging medical terminology use (C), or relying solely on non-verbal cues (D) may result in underreporting or misinterpretation of pain. Effective therapeutic communication involves adapting assessment methods to align with the patient's cultural norms and preferences, thereby enhancing trust and accuracy in reporting symptoms.

Question 73: Correct Answer: C) Advising her to follow a balanced diet low in saturated fats and high in fiber.
Rationale: A balanced diet low in saturated fats and high in fiber is fundamental for preventing chronic diseases such as cardiovascular disease, diabetes, and certain cancers. While annual mammograms (Option A) are important, they are secondary prevention measures. Annual influenza vaccinations (Option B) are also important but target infectious diseases rather than chronic conditions. Regular blood glucose screening (Option D) is more relevant for individuals with risk factors or symptoms of diabetes. Thus, dietary modification (Option C) is the most appropriate primary prevention strategy for Maria.

Question 74: Correct Answer: A) Prescribing a proton pump inhibitor concurrently
Rationale: NSAIDs can exacerbate peptic ulcer disease by inhibiting prostaglandin synthesis, which protects the gastric mucosa. Co-prescribing a proton pump inhibitor reduces gastric acid secretion and minimizes ulcer risk. Monitoring blood pressure (B), fluid intake (C), and liver function tests (D) are important but do not directly address the primary risk of gastrointestinal complications associated with NSAID use in patients with peptic ulcer disease.

Question 75: Correct Answer: C) Clarifying the specific question or need for the consult
Rationale: Clarifying the specific question or need for the consult is crucial as it ensures that all team members understand the primary reason for the consultation and can provide targeted expertise. While identifying the primary care physician (A), reviewing the patient's complete medical history (B), and scheduling a multidisciplinary team meeting (D) are important steps, they are secondary to establishing a clear purpose for the consultation. This clarity helps streamline communication and fosters focused, efficient collaboration among healthcare professionals.

Question 76: Correct Answer: A) Educating the patient on medication adherence
Rationale: Educating patients on medication adherence is pivotal in managing chronic heart failure and preventing hospital readmissions. While scheduling follow-up appointments (B), implementing dietary modifications (C), and encouraging physical activity (D) are essential components of comprehensive care, adherence to prescribed medications directly impacts disease progression and symptom control. Research supports that proper medication management significantly reduces readmission rates, underscoring its priority in care planning.

Question 77: Correct Answer: B) AUDIT-C
Rationale: The AUDIT-C (Alcohol Use Disorders Identification Test - Consumption) is a validated screening tool specifically designed to identify alcohol use disorders. It is widely used in clinical settings due to its high sensitivity and specificity. The CAGE Questionnaire (A) is useful but less comprehensive than the AUDIT-C. The CIWA-Ar (C) is used for assessing the severity of alcohol withdrawal, not for initial screening. The T-ACE (D) is tailored more towards pregnant women, making it less suitable for the general medical-surgical population.

Question 78: Correct Answer: B) Low-dose computed tomography (LDCT) annually
Rationale: LDCT annually is recommended for high-risk individuals, such as long-term smokers aged 55-80, due to its higher sensitivity and specificity in detecting early-stage lung cancer. Chest X-ray (A) has lower sensitivity and does not reduce mortality rates. Sputum cytology (C) has limited effectiveness and is not routinely recommended. MRI of the chest (D), while detailed, is not standard practice for lung cancer screening due to cost and lack of evidence supporting its routine use.

Question 79: Correct Answer: A) Social support network
Rationale: A strong social support network is crucial in understanding how a patient copes with stress and adversity. While financial status, physical health, and employment history can influence coping, they do not directly provide insight into the patient's coping mechanisms as effectively as their social connections and support systems.

Question 80: Correct Answer: D) Decreased Cardiac Output
Rationale: Decreased cardiac output is critical in congestive heart failure as it directly affects the heart's ability to pump blood efficiently. While "Activity Intolerance" (A), "Fluid Volume Excess" (B), and "Impaired Gas Exchange" (C) are relevant, they are secondary to the primary issue of decreased cardiac output. Effective management of cardiac output can mitigate other symptoms and improve overall patient outcomes.

Question 81: Correct Answer: C) Discuss potential home modifications and safety measures.
Rationale: Discussing home modifications and safety measures directly addresses mobility concerns by creating a safer environment, promoting independence, and involving the family in practical solutions. Option A is dismissive of

immediate concerns. Option B offers professional support but may not address all safety issues at home. Option D suggests external help without empowering the family or considering long-term sustainability.

Question 82: Correct Answer: B) Chest pain on exertion
Rationale: Chest pain on exertion is a classic symptom of angina pectoris, often associated with cardiovascular issues such as coronary artery disease. A persistent cough (Option A) may be related to respiratory conditions, frequent headaches (Option C) could indicate neurological or vascular issues, and unexplained weight loss (Option D) might suggest metabolic or oncological problems. The key difference lies in the direct association of chest pain on exertion with the heart's oxygen demand and supply imbalance.

Question 83: Correct Answer: D) Patient's literacy level
Rationale: Patient's literacy level is crucial for accurate assessment during the evaluation phase as it directly affects their ability to comprehend and follow instructions. Nurse's time constraints (Option A), while impactful, can be managed with efficient planning. Fear or anxiety (Option B) may interfere but can be alleviated through reassurance techniques. Use of medical jargon by the nurse (Option C), though problematic, can be corrected with plain language. Literacy level fundamentally determines the patient's capability to understand health information, making it a significant barrier.

Question 84: Correct Answer: A) Daily weight monitoring
Rationale: Daily weight monitoring is crucial for CHF patients as it helps detect fluid retention early, allowing for prompt intervention to prevent exacerbations. Weekly telehealth check-ins (B) and monthly medication reviews (C), while useful, do not offer the immediate detection of changes in condition that daily monitoring provides. Quarterly cardiac rehabilitation sessions (D), though beneficial for long-term management, are too infrequent to catch acute changes.

Question 85: Correct Answer: C) Trail Making Test Part B
Rationale: The Trail Making Test Part B specifically evaluates executive function, including task-switching ability and cognitive flexibility. The MMSE (A) assesses general cognitive impairment but not executive function specifically. The GCS (B) measures consciousness level, not detailed cognitive abilities. The Rancho Los Amigos Scale (D) assesses recovery levels post-brain injury but does not focus on executive function.

Question 86: Correct Answer: B) Aortic stenosis
Rationale: A systolic murmur best heard at the second right intercostal space suggests aortic stenosis, characterized by narrowing of the aortic valve leading to turbulent blood flow during systole. Mitral valve prolapse (Option A) typically produces a mid-systolic click and late systolic murmur heard at the apex. Tricuspid regurgitation (Option C) presents with a holosystolic murmur heard best at the lower left sternal border. Pulmonary hypertension (Option D) may cause various auscultatory findings but not specifically a murmur localized to the second right intercostal space.

Question 87: Correct Answer: C) Assessing the complexity of the patient's condition
Rationale: The complexity of the patient's condition is crucial in determining whether it is safe to delegate a task to a UAP. While ensuring previous experience (A), job description alignment (B), and recent training (D) are important, they do not override the need to assess if the patient's condition requires more advanced nursing judgment and intervention, which cannot be safely delegated to UAPs.

Question 88: Correct Answer: B) Maria's incision site will show no signs of infection within one week.
Rationale: The correct answer is B). This outcome specifically addresses the prevention of infection, a common postoperative complication. Option A), while important for recovery, does not directly measure complication prevention. Option C), although beneficial for respiratory function, does not address infection risk specifically. Option D), while relevant to pain management, does not focus on preventing complications like infection.

Question 89: Correct Answer: C) History of previous overdose
Rationale: A history of previous overdose is the most significant predictor of future overdose risk and should be prioritized during assessment. Duration (A) and frequency (B) are important but do not directly correlate with overdose risk as strongly as past incidents. Concurrent use of benzodiazepines (D), while increasing risk due to synergistic effects, still does not outweigh the predictive value of a previous overdose history.

Question 90: Correct Answer: C) Setting specific, achievable goals with the patient
Rationale: Setting specific, achievable goals with patients is grounded in goal-setting theory and has been shown to enhance motivation and adherence to self-management behaviors. Educating patients (A), involving family members (B), and providing continuous professional monitoring (D) are important but do not directly empower patients to take control of their health. Goal-setting allows for measurable progress and fosters a sense of accomplishment, which is crucial for sustaining long-term behavior changes.

Question 91: Correct Answer: A) Abdominal ultrasound
Rationale: An abdominal ultrasound is the first-line imaging study for evaluating liver abnormalities due to its ability to visualize liver structure and detect biliary obstructions or masses non-invasively. MRI (B), while detailed, is usually reserved for further evaluation if ultrasound findings are inconclusive or more detail is needed. CT scan (C), though useful for detailed cross-sectional images, involves radiation exposure and is not typically the initial choice for liver evaluation. HIDA scan (D), specific for bile duct patency assessment, follows after ultrasound if biliary obstruction is suspected but not confirmed by ultrasound.

Question 92: Correct Answer: B) Serum lipase
Rationale: Serum lipase is the most indicative laboratory test for acute pancreatitis due to its higher specificity and longer elevation duration compared to serum amylase. While serum amylase can also be elevated, it is less specific and can rise in other conditions. LFTs assess liver function but are not specific to pancreatitis. CBC may show elevated white blood cells due to inflammation but does not directly diagnose pancreatitis. Thus, serum lipase remains the gold standard.

Question 93: Correct Answer: D) Computed Tomography Pulmonary Angiography (CTPA)
Rationale: Computed Tomography Pulmonary Angiography (CTPA) is the gold standard for diagnosing pulmonary embolism due to its high sensitivity and specificity. Chest X-ray (Option A) can rule out other causes but cannot confirm PE. The D-dimer test (Option B), while useful for ruling out PE, lacks specificity. Ventilation-perfusion (V/Q) scan (Option C), though useful, has been largely supplanted by CTPA due to its lower accuracy compared to CTPA.

Question 94: Correct Answer: B) Using teach-back method to confirm David's understanding
Rationale: The teach-back method (Option B) ensures that David comprehends the information by having him repeat it back in his own words. This technique confirms understanding and allows for clarification if needed. Providing pamphlets (Option A), giving dietary lists (Option C), and scheduling follow-ups (Option D), while useful, do not actively engage David in the learning process or verify his comprehension. The teach-back method is recognized as an effective strategy for enhancing patient education and promoting adherence to lifestyle modifications through active participation.

Question 95: Correct Answer: B) Hypocalcemia
Rationale: Hypocalcemia is characterized by symptoms such as confusion, muscle weakness, and ECG changes like prolonged QT interval. While hypokalemia can cause muscle weakness and ECG changes, it typically presents with U

waves rather than prolonged QT intervals. Hypermagnesemia also affects neuromuscular function but usually causes bradycardia or hypotension rather than QT prolongation. Hyperphosphatemia can lead to secondary hypocalcemia but does not directly cause these symptoms. The direct relationship between low calcium levels and prolonged QT interval makes hypocalcemia the correct answer.

Question 96: Correct Answer: B) Installing a walk-in shower and providing a shower chair

Rationale: Installing a walk-in shower and providing a shower chair (Option B) allows Mrs. Smith to bathe more safely and independently by minimizing fall risks. Close supervision (Option A) can be helpful but might reduce her sense of autonomy. Bathing her entirely (Option C) removes her independence, which can negatively impact self-esteem. Limiting baths (Option D) might compromise hygiene without addressing safety concerns directly. Therefore, Option B offers the best balance between safety and autonomy.

Question 97: Correct Answer: B) Auditory

Rationale: Mr. Lee's difficulty with reading alone and preference for discussions or hearing explanations suggest an auditory learning style, where listening plays a crucial role in comprehension and retention of information. Visual learners (A) rely on images, kinesthetic learners (C) on physical activities, and read/write learners (D) on text-based resources. Thus, auditory (B) best fits Mr. Lee's described learning preference.

Question 98: Correct Answer: A) Administering prophylactic antibiotics within 60 minutes before incision

Rationale: Administering prophylactic antibiotics within 60 minutes before incision is crucial to ensure adequate tissue levels during surgery, thereby significantly reducing SSIs. While maintaining normothermia (B), using chlorhexidine-alcohol (C), and ensuring tight glucose control (D) are important, they are secondary to timely antibiotic administration. Normothermia reduces infection risk but is less immediate than antibiotics. Chlorhexidine-alcohol is effective but not as critical as antibiotic timing. Tight glucose control minimizes infection risk but doesn't directly address perioperative bacterial load like antibiotics.

Question 99: Correct Answer: B) Administer naloxone as per protocol

Rationale: Administering naloxone reverses opioid-induced sedation and respiratory depression, providing an immediate life-saving intervention. Calling the physician (Option A), while important, delays urgent treatment. Decreasing the opioid dosage (Option C) addresses the cause but is not an immediate remedy for sedation and respiratory depression. Increasing monitoring frequency (Option D), though essential, does not counteract the acute effects of opioid overdose as effectively as naloxone.

Question 100: Correct Answer: D) Clinical judgment

Rationale: Clinical judgment is essential for accurately assessing patient outcomes because it involves synthesizing data, interpreting results, and making informed decisions. Critical thinking (A), while important, supports clinical judgment rather than replacing it. Documentation accuracy (B) ensures records are correct but does not assess outcomes directly. Patient interviewing techniques (C) gather information but do not encompass the comprehensive assessment needed in evaluation.

Question 101: Correct Answer: B) Current medications

Rationale: Assessing current medications is crucial in patients with chronic illnesses to understand their ongoing treatments and potential drug interactions. While family medical history (A), past surgical history (C), and social history (D) are important, they do not provide immediate insights into current management and potential complications like current medications do. Knowing a patient's medication regimen helps in identifying possible side effects, adherence issues, and interactions that could affect their condition.

Question 102: Correct Answer: B) Maintain a consistent intake of green leafy vegetables to avoid fluctuations in INR levels.

Rationale: Green leafy vegetables are high in vitamin K, which can antagonize the effects of warfarin. Maintaining a consistent intake helps stabilize INR levels. Increasing intake (Option A) could reduce warfarin's effectiveness, while eliminating them (Option C) is unnecessary and impractical. Consuming them occasionally (Option D) could cause fluctuations in INR levels.

Question 103: Correct Answer: A) Ineffective Breathing Pattern

Rationale: Ineffective breathing pattern is crucial in COPD management as it directly affects oxygenation and ventilation. While "Risk for Infection" (B), "Activity Intolerance" (C), and "Imbalanced Nutrition" (D) are important, they are secondary concerns. Prioritizing effective breathing patterns helps maintain adequate oxygen levels, reducing the risk of further complications and enhancing overall health stability in COPD patients.

Question 104: Correct Answer: C) Education on recognizing early signs of exacerbation.

Rationale: Prioritizing education on recognizing early signs of exacerbation is crucial because timely intervention can prevent hospital readmissions and further complications in COPD patients like Ms. Lee. Proper inhaler technique (A), smoking cessation programs (B), and guidance on physical activity limitations (D) are also important but secondary to ensuring she can identify and respond promptly to worsening symptoms, which directly impacts her immediate health status.

Question 105: Correct Answer: C) Palpation

Rationale: Palpation is crucial in evaluating acute abdominal pain as it helps identify areas of tenderness, masses, or organomegaly. In Mr. Johnson's case, guarding and rebound tenderness suggest peritoneal irritation, which palpation can further delineate. Percussion (Option A) helps assess fluid or gas but is less specific for acute pain localization. Auscultation (Option B) identifies bowel sounds but does not directly evaluate pain. Inspection (Option D) provides visual clues but lacks the tactile feedback necessary for assessing tenderness.

Question 106: Correct Answer: C) Utilizing digital health interventions like mobile apps

Rationale: Digital health interventions, such as mobile apps, have been shown to significantly improve self-management in patients with chronic illnesses by providing real-time feedback, personalized reminders, and educational resources. While detailed written instructions (A), regular follow-up phone calls (B), and peer support groups (D) are also beneficial, they lack the immediacy and personalization that digital tools offer. Mobile apps can integrate various self-management strategies, making them more effective in promoting adherence and behavior change.

Question 107: Correct Answer: A) Presenting evidence-based research to support the proposed treatment plan.

Rationale: Presenting evidence-based research (Option A) aligns with the professional role of a nurse in advocating for patients by ensuring that decisions are grounded in scientific evidence. Option B is incorrect as it does not demonstrate critical thinking or advocacy. Option C shows poor delegation and abdication of responsibility. Option D, while important, does not encompass the comprehensive role of a nurse in multidisciplinary decision-making.

Question 108: Correct Answer: C) Renal impairment

Rationale: The combination of lisinopril (an ACE inhibitor) and ibuprofen (a nonsteroidal anti-inflammatory drug) can lead to reduced renal function due to their combined effects on renal blood flow and glomerular filtration rate. Hyperkalemia (A), hypotension (B), and gastrointestinal bleeding (D) are potential side effects but are less directly related to this specific interaction. Monitoring renal function is essential in patients taking both medications to prevent nephrotoxicity.

Question 109: Correct Answer: C) Executive function

Rationale: The MoCA includes tasks specifically designed to assess executive functions such as planning, organization, and problem-solving, which are not comprehensively evaluated by the MMSE. While both tests cover language (A), attention (B), and memory recall (D), MoCA's inclusion of executive function tasks makes it more suitable for detecting mild cognitive impairment where executive dysfunction might be present. Incorrect options overlap with both tests but do not highlight MoCA's unique advantage.

Question 110: Correct Answer: C) Hypokalemia

Rationale: Prolonged nasogastric suctioning often results in hypokalemia due to the loss of gastric contents rich in potassium. Hyperkalemia (A) is unlikely as potassium is lost, not retained. Hypocalcemia (B) can occur but is less common compared to hypokalemia. Hypernatremia (D) might occur if water loss exceeds sodium loss, but hypokalemia remains the primary concern.

Question 111: Correct Answer: A) Cytochrome P450

Rationale: The Cytochrome P450 enzyme system is the most commonly involved in drug metabolism and potential interactions. It plays a key role in metabolizing many medications, making it essential for assessing drug interactions. The Renin-Angiotensin System (B), Sodium-Potassium Pump (C), and Glutathione S-transferase (D) are involved in other physiological processes but are not primarily responsible for drug metabolism. Understanding Cytochrome P450's role helps predict how different drugs might interact when co-administered.

Question 112: Correct Answer: B) Report Nurse Mike's behavior to the nursing supervisor immediately.

Rationale: Reporting unethical behavior such as falsifying documentation is crucial for patient safety and maintaining professional integrity. Confronting Nurse Mike privately (Option A) may not ensure proper resolution or accountability. Correcting documentation errors herself (Option C) could implicate Sarah in unethical practices, while ignoring the situation (Option D) neglects her duty to uphold ethical standards in nursing.

Question 113: Correct Answer: D) CT pulmonary angiography

Rationale: CT pulmonary angiography is the gold standard for diagnosing pulmonary embolism, providing detailed images of blood vessels in the lungs. A chest X-ray can identify other causes of symptoms but not confirm a PE. An ECG may show signs of right heart strain but is not diagnostic for PE. The D-dimer assay can indicate clot presence but lacks specificity and cannot confirm PE alone. Thus, CT pulmonary angiography provides definitive diagnosis through direct visualization.

Question 114: Correct Answer: B) Collect a stool sample for Clostridium difficile testing.

Rationale: Collecting a stool sample for Clostridium difficile testing is crucial in diagnosing antibiotic-associated diarrhea caused by C. difficile overgrowth. Discontinuing all antibiotics (Option A) might be harmful without proper diagnosis and guidance from a healthcare provider. Increasing fluid intake (Option C) helps manage dehydration but does not address the cause of symptoms. Antidiarrheal medication (Option D), without identifying C. difficile, could worsen the condition by retaining toxins in the colon. Accurate diagnosis ensures appropriate treatment and infection control measures are implemented effectively.

Question 115: Correct Answer: B) Inspecting surgical site for signs of infection

Rationale: Inspecting the surgical site for signs of infection is crucial for early detection of complications like hemorrhage or infection. Monitoring blood pressure trends (Option A), measuring body temperature regularly (Option C), and assessing pain levels frequently (Option D) are important but do not provide direct visual evidence that could indicate immediate postoperative complications like inspecting the surgical site does.

Question 116: Correct Answer: A) Randomized controlled trials (RCTs)

Rationale: RCTs provide the highest level of evidence due to their design, which minimizes bias and allows for causal inference. Cohort studies (B) and case-control studies (C), while valuable, are observational and thus more prone to biases. Expert opinion (D), though useful, is considered the lowest level of evidence as it lacks empirical support.

Question 117: Correct Answer: C) Implementing strict neutropenic precautions

Rationale: Strict neutropenic precautions are essential for immunocompromised patients to prevent infections by minimizing exposure to pathogens. This includes measures like wearing masks, limiting fresh flowers/plants, and thorough hand hygiene practices by everyone entering the room. Option A (disinfecting surfaces), while important, is part of broader neutropenic precautions but alone isn't sufficient. Option B (restricting visitors), though helpful, doesn't encompass all necessary precautions. Option D (high-protein diet), supports general health but does not directly prevent infections in immunocompromised individuals.

Question 118: Correct Answer: C) Offer to demonstrate proper medication administration techniques.

Rationale: Demonstrating medication administration techniques empowers the caregiver with practical skills and confidence, directly addressing his immediate concern. Option A provides information but lacks interactive guidance. Option B offers external help but may not be immediately available or sustainable long-term. Option D provides emotional support but doesn't directly address his current need for medication management skills.

Question 119: Correct Answer: A) Respect and dignity

Rationale: Respect and dignity are foundational principles of patient- and family-centered care, ensuring that patients' values, beliefs, and preferences are honored. While information sharing (B), collaboration (C), and participation (D) are also critical, they all stem from the core principle of respect and dignity. Without this foundation, true collaboration, effective information sharing, and meaningful participation cannot occur. Information sharing focuses on communication, collaboration emphasizes teamwork, and participation involves active engagement; however, respect and dignity underpin all these aspects by fostering a trusting environment.

Question 120: Correct Answer: B) Trousseau's sign

Rationale: Hypocalcemia can cause neuromuscular irritability, which Trousseau's sign detects by inducing carpal spasm with a blood pressure cuff. Chvostek's sign (A), while also indicative of hypocalcemia, is less specific than Trousseau's sign for assessing latent tetany. Deep tendon reflexes (C) are less reliable for early hypocalcemia detection. Babinski's reflex (D) is unrelated to calcium levels and more indicative of neurological issues.

Question 121: Correct Answer: A) The Iowa Model of Evidence-Based Practice

Rationale: The Iowa Model is widely recognized for its comprehensive approach to integrating EBP into nursing care, involving specific steps from assessing needs to evaluating outcomes. The Stetler Model (B), Johns Hopkins Model (C), and ACE Star Model (D), while effective, have different frameworks or focuses. The Iowa Model's structured methodology makes it particularly suitable for systematic implementation in clinical settings.

Question 122: Correct Answer: B) Organize regular team meetings to discuss challenges and share tips.

Rationale: Regular team meetings create an open forum for addressing issues collaboratively and sharing solutions, promoting collective problem-solving and support. Individual training sessions (A), while helpful, don't foster teamwork; reporting inefficiencies (C) might lead to top-down solutions without input from those affected; assigning tech-savvy staff

(D), though useful short-term, doesn't build overall competency or teamwork. Thus, option B is correct as it enhances interdisciplinary collaboration by leveraging collective knowledge and experience.

Question 123: Correct Answer: C) Pharmacotherapy combined with behavioral counseling

Rationale: Combining pharmacotherapy with behavioral counseling addresses both the physical addiction to nicotine and the psychological aspects of smoking cessation. Nicotine replacement therapy (A) alone focuses only on physical dependence. Behavioral counseling (B), while helpful, may not be sufficient without addressing physical cravings. Public health campaigns (D), though important for awareness, do not provide individualized support needed for effective cessation. The combination approach offers a more comprehensive solution by integrating both medical and psychological support mechanisms.

Question 124: Correct Answer: C) Incorporating non-pharmacological methods such as guided imagery and relaxation techniques.

Rationale: Non-pharmacological methods like guided imagery and relaxation techniques are crucial in managing pain while minimizing opioid use, especially for patients with a history of substance abuse. Option A (scheduled acetaminophen and NSAIDs) is effective but may not be sufficient alone. Option B (PCA with low-dose opioids) still involves opioids, which should be avoided given the patient's history. Option D (combination of acetaminophen and low-dose opioids as needed) also includes opioids, increasing the risk of dependency. Therefore, option C is prioritized for its effectiveness in pain management without relying on opioids.

Question 125: Correct Answer: C) Inspecting feet daily for injuries

Rationale: Inspecting feet daily for injuries is essential for diabetic patients to prevent complications such as infections or ulcers, which can lead to severe outcomes including amputation. Soaking feet daily in warm water (A) can cause skin maceration and should be avoided. Walking barefoot at home (B) increases the risk of injury and infection. Using over-the-counter corn removers (D) can cause chemical burns or damage due to neuropathy and should be avoided without professional advice.

MEDSURG-BC Exam Practice Questions [SET 4]

Question 1: In a patient receiving opioid therapy for chronic pain management, which of the following symptoms would most likely indicate opioid-induced hyperalgesia?
A) Constipation
B) Increased sensitivity to pain
C) Sedation
D) Respiratory depression

Question 2: Mr. Johnson, a 65-year-old male, presents with complaints of shortness of breath and fatigue over the past two weeks. During the review of systems, he mentions experiencing increased nocturia and mild ankle swelling. Which system should be further evaluated to identify the underlying cause of his symptoms?
A) Respiratory system
B) Cardiovascular system
C) Renal system
D) Endocrine system

Question 3: Maria, a 65-year-old female with a history of hypertension and diabetes, presents with sudden onset of right-sided weakness and difficulty speaking. Her CT scan reveals an ischemic stroke in the left middle cerebral artery territory. What is the most appropriate initial intervention?
A) Administer aspirin
B) Administer tissue plasminogen activator (tPA)
C) Start heparin infusion
D) Perform carotid endarterectomy

Question 4: During a postoperative evaluation, you notice that Mr. Lee, who underwent abdominal surgery, has not met his expected pain management outcomes despite following the prescribed regimen. What is the next best step in planning further care?
A) Increase the dosage of current pain medications.
B) Reassess the patient's pain using a different scale.
C) Consult with the pain management team for alternative therapies.
D) Educate the patient on non-pharmacological pain relief techniques.

Question 5: In managing obesity through lifestyle modifications, which approach has shown the greatest efficacy according to contemporary research?
A) Adopting a low-carbohydrate diet
B) Incorporating intermittent fasting
C) Following a balanced, calorie-restricted diet combined with regular physical activity
D) Utilizing meal replacement shakes

Question 6: Nurse Jamie is working on a busy medical-surgical unit and needs to delegate tasks to ensure all patients receive timely care. She decides to delegate the task of monitoring vital signs for a post-operative patient, Mr. Smith, who is stable but requires frequent checks. To whom should Nurse Jamie delegate this task?
A) A licensed practical nurse (LPN)
B) A certified nursing assistant (CNA)
C) Another registered nurse (RN)
D) A student nurse

Question 7: Mr. Lee is admitted with suspected sepsis. Nurse Emma must perform an initial assessment. Which skill should she prioritize to identify early signs of sepsis?
A) Measure body temperature
B) Monitor urine output
C) Check blood pressure
D) Conduct a thorough skin assessment

Question 8: In the context of self-management education, which method is considered most effective for improving patient outcomes?
A) Traditional face-to-face educational sessions
B) Interactive online learning modules
C) Distribution of printed educational materials
D) Group workshops led by healthcare professionals

Question 9: Mr. Lee, a 72-year-old patient with chronic obstructive pulmonary disease (COPD), requires modifications in his care plan to prevent exacerbations during his hospital stay for pneumonia. Which environmental modification should the nurse prioritize?
A) Maintain room temperature at 75°F (24°C).
B) Ensure continuous humidification of inspired air.
C) Limit fluid intake to prevent fluid overload.
D) Keep the head of the bed elevated at 30 degrees.

Question 10: Emily, a 35-year-old female with a history of thrombocytopenia, is scheduled for surgery. Which blood product should be administered to optimize her platelet count preoperatively?
A) Packed red blood cells (PRBCs)
B) Fresh frozen plasma (FFP)
C) Platelet concentrates
D) Cryoprecipitate

Question 11: Nurse Emily is tasked with developing a protocol for postoperative pain management in a surgical unit. She finds conflicting evidence about using multimodal analgesia versus opioid monotherapy. What should be her primary consideration when deciding which approach to implement?
A) Patient preferences and values regarding pain management.
B) The cost-effectiveness of each analgesic regimen.
C) The historical practices of pain management in her unit.
D) Recommendations from pharmaceutical representatives.

Question 12: Which laboratory finding is most indicative of acute pancreatitis?
A) Elevated serum amylase
B) Elevated serum lipase
C) Elevated alanine aminotransferase (ALT)
D) Elevated aspartate aminotransferase (AST)

Question 13: Which of the following strategies is considered most effective for smoking cessation according to recent studies?
A) Nicotine replacement therapy alone
B) Behavioral counseling alone
C) A combination of nicotine replacement therapy and behavioral counseling
D) Gradual reduction in cigarette use without additional support

Question 14: Mr. Lee is on digoxin for heart failure and has recently started taking verapamil for atrial fibrillation. What potential adverse effect should the nurse monitor closely?
A) Bradycardia
B) Tachycardia

C) Hypertension
D) Hypercalcemia

Question 15: Ms. Smith, a 60-year-old woman with osteoarthritis, expresses interest in non-pharmacologic treatments to manage her symptoms. Which complementary therapy has the strongest evidence supporting its effectiveness in reducing osteoarthritis pain?
A) Tai Chi
B) Reiki
C) Magnet Therapy
D) Crystal Healing

Question 16: Which of the following is the most effective method for assessing a patient's understanding of their post-operative care plan?
A) Verbal questioning
B) Written questionnaire
C) Teach-back method
D) Visual aids

Question 17: Which assessment skill is most critical for a nurse when evaluating a patient with suspected deep vein thrombosis (DVT)?
A) Palpation of peripheral pulses
B) Measurement of calf circumference
C) Auscultation of heart sounds
D) Inspection for skin discoloration

Question 18: Emily, a 45-year-old patient with newly diagnosed type 2 diabetes, is struggling to adhere to her medication regimen. During a follow-up visit, she mentions that she often forgets to take her medication and feels overwhelmed by the dietary changes. What is the most significant barrier to Emily's adherence?
A) Lack of understanding of the disease process
B) Complexity of the medication regimen
C) Psychological resistance to lifestyle changes
D) Inadequate support system

Question 19: John, a 60-year-old male patient with chronic pain, frequently visits the clinic with complaints of worsening pain despite medication adherence. He appears withdrawn and has poor eye contact during consultations. Upon further questioning, he reveals his caregiver often withholds medication as punishment. What is the most appropriate nursing intervention?
A) Increase his pain medication dosage.
B) Educate John on proper medication use.
C) Report suspected abuse to adult protective services.
D) Schedule more frequent follow-up appointments.

Question 20: Mrs. Johnson, a 72-year-old patient with chronic heart failure, has been admitted due to fluid overload. During the evaluation phase of her care plan, which indicator would best reflect the effectiveness of the interventions implemented?
A) Decreased peripheral edema.
B) Improved respiratory rate.
C) Reduced daily weight measurements.
D) Enhanced patient-reported quality of life.

Question 21: Which of the following is a key component of a restraint-free environment in medical-surgical nursing?
A) Regularly scheduled toileting and hydration.
B) Use of bed alarms to alert staff to patient movement.
C) Administering sedatives to calm agitated patients.
D) Applying soft wrist restraints as a precautionary measure.

Question 22: Which neurotransmitter system is primarily implicated in the reinforcing effects of substance use disorders?
A) Serotonin
B) Dopamine
C) GABA
D) Glutamate

Question 23: When a patient expresses anger about their treatment plan, which response best demonstrates therapeutic communication?
A) "I understand you're upset. Let's talk about what's bothering you."
B) "You need to calm down; this is for your own good."
C) "Many patients feel this way initially but adjust over time."
D) "It's normal to feel this way, but we have to follow the plan."

Question 24: Mrs. Thompson, a 68-year-old patient with chronic osteoarthritis, is seeking non-pharmacologic treatments to manage her pain. Which of the following interventions is most likely to provide significant pain relief based on current evidence?
A) Acupuncture
B) Aromatherapy
C) Cognitive Behavioral Therapy (CBT)
D) Hydrotherapy

Question 25: What is the primary role of a medical-surgical nurse in advocating for patient safety during a multidisciplinary team meeting?
A) Ensuring that all team members follow hospital policies
B) Communicating the patient's preferences and concerns
C) Monitoring the implementation of evidence-based practices
D) Documenting all discussions and decisions made during the meeting

Question 26: When implementing a nursing intervention for pain management in postoperative patients, which factor should be prioritized to ensure its effectiveness?
A) The patient's verbal report of pain intensity
B) The type and dosage of analgesics prescribed
C) The timing of medication administration
D) The patient's previous response to pain treatments

Question 27: Mr. Johnson, a 58-year-old male with a history of hypertension and diabetes, presents to the emergency department with confusion and weakness. His lab results show a serum sodium level of 125 mEq/L. What is the most appropriate initial nursing intervention?
A) Administer hypertonic saline.
B) Restrict water intake.
C) Administer isotonic saline.
D) Encourage oral fluid intake.

Question 28: David, a 29-year-old male with a history of opioid use disorder, presents with muscle aches, diarrhea, and anxiety after stopping heroin use two days ago. Which assessment finding would confirm opioid withdrawal?
A) Bradycardia
B) Hypotension
C) Mydriasis
D) Hyperthermia

Question 29: During the assessment of an elderly patient, which sign is most suggestive of elder abuse?
A) Poor personal hygiene
B) Weight loss due to malnutrition
C) Sudden changes in behavior or mood
D) Lack of mobility aids despite apparent need

Question 30: Which of the following is the most critical

first step in implementing evidence-based practice (EBP) in a clinical setting?
A) Conducting a comprehensive literature review
B) Formulating a clear clinical question
C) Evaluating the outcomes of current practices
D) Integrating patient preferences and values

Question 31: Michael, a 58-year-old male post-operative patient following an abdominal surgery, reports severe pain at the incision site and has a fever of 101°F. His wound appears red and swollen. Which nursing diagnosis should be prioritized?
A) Acute Pain
B) Hyperthermia
C) Risk for Infection
D) Impaired Tissue Integrity

Question 32: Ms. Lee, an 80-year-old patient with early-stage dementia, often becomes agitated in the evenings. Which diversional activity is most suitable to help calm her during these times?
A) Playing soft classical music
B) Encouraging her to engage in light gardening
C) Providing coloring books and crayons
D) Watching nature documentaries on television

Question 33: Which outcome best reflects the success of a discharge planning protocol for heart failure patients?
A) Reduction in 30-day readmission rates
B) Increase in follow-up appointment adherence
C) Improvement in self-care behavior scores
D) Enhancement of quality of life measures

Question 34: In managing osteoarthritis, which non-pharmacologic intervention is supported by evidence for improving joint function and reducing pain?
A) Weight loss
B) Tai Chi
C) Ultrasound therapy
D) Massage therapy

Question 35: A patient presents with muscle weakness, lethargy, and ECG changes showing a prolonged QT interval. Which electrolyte imbalance should be suspected?
A) Hypermagnesemia
B) Hypocalcemia
C) Hypercalcemia
D) Hyponatremia

Question 36: Nurse James is educating Mr. Lee, who has recently been prescribed anticoagulant therapy following a stroke. Mr. Lee is concerned about potential side effects and interactions with his current medications. What should Nurse James emphasize during their discussion?
A) The importance of regular blood tests to monitor therapy effectiveness.
B) A list of foods high in vitamin K that should be avoided.
C) The need for immediate medical attention if experiencing unusual bleeding or bruising.
D) Ensuring consistent medication timing each day.

Question 37: Which of the following tasks is most appropriate for a medical-surgical nurse to delegate to a licensed practical nurse (LPN) in a postoperative care setting?
A) Administering IV push medications
B) Conducting initial patient assessments
C) Monitoring vital signs
D) Developing a comprehensive discharge plan

Question 38: Which skill is paramount when developing a nursing care plan that addresses both physical and psychosocial needs of a patient?
A) Holistic assessment
B) Evidence-based practice
C) Multidisciplinary collaboration
D) Time management

Question 39: A patient presents with a serum potassium level of 6.2 mEq/L. Which immediate intervention should the nurse prioritize to address this abnormal value?
A) Administer sodium bicarbonate intravenously
B) Administer calcium gluconate intravenously
C) Administer insulin and glucose intravenously
D) Administer furosemide intravenously

Question 40: Which blood product is most appropriate for a patient with a deficiency in clotting factors due to liver disease?
A) Fresh Frozen Plasma (FFP)
B) Platelets
C) Cryoprecipitate
D) Packed Red Blood Cells (PRBCs)

Question 41: Which nursing diagnosis should be prioritized for a post-operative patient who is experiencing acute pain, has an elevated heart rate, and is at risk for infection?
A) Risk for Infection
B) Acute Pain
C) Impaired Physical Mobility
D) Ineffective Airway Clearance

Question 42: John, a 55-year-old male with a history of chronic obstructive pulmonary disease (COPD), presents to the emergency department with increased shortness of breath, productive cough, and fever. Which of the following interventions should be prioritized in managing his acute exacerbation?
A) Administering intravenous antibiotics immediately
B) Initiating non-invasive positive pressure ventilation (NIPPV)
C) Providing supplemental oxygen to maintain SpO2 between 88-92%
D) Administering a high dose of systemic corticosteroids

Question 43: Mr. Lee, a 55-year-old man with diabetic neuropathy, has been prescribed pregabalin for his chronic pain but reports dizziness and somnolence affecting his daily activities. What is the best course of action?
A) Discontinue pregabalin immediately.
B) Reduce the dosage of pregabalin gradually.
C) Switch to another medication like duloxetine.
D) Advise Mr. Lee to tolerate these side effects as they will diminish over time.

Question 44: Sarah, a 72-year-old female with type 2 diabetes mellitus, presents with a non-healing foot ulcer. Her blood glucose levels have been consistently high despite medication adherence. Which nursing diagnosis should be prioritized?
A) Risk for Infection
B) Imbalanced Nutrition: Less than Body Requirements
C) Impaired Skin Integrity
D) Ineffective Health Maintenance

Question 45: Which of the following sources is most reliable for obtaining evidence-based guidelines for medical-surgical nursing practice?
A) Peer-reviewed journal articles
B) Nursing textbooks
C) Online medical forums

D) Continuing education workshops

Question 46: A 55-year-old patient named Mr. Johnson is scheduled for discharge after a partial colectomy. As part of the discharge planning, the nurse needs to provide education on wound care and signs of infection. Which approach is most effective for ensuring Mr. Johnson understands and retains this information?
A) Providing written instructions and a demonstration
B) Giving a verbal explanation and asking him to repeat it back
C) Using a video tutorial followed by a Q&A session
D) Scheduling a follow-up call to review instructions

Question 47: Ms. Rodriguez, a 52-year-old female with a history of type 2 diabetes, reports tingling and numbness in her feet during her review of systems. She also mentions occasional dizziness and blurred vision. Which complication should be primarily considered?
A) Diabetic retinopathy
B) Peripheral neuropathy
C) Autonomic neuropathy
D) Diabetic nephropathy

Question 48: Sarah, a nurse educator, is developing a training module on evidence-based practice for her colleagues. Which supporting material would be most effective in facilitating their learning?
A) A comprehensive textbook on evidence-based practice
B) Case studies demonstrating successful implementation of evidence-based practice
C) An online forum for discussing evidence-based practice concepts
D) Lecture notes summarizing key principles of evidence-based practice

Question 49: Mrs. Thompson, a 78-year-old female with a history of hypertension and diabetes, is being discharged after a successful surgery. As part of discharge planning, what is the most crucial consideration for her home care plan?
A) Ensuring she has access to transportation for follow-up appointments.
B) Arranging for home health services to monitor her blood pressure and glucose levels.
C) Educating her about potential surgical site infections.
D) Providing dietary counseling to manage her diabetes.

Question 50: Nurse John is implementing a new evidence-based protocol for preventing pressure ulcers in bedridden patients. He encounters resistance from some staff members who are accustomed to older methods. What is the most effective strategy he should use to promote adherence to the new protocol?
A) Mandate immediate compliance without discussion.
B) Provide education sessions highlighting evidence supporting the new protocol.
C) Allow staff members to choose between old and new methods.
D) Implement changes gradually without formal training.

Question 51: Nurse Alex is reviewing a clinical guideline for the management of sepsis in adult patients. The guideline recommends the use of a specific antibiotic regimen based on recent meta-analyses. Which step should Nurse Alex take next to ensure evidence-based practice in implementing this guideline?
A) Apply the guideline directly to all sepsis patients.
B) Evaluate the applicability of the guideline to the specific patient population.
C) Use personal clinical experience to decide on antibiotic use.
D) Seek approval from the hospital's administration before implementation.

Question 52: Ms. Lee, a 70-year-old woman with heart failure and chronic kidney disease, takes multiple prescriptions including diuretics and ACE inhibitors. She experiences sudden weight gain and swelling in her legs. What should be the nurse's priority action?
A) Evaluate her adherence to the prescribed diuretic regimen.
B) Recommend reducing salt intake immediately.
C) Increase the dose of ACE inhibitors as per protocol.
D) Schedule an urgent echocardiogram.

Question 53: Maria, a 45-year-old diabetic patient, presents with a non-healing foot ulcer. What should be the primary focus in her nursing care plan to promote wound healing?
A) Ensuring strict blood glucose control and regular wound assessments
B) Increasing carbohydrate intake to boost energy levels
C) Advising complete bed rest to avoid pressure on the foot
D) Applying antiseptic ointments without changing dressings frequently

Question 54: Which of the following behaviors is most indicative of emotional abuse in a patient during a psychosocial assessment?
A) Frequent unexplained injuries
B) Consistent belittling or humiliation by a partner
C) Unexplained financial difficulties
D) Isolation from friends and family

Question 55: In preparing for discharge planning for Mr. Lee, who has multiple chronic conditions, what should Nurse Maria prioritize in her professional role?
A) Ensuring all prescriptions are filled before discharge.
B) Coordinating follow-up appointments with specialists.
C) Educating Mr. Lee on managing his conditions at home.
D) Arranging transportation for Mr. Lee from the hospital.

Question 56: Maria, a 30-year-old woman, reports severe abdominal pain radiating to her back along with nausea and vomiting for the past 24 hours. Physical examination reveals tenderness in the epigastric region and positive Cullen's sign. What is the most likely diagnosis?
A) Acute Cholecystitis
B) Acute Pancreatitis
C) Peptic Ulcer Disease
D) Appendicitis

Question 57: Mr. Smith, a 58-year-old male with a history of hypertension and diabetes, presents with chest pain and shortness of breath. His troponin levels are elevated. Which additional diagnostic test should be prioritized to confirm myocardial infarction?
A) Electrocardiogram (ECG)
B) Chest X-ray
C) Echocardiogram
D) Cardiac catheterization

Question 58: Mr. Johnson, a 65-year-old male with a history of chronic obstructive pulmonary disease (COPD), presents with increased shortness of breath, productive cough, and wheezing. During the assessment, which diagnostic test would be most appropriate to evaluate the severity of his respiratory compromise?
A) Chest X-ray
B) Arterial blood gas (ABG) analysis
C) Pulmonary function tests (PFTs)
D) Sputum culture

Question 59: Which of the following vaccines should be administered to pregnant women during each pregnancy to protect both mother and infant from pertussis?
A) MMR (Measles, Mumps, Rubella)
B) Varicella
C) Tdap (Tetanus, diphtheria, and pertussis)
D) HPV (Human Papillomavirus)

Question 60: Mrs. Garcia, a 55-year-old diabetic patient, is recovering from a below-the-knee amputation. The nurse must modify her diet to promote wound healing and manage blood glucose levels. Which dietary modification should be prioritized?
A) High-protein diet with controlled carbohydrate intake.
B) Low-fat diet with increased fiber intake.
C) High-carbohydrate diet with reduced protein intake.
D) Low-sodium diet with moderate protein intake.

Question 61: In therapeutic communication, what is the primary purpose of using reflective listening?
A) To offer solutions to the patient's problems
B) To demonstrate understanding and empathy
C) To gather detailed medical history
D) To redirect the conversation back to medical facts

Question 62: Sarah, a 45-year-old patient, is admitted with severe anemia and requires a blood transfusion. Which of the following assessments is most crucial before administering packed red blood cells (PRBCs)?
A) Checking the patient's vital signs
B) Verifying the patient's blood type and crossmatch
C) Ensuring the patient has signed an informed consent
D) Monitoring the patient's urine output

Question 63: Ms. Garcia, a 60-year-old woman with rheumatoid arthritis, complains of increased difficulty concentrating and remembering daily tasks over the past few months. You suspect cognitive impairment related to her chronic condition. Which diagnostic test would best help differentiate between depression-related cognitive impairment and early dementia?
A) Geriatric Depression Scale (GDS)
B) Neuropsychological testing
C) Electroencephalogram (EEG)
D) Brain MRI

Question 64: Ms. Lee, a 45-year-old female with hypertension, reports experiencing severe headaches and visual disturbances. During your assessment, her blood pressure reads 190/110 mmHg. What would be your priority nursing diagnosis?
A) Risk for stroke related to elevated blood pressure
B) Acute pain related to severe headache
C) Impaired vision related to hypertensive retinopathy
D) Risk for ineffective cerebral tissue perfusion related to hypertension

Question 65: Sarah, a medical-surgical nurse, is part of an interdisciplinary team caring for a post-operative patient experiencing complications. During a team meeting, conflicting opinions arise regarding pain management strategies. How should Sarah facilitate effective collaboration among team members?
A) Suggest a vote to determine the best pain management strategy.
B) Encourage each team member to present evidence-based practices supporting their opinion.
C) Recommend deferring to the surgeon's preference as they have primary responsibility.
D) Propose implementing a trial period for each suggested strategy.

Question 66: When assessing a patient's risk for suicide, which aspect of their psychiatric history is most critical to evaluate?
A) History of anxiety disorders
B) History of bipolar disorder
C) History of psychotic episodes
D) History of personality disorders

Question 67: When educating a patient about managing their chronic illness, which educational strategy is considered most beneficial according to contemporary research?
A) One-on-one education sessions
B) Group education classes
C) Interactive digital modules
D) Printed educational materials

Question 68: When implementing a care plan for a postoperative patient, which of the following skills is most critical to prevent surgical site infection?
A) Sterile dressing changes
B) Hand hygiene compliance
C) Proper wound irrigation technique
D) Timely administration of antibiotics

Question 69: During the initial assessment of Mrs. Smith, who presents with shortness of breath and chest discomfort, which skill is most critical for Nurse Jamie to utilize to determine the immediate cause?
A) Auscultate lung sounds
B) Measure oxygen saturation levels
C) Obtain an electrocardiogram (ECG)
D) Assess for jugular vein distention

Question 70: Mr. Johnson, a 68-year-old patient with a history of hypertension and diabetes, presents with a sudden onset of confusion and slurred speech. His vital signs are as follows: BP 180/110 mmHg, HR 100 bpm, RR 22 breaths/min, and SpO2 95%. What is the most critical vital sign that requires immediate intervention?
A) Blood Pressure
B) Heart Rate
C) Respiratory Rate
D) Oxygen Saturation

Question 71: Which diagnostic test is most appropriate for confirming a diagnosis of pulmonary embolism?
A) Chest X-ray
B) D-dimer assay
C) Ventilation-perfusion (V/Q) scan
D) Spiral CT angiography

Question 72: Ms. Garcia, a 42-year-old patient diagnosed with hypertension, expresses difficulty in adhering to her medication regimen due to forgetfulness. What is the most effective teaching intervention for the nurse to implement?
A) Educate Ms. Garcia about the importance of medication adherence.
B) Suggest she uses a daily pill organizer.
C) Recommend setting up reminders on her smartphone.
D) Involve a family member in managing her medications.

Question 73: Which screening test is most appropriate for early detection of colorectal cancer in average-risk adults aged 50-75 years?
A) Fecal Immunochemical Test (FIT)
B) Colonoscopy every 10 years
C) Flexible Sigmoidoscopy every 5 years
D) Double-contrast Barium Enema every 5 years

Question 74: A patient named Mr. Lee has been diagnosed with Type 2 diabetes mellitus and needs education on self-management practices. Which

approach is most likely to enhance his adherence to lifestyle changes?
A) Provide a list of dietary restrictions and exercise recommendations.
B) Enroll him in a diabetes self-management education (DSME) program.
C) Give him pamphlets on diabetes management during his discharge.
D) Schedule regular follow-up visits with his endocrinologist.

Question 75: In interdisciplinary healthcare team collaboration, which aspect should a medical-surgical nurse consider most critical when delegating tasks?
A) The educational background of team members
B) The workload distribution among team members
C) The legal scope of practice for each team member
D) The interpersonal relationships within the team

Question 76: When educating a patient about lifestyle modifications for hypertension management, which approach is most likely to result in long-term adherence?
A) Providing a detailed diet plan and exercise schedule
B) Encouraging small, incremental changes tailored to the patient's preferences
C) Referring the patient to a nutritionist and personal trainer
D) Emphasizing the risks of non-compliance

Question 77: John, a 65-year-old male with a history of chronic obstructive pulmonary disease (COPD), presents to the emergency department with increased shortness of breath and productive cough. Upon assessment, his vital signs are: BP 145/90 mmHg, HR 110 bpm, RR 28 breaths/min, and SpO2 85% on room air. Which nursing diagnosis should be prioritized?
A) Ineffective Airway Clearance
B) Impaired Gas Exchange
C) Activity Intolerance
D) Anxiety

Question 78: Ms. Lee, a 30-year-old nurse working in a hospital setting, seeks advice on vaccinations to protect herself and her patients from infectious diseases. Which vaccination should she ensure is up-to-date to minimize transmission risks in the healthcare environment?
A) Hepatitis A vaccine
B) Hepatitis B vaccine
C) Rabies vaccine
D) Typhoid vaccine

Question 79: When evaluating a patient's respiratory rate, which of the following factors can most significantly affect the accuracy of your assessment?
A) Patient's level of consciousness
B) Use of supplemental oxygen
C) Patient's position during assessment
D) Recent physical activity

Question 80: Which of the following medications is most appropriate for managing neuropathic pain in a patient with diabetic peripheral neuropathy?
A) Ibuprofen
B) Gabapentin
C) Acetaminophen
D) Oxycodone

Question 81: In assessing a patient with suspected fluid volume deficit, which clinical indicator is considered the most reliable measure of extracellular fluid volume status?
A) Skin turgor
B) Blood pressure
C) Serum sodium level
D) Central venous pressure (CVP)

Question 82: When managing a postoperative patient's pain, which skill should a medical-surgical nurse prioritize to ensure effective pain management?
A) Administering prescribed analgesics on schedule
B) Educating the patient about pain management techniques
C) Assessing pain using a standardized pain scale
D) Encouraging the patient to report pain early

Question 83: A 68-year-old patient named Mr. Thompson has been admitted for congestive heart failure (CHF) exacerbation. The nurse is developing a care plan and needs to modify the patient's activity level. Which modification should be prioritized to optimize Mr. Thompson's cardiac function while minimizing fatigue?
A) Encourage ambulation three times a day for 15 minutes each.
B) Schedule physical therapy sessions twice daily.
C) Implement bed rest with bathroom privileges.
D) Allow unrestricted activity as tolerated by the patient.

Question 84: Which of the following vaccines is specifically recommended for adults aged 50 years and older to prevent shingles?
A) Hepatitis A
B) Shingrix
C) Meningococcal ACWY
D) Rabies

Question 85: During a respiratory assessment, which finding most strongly suggests the presence of pleural effusion?
A) Dullness to percussion over affected area
B) Hyperresonance to percussion over affected area
C) Increased tactile fremitus over affected area
D) Wheezing on auscultation over affected area

Question 86: John, a 50-year-old diabetic patient, has been experiencing frequent hypoglycemic episodes. The nurse aims to reduce these episodes as part of his care plan. Which outcome best reflects effective nursing intervention?
A) John will report fewer dizziness episodes.
B) John's HbA1c level will be maintained below 7% over the next six months.
C) John's blood glucose levels will remain between 70-130 mg/dL before meals.
D) John will attend diabetes management classes regularly.

Question 87: During a routine physical assessment, a 65-year-old patient named Mr. Johnson reports experiencing frequent dizziness and occasional fainting spells. Which system should the nurse prioritize in her review to determine the underlying cause?
A) Cardiovascular system
B) Respiratory system
C) Gastrointestinal system
D) Musculoskeletal system

Question 88: What is the most appropriate initial step a nurse should take when considering the use of physical restraints on a patient exhibiting aggressive behavior?
A) Apply the restraints immediately to prevent harm.
B) Assess the patient's underlying causes of aggression.
C) Notify the physician for an order to apply restraints.
D) Document the patient's aggressive behavior in the medical record.

Question 89: Which educational strategy is most effective for improving patient adherence to a postoperative care plan in a diverse patient population?
A) Lecture-based sessions

B) Interactive workshops
C) Written instructional materials
D) Multimedia presentations

Question 90: When evaluating a patient's health history, which aspect is essential for identifying potential hereditary conditions?
A) Social habits
B) Family medical history
C) Past surgical history
D) Immunization records

Question 91: Mary, a 45-year-old female, is recovering from knee replacement surgery. She develops redness, warmth, and swelling in her calf on postoperative day three. Which action should the nurse prioritize?
A) Apply warm compresses to the affected area.
B) Elevate the leg and apply compression stockings.
C) Assess for signs of deep vein thrombosis (DVT).
D) Encourage increased fluid intake.

Question 92: Mr. Lee, a 72-year-old male with COPD, presents with shortness of breath and his ABG results show pH 7.30, PaCO2 55 mmHg, and HCO3- 28 mEq/L. What is the primary nursing intervention?
A) Increase oxygen flow rate.
B) Prepare for intubation.
C) Encourage pursed-lip breathing.
D) Administer sodium bicarbonate.

Question 93: Which non-pharmacologic treatment is most effective in reducing chronic lower back pain according to contemporary research?
A) Acupuncture
B) Yoga
C) Cognitive Behavioral Therapy (CBT)
D) Physical Therapy

Question 94: When evaluating the effectiveness of a nursing care plan, which method provides the most comprehensive assessment?
A) Reviewing patient satisfaction surveys
B) Monitoring changes in clinical indicators
C) Conducting regular interdisciplinary team meetings
D) Performing continuous patient assessments

Question 95: Which electrolyte imbalance is most commonly associated with the development of cardiac arrhythmias in patients with chronic kidney disease (CKD)?
A) Hyperkalemia
B) Hypocalcemia
C) Hypernatremia
D) Hypomagnesemia

Question 96: In evaluating the effectiveness of a patient education program on diabetes management, which method provides the most reliable data?
A) Patient self-reports
B) Pre- and post-test assessments
C) Patient satisfaction surveys
D) Randomized controlled trials (RCTs)

Question 97: When evaluating the effectiveness of restraints, which indicator would best demonstrate successful implementation?
A) Decrease in patient falls after applying restraints.
B) Patient's vital signs remain stable during restraint use.
C) Reduction in episodes of aggressive behavior with minimal restraint use.
D) Increased documentation of restraint application in patient records.

Question 98: What is the primary reason for using chlorhexidine-impregnated dressings on central venous catheters?
A) To reduce the incidence of bloodstream infections
B) To prevent local skin irritation at the insertion site
C) To minimize allergic reactions to adhesive materials
D) To promote faster healing of the insertion site

Question 99: Emily, a 17-year-old patient diagnosed with Type 1 diabetes, struggles with adhering to her treatment regimen while trying to fit in with her peers at school. Which developmental stage is Emily experiencing according to Erikson's psychosocial theory?
A) Identity vs. Role Confusion
B) Intimacy vs. Isolation
C) Autonomy vs. Shame and Doubt
D) Initiative vs. Guilt

Question 100: Sarah, a 65-year-old patient with congestive heart failure (CHF), has been admitted to the hospital. As part of her care plan, the nurse sets an outcome to improve her cardiac output. Which of the following is the most appropriate measurable outcome for Sarah?
A) Sarah will report no shortness of breath.
B) Sarah's heart rate will remain below 100 beats per minute.
C) Sarah's ejection fraction will improve by 10% within three months.
D) Sarah will adhere to a low-sodium diet.

Question 101: Mary, a 58-year-old diabetic patient, presents with a non-healing foot ulcer. What is the most critical intervention to promote wound healing?
A) Ensuring strict blood glucose control
B) Applying a hydrocolloid dressing
C) Administering prophylactic antibiotics
D) Elevating the affected foot

Question 102: Which of the following cognitive assessment tools includes a component specifically designed to evaluate visuospatial abilities?
A) Mini-Mental State Examination (MMSE)
B) Saint Louis University Mental Status Exam (SLUMS)
C) Montreal Cognitive Assessment (MoCA)
D) Geriatric Depression Scale (GDS)

Question 103: When evaluating the outcome of an educational intervention for diabetic patients, which indicator is most relevant?
A) Decrease in HbA1c levels
B) Increase in knowledge test scores
C) Reduction in hospital readmissions
D) Improvement in dietary habits

Question 104: Mrs. Thompson, a post-operative patient, is becoming increasingly agitated and attempting to pull out her surgical drains. The healthcare team decides that restraints might be necessary. What should be included in the care plan to ensure patient safety while using restraints?
A) Check restraint tightness every 4 hours.
B) Provide range-of-motion exercises every 2 hours.
C) Monitor vital signs once per shift.
D) Allow family members to adjust restraints as needed.

Question 105: What is the primary benefit of implementing bedside shift reports in a medical-surgical unit?
A) Enhancing nurse accountability
B) Improving patient safety
C) Increasing staff satisfaction

D) Promoting family involvement

Question 106: Nurse Emily is caring for a patient, Mr. Johnson, who has terminal cancer. Mr. Johnson expresses a desire to discontinue treatment and pursue palliative care, but his family insists on continuing aggressive treatment. What is the most ethically appropriate action for Nurse Emily?
A) Respect the family's wishes and continue aggressive treatment.
B) Advocate for Mr. Johnson's autonomy and support his decision to pursue palliative care.
C) Refer the case to the hospital ethics committee without taking sides.
D) Follow the physician's orders regardless of Mr. Johnson's wishes.

Question 107: Sarah, a 45-year-old patient with chronic kidney disease (CKD), is prescribed a new medication. Which of the following considerations is most critical for ensuring safe medication administration in Sarah's case?
A) Adjusting the dosage based on Sarah's weight
B) Monitoring liver function tests regularly
C) Assessing renal function and adjusting dosage accordingly
D) Evaluating potential drug-drug interactions

Question 108: Which of the following modifications is most appropriate for a patient with chronic obstructive pulmonary disease (COPD) to enhance their respiratory function during activities of daily living (ADLs)?
A) Encourage deep breathing exercises.
B) Implement pursed-lip breathing techniques.
C) Increase fluid intake to thin secretions.
D) Provide supplemental oxygen continuously.

Question 109: In an interdisciplinary healthcare team, which factor is most critical for ensuring effective collaboration and optimal patient care?
A) Clear role definitions
B) Equal participation in decision-making
C) Shared goals and vision
D) Frequent informal interactions

Question 110: Mr. Lee, who has recently suffered a stroke, is experiencing difficulty with dressing himself due to hemiparesis on his right side. Which strategy would be most beneficial in helping him regain independence in dressing?
A) Encouraging him to dress using only his unaffected side
B) Teaching him one-handed dressing techniques using adaptive clothing
C) Dressing him completely until he regains full function
D) Using Velcro fasteners instead of buttons or zippers on his clothing

Question 111: When selecting a mechanical ventilator for a patient with acute respiratory distress syndrome (ARDS), which mode is most appropriate to ensure lung-protective ventilation?
A) Volume-controlled ventilation
B) Pressure-controlled ventilation
C) High-frequency oscillatory ventilation
D) Synchronized intermittent mandatory ventilation (SIMV)

Question 112: David, a 45-year-old patient with a history of deep vein thrombosis (DVT), complains of sudden severe abdominal pain and vomiting two days post-colectomy surgery. Which potential complication should be suspected?
A) Mesenteric ischemia due to arterial embolism
B) Gastrointestinal perforation
C) Acute pancreatitis
D) Small bowel obstruction

Question 113: Which of the following factors is most strongly associated with an increased risk of suicide in patients with major depressive disorder?
A) Social isolation
B) Family history of suicide
C) Substance abuse
D) Previous suicide attempt

Question 114: Patient Maria, a 45-year-old female with a history of heart failure, presents with shortness of breath and peripheral edema. Her lab results reveal a potassium level of 5.8 mEq/L. Which intervention should be prioritized?
A) Administer loop diuretics
B) Administer potassium-sparing diuretics
C) Initiate dialysis immediately
D) Encourage high-potassium foods

Question 115: Patient John, a 65-year-old male with a history of chronic kidney disease, presents with confusion and muscle weakness. His lab results show serum sodium of 125 mEq/L. Which of the following is the most appropriate initial intervention?
A) Administer hypertonic saline
B) Restrict water intake
C) Administer isotonic saline
D) Encourage oral sodium intake

Question 116: Which of the following interventions is most effective in reducing cardiovascular risk in patients with hypertension through lifestyle modifications?
A) Reducing sodium intake to less than 2,300 mg per day
B) Engaging in moderate-intensity aerobic physical activity for at least 150 minutes per week
C) Limiting alcohol consumption to no more than one drink per day for women and two drinks per day for men
D) Increasing dietary potassium intake to counteract sodium's effects

Question 117: Which electrolyte imbalance is most commonly associated with the use of loop diuretics like furosemide?
A) Hyperkalemia
B) Hypokalemia
C) Hypercalcemia
D) Hyponatremia

Question 118: Which of the following strategies is most effective in promoting health and wellness among patients with chronic diseases according to contemporary research?
A) Implementing community-based exercise programs
B) Providing individualized dietary plans
C) Conducting regular health education seminars
D) Utilizing telehealth for continuous monitoring

Question 119: Which of the following strategies is most effective in minimizing the risk of adverse drug interactions in polypharmacy among elderly patients?
A) Reviewing medications annually
B) Utilizing a comprehensive medication review (CMR)
C) Encouraging self-medication management
D) Reducing the number of prescribed medications

Question 120: Which of the following is the most appropriate initial intervention for a patient suspected of having a pulmonary embolism (PE) postoperatively?
A) Administering aspirin
B) Initiating intravenous heparin

C) Performing a chest X-ray
D) Starting oral anticoagulants

Question 121: In the context of managing chronic pain, which CAM therapy has shown the most consistent results according to recent systematic reviews?
A) Chiropractic care
B) Herbal supplements
C) Mindfulness meditation
D) Homeopathy

Question 122: Nurse Emily is taking a health history from Mr. Thompson, who has been diagnosed with chronic obstructive pulmonary disease (COPD). To understand how well he manages his condition, which question should she ask?
A) "How often do you use your inhaler?"
B) "Do you have any pets at home?"
C) "Have you traveled recently?"
D) "What medications are you currently taking?"

Question 123: In a patient with chronic obstructive pulmonary disease (COPD), which physical assessment finding is most characteristic?
A) Barrel chest
B) Clubbing of fingers
C) Pitting edema
D) Splenomegaly

Question 124: Which of the following factors can cause a falsely low blood pressure reading during manual measurement?
A) Using a cuff that is too small
B) Placing the arm above heart level
C) Deflating the cuff too slowly
D) Measuring blood pressure after exercise

Question 125: John, a 45-year-old male, presents with acute chest pain radiating to his left arm, shortness of breath, and diaphoresis. His ECG shows ST-segment elevation in leads II, III, and aVF. Which diagnosis is most likely?
A) Stable Angina
B) Non-ST Elevation Myocardial Infarction (NSTEMI)
C) ST-Elevation Myocardial Infarction (STEMI)
D) Unstable Angina

ANSWER WITH DETAILED EXPLANATION SET [4]

Question 1: Correct Answer: B) Increased sensitivity to pain
Rationale: Opioid-induced hyperalgesia (OIH) is characterized by an increased sensitivity to pain despite ongoing opioid use. This paradoxical response occurs due to neuroplastic changes in the central nervous system. Constipation (A), sedation (C), and respiratory depression (D) are common opioid side effects but do not indicate OIH. The phenomenon of OIH involves NMDA receptor activation and descending facilitation pathways, distinguishing it from other side effects. Recognizing increased pain sensitivity as a sign of OIH is crucial for adjusting treatment plans.

Question 2: Correct Answer: B) Cardiovascular system
Rationale: The cardiovascular system should be further evaluated because symptoms such as shortness of breath, fatigue, nocturia, and ankle swelling are indicative of congestive heart failure (CHF). CHF can lead to fluid accumulation in the lungs (causing shortness of breath), and peripheral edema (ankle swelling). Nocturia can result from increased renal perfusion when lying down. While the respiratory system (A) might explain shortness of breath, it does not account for nocturia or ankle swelling. The renal system (C) could explain nocturia but not the other symptoms comprehensively. The endocrine system (D) is less likely to present with this specific combination of symptoms.

Question 3: Correct Answer: B) Administer tissue plasminogen activator (tPA)
Rationale: tPA is the treatment of choice for acute ischemic stroke within the first few hours of symptom onset to dissolve clots and restore blood flow. Aspirin (A), while important for long-term management, is not as effective acutely as tPA. Heparin infusion (C) is not typically used in the acute phase due to bleeding risk. Carotid endarterectomy (D) is a surgical procedure for preventing future strokes but is not an initial intervention.

Question 4: Correct Answer: B) Reassess the patient's pain using a different scale.
Rationale: Reassessing Mr. Lee's pain using a different scale ensures accurate evaluation of his pain levels and helps identify if current assessments were inadequate or inappropriate. Increasing dosage (A), consulting with specialists (C), or educating on alternative techniques (D) may be necessary later but first require accurate reassessment to guide appropriate adjustments in care planning and implementation effectively.

Question 5: Correct Answer: C) Following a balanced, calorie-restricted diet combined with regular physical activity
Rationale: Following a balanced, calorie-restricted diet combined with regular physical activity is the most effective approach for managing obesity. This combination promotes sustainable weight loss by addressing both caloric intake and energy expenditure. While low-carbohydrate diets (A), intermittent fasting (B), and meal replacement shakes (D) can be effective short-term strategies, they often lack sustainability and comprehensive benefits seen with balanced diets and exercise. Contemporary research emphasizes the importance of a holistic approach that includes both dietary management and physical activity for long-term success.

Question 6: Correct Answer: A) A licensed practical nurse (LPN)
Rationale: Delegating the task of monitoring vital signs to an LPN is appropriate as LPNs are trained and licensed to perform this task independently. While CNAs can also monitor vital signs, they may require more supervision compared to LPNs. An RN could perform the task but would be better utilized for more complex patient care activities. Student nurses are still in training and require direct supervision, making them less ideal for delegation in this scenario.

Question 7: Correct Answer: C) Check blood pressure
Rationale: Hypotension is a critical early sign of sepsis indicating potential septic shock, necessitating prompt intervention. While measuring body temperature (Option A), monitoring urine output (Option B), and conducting a skin assessment (Option D) are important components of sepsis evaluation, they do not provide immediate insight into hemodynamic stability like blood pressure does.

Question 8: Correct Answer: B) Interactive online learning modules
Rationale: Interactive online learning modules are highly effective for improving patient outcomes because they offer flexibility, accessibility, and engagement through multimedia content. Traditional face-to-face sessions (A), printed materials (C), and group workshops (D) can be useful but often lack the interactive elements that enhance understanding and retention. Online modules can be tailored to individual learning paces and styles, making them a superior option for comprehensive self-management education.

Question 9: Correct Answer: B) Ensure continuous humidification of inspired air.
Rationale: Continuous humidification of inspired air helps maintain airway moisture, reducing the risk of mucus plugging and exacerbations in COPD patients like Mr. Lee. Maintaining room temperature at 75°F (Option A), limiting fluid intake (Option C), or keeping the head of the bed elevated at 30 degrees (Option D), although beneficial in certain contexts, do not directly address airway hydration which is critical in preventing COPD exacerbations during pneumonia recovery.

Question 10: Correct Answer: C) Platelet concentrates
Rationale: Platelet concentrates are specifically used to increase platelet counts in patients with thrombocytopenia, which is critical before surgery to prevent excessive bleeding. PRBCs (A), FFP (B), and cryoprecipitate (D) do not primarily address low platelet counts. Platelet concentrates directly target the deficiency in platelet numbers, optimizing Emily's condition for surgery by reducing bleeding risk.

Question 11: Correct Answer: A) Patient preferences and values regarding pain management.
Rationale: Prioritizing patient preferences ensures that care is patient-centered and aligned with individual needs, which is a core principle of evidence-based practice. Cost-effectiveness (B), while important, comes secondary to patient-centered care. Historical practices (C) may not reflect current best evidence, and pharmaceutical recommendations (D) could be biased. This focus on patient values is supported by contemporary research promoting personalized care.

Question 12: Correct Answer: B) Elevated serum lipase
Rationale: Elevated serum lipase is the most specific and sensitive marker for acute pancreatitis, as it remains elevated longer than amylase and is more pancreas-specific. While elevated serum amylase (Option A) can also indicate acute pancreatitis, it can be elevated in other conditions like mumps. Elevated ALT (Option C) and AST (Option D) are more indicative of liver damage rather than pancreatic issues, making them less specific for diagnosing acute pancreatitis.

Question 13: Correct Answer: C) A combination of nicotine replacement therapy and behavioral counseling
Rationale: A combination of nicotine replacement therapy and behavioral counseling is considered the most effective strategy for smoking cessation. This dual approach addresses both the physical addiction to nicotine and the behavioral aspects of smoking, leading to higher success rates. Nicotine replacement therapy alone (A) or behavioral counseling alone (B) are beneficial but less effective when used independently. Gradual reduction in cigarette use

without additional support (D) often lacks structure and professional guidance, making it less successful. Recent studies highlight the synergistic effect of combining pharmacological support with behavioral interventions.

Question 14: Correct Answer: A) Bradycardia

Rationale: Verapamil can increase digoxin levels by inhibiting its clearance, leading to bradycardia due to enhanced effects on cardiac conduction. Tachycardia (Option B), hypertension (Option C), and hypercalcemia (Option D) are not typical interactions between digoxin and verapamil; in fact, verapamil generally lowers blood pressure rather than increasing it.

Question 15: Correct Answer: A) Tai Chi

Rationale: Tai Chi has substantial evidence supporting its effectiveness in reducing osteoarthritis pain through improved joint function and reduced inflammation, as evidenced by multiple randomized controlled trials. Reiki is primarily used for stress reduction and lacks robust evidence for osteoarthritis pain relief. Magnet therapy and crystal healing are considered pseudoscientific with insufficient empirical support for managing osteoarthritis symptoms effectively.

Question 16: Correct Answer: C) Teach-back method

Rationale: The teach-back method is the most effective way to assess a patient's understanding because it requires them to explain the care plan in their own words, ensuring comprehension. Verbal questioning and written questionnaires may not fully reveal misunderstandings, while visual aids support learning but do not confirm understanding. The teach-back method allows for immediate clarification and reinforcement, making it superior for ensuring patient knowledge retention.

Question 17: Correct Answer: B) Measurement of calf circumference

Rationale: Measurement of calf circumference is crucial in assessing suspected DVT because it can indicate swelling, which is a common sign of DVT. Palpation of peripheral pulses (Option A) and auscultation of heart sounds (Option C) are essential skills but less specific to DVT. Inspection for skin discoloration (Option D) can help identify other conditions but isn't as directly indicative of DVT as measurement of calf circumference.

Question 18: Correct Answer: B) Complexity of the medication regimen

Rationale: The complexity of the medication regimen is often a significant barrier to adherence, especially in newly diagnosed patients like Emily. While psychological resistance and lack of understanding are also barriers, they are secondary to the immediate challenge of managing a complex regimen. An inadequate support system can contribute but is less directly impactful compared to regimen complexity. Simplifying her medication schedule could enhance adherence.

Question 19: Correct Answer: C) Report suspected abuse to adult protective services.

Rationale: The most appropriate nursing intervention is to report suspected abuse to adult protective services (Option C). This ensures that John receives protection from potential harm and that his situation is investigated by authorities trained in handling such cases. Increasing his medication dosage (Option A) or scheduling more frequent appointments (Option D) addresses symptoms but not the underlying issue of abuse. Educating John on proper medication use (Option B) is redundant since he already adheres to his regimen; the problem lies with his caregiver's actions.

Question 20: Correct Answer: C) Reduced daily weight measurements.

Rationale: Reduced daily weight measurements are a direct indicator of fluid balance and effectiveness in managing fluid overload in heart failure patients like Mrs. Johnson. While decreased peripheral edema (A), improved respiratory rate (B), and enhanced quality of life (D) are significant, daily weights provide precise, quantifiable data on fluid status changes. Weight reduction correlates closely with effective fluid management interventions.

Question 21: Correct Answer: A) Regularly scheduled toileting and hydration.

Rationale: The correct answer is A) Regularly scheduled toileting and hydration. Ensuring basic needs are met can prevent behaviors that might otherwise lead to restraint use, promoting a restraint-free environment. This strategy is supported by evidence-based practices focusing on non-restraint interventions. Option B, while useful, does not address basic needs directly. Option C involves medication, which should be used cautiously and not as a primary intervention for agitation. Option D contradicts the concept of a restraint-free environment by using restraints preemptively rather than addressing potential causes.

Question 22: Correct Answer: B) Dopamine

Rationale: Dopamine plays a critical role in the brain's reward system and is heavily implicated in the reinforcing effects of substances, making it central to substance use disorders. Serotonin (A), while involved in mood regulation, does not primarily drive reinforcement. GABA (C), an inhibitory neurotransmitter, affects anxiety and sedation rather than reinforcement. Glutamate (D), an excitatory neurotransmitter, plays a role in learning and memory but is not the primary driver of reinforcement in substance use.

Question 23: Correct Answer: A) "I understand you're upset. Let's talk about what's bothering you."

Rationale: Validating the patient's feelings and inviting them to discuss their concerns (A) shows empathy and promotes an open dialogue. Telling the patient to calm down (B) can be dismissive, suggesting future adjustment (C) doesn't address immediate emotions, and normalizing feelings while insisting on the plan (D) lacks empathy. Thus, acknowledging and exploring the patient's feelings is key.

Question 24: Correct Answer: A) Acupuncture

Rationale: Acupuncture has been shown through various studies to significantly reduce pain in patients with osteoarthritis by stimulating specific points on the body, which may release endorphins and improve blood flow. While aromatherapy (B) can provide relaxation, its direct impact on pain relief is less supported by evidence. Cognitive Behavioral Therapy (CBT) (C) helps in managing the psychological aspects of chronic pain but does not directly alleviate physical symptoms. Hydrotherapy (D), though beneficial for joint mobility and overall well-being, does not have as strong evidence for direct pain relief compared to acupuncture.

Question 25: Correct Answer: B) Communicating the patient's preferences and concerns

Rationale: The primary role of a medical-surgical nurse in advocating for patient safety is to communicate the patient's preferences and concerns. This ensures that care is patient-centered and respects individual needs. While ensuring adherence to hospital policies (Option A), monitoring evidence-based practices (Option C), and documenting discussions (Option D) are important, they do not directly address patient advocacy as effectively as communicating patient preferences does.

Question 26: Correct Answer: A) The patient's verbal report of pain intensity

Rationale: Prioritizing the patient's verbal report of pain intensity is essential because it provides real-time feedback on their current pain level, guiding appropriate intervention adjustments. While the type and dosage of analgesics (B), timing of medication administration (C), and previous responses to treatments (D) are significant considerations, they must be tailored based on the patient's current subjective experience of pain. Effective pain management hinges on addressing what the patient feels at the moment rather than solely relying on predetermined factors.

Question 27: Correct Answer: B) Restrict water intake.

Rationale: The initial approach to hyponatremia (serum

sodium <135 mEq/L) involves restricting water intake to prevent further dilution of sodium. Hypertonic saline (A) is reserved for severe cases or symptomatic hyponatremia. Isotonic saline (C) may be used in hypovolemic hyponatremia but isn't the first step here. Encouraging oral fluid intake (D) would worsen hyponatremia by further diluting serum sodium levels.

Question 28: Correct Answer: C) Mydriasis

Rationale: Mydriasis (pupil dilation) is a classic sign of opioid withdrawal along with symptoms like muscle aches and diarrhea. Bradycardia (A), hypotension (B), and hyperthermia (D) are not typical of opioid withdrawal; rather, opioid intoxication can cause bradycardia and hypotension while hyperthermia may indicate other conditions such as infections or stimulant overdose. The presence of mydriasis in this context supports the diagnosis of opioid withdrawal.

Question 29: Correct Answer: C) Sudden changes in behavior or mood

Rationale: Sudden changes in behavior or mood are strong indicators of elder abuse, reflecting psychological trauma. Poor personal hygiene (A), weight loss due to malnutrition (B), and lack of mobility aids (D) could result from neglect but do not directly confirm abuse. Behavioral changes are more directly linked to the emotional and psychological effects of abuse, making it a more definitive sign when assessing elder patients for potential mistreatment.

Question 30: Correct Answer: B) Formulating a clear clinical question

Rationale: Formulating a clear clinical question is the foundational step in EBP, guiding the entire process. Without a well-defined question, subsequent steps like literature review and evaluation lack direction. Conducting a comprehensive literature review (A) comes after formulating the question. Evaluating current practices (C) and integrating patient preferences (D), while important, are subsequent steps that rely on having a clear question to address.

Question 31: Correct Answer: D) Impaired Tissue Integrity

Rationale: Prioritizing "Impaired Tissue Integrity" is crucial due to signs of potential wound infection (redness, swelling, fever). This diagnosis addresses both the physical state of the tissue and underlying issues contributing to pain and fever. While "Acute Pain" (Option A), "Hyperthermia" (Option B), and "Risk for Infection" (Option C) are important, focusing on tissue integrity directly impacts all these aspects by addressing the root cause of symptoms.

Question 32: Correct Answer: A) Playing soft classical music

Rationale: Soft classical music has been shown to have calming effects on patients with dementia by reducing agitation and promoting relaxation through auditory stimulation. Light gardening (B), while therapeutic during the day, may not be practical or safe in the evening when agitation peaks. Coloring books (C), though beneficial for some dementia patients, may not be effective during periods of agitation. Nature documentaries on television (D), although visually soothing, may not provide the same consistent calming effect as soft classical music (A).

Question 33: Correct Answer: A) Reduction in 30-day readmission rates

Rationale: Reduction in 30-day readmission rates is a direct and measurable indicator of effective discharge planning. B (Increase in follow-up appointment adherence), C (Improvement in self-care behavior scores), and D (Enhancement of quality of life measures) are important but less direct. Readmission rates are widely used to evaluate discharge protocols' effectiveness, supported by evidence-based practice guidelines.

Question 34: Correct Answer: A) Weight loss

Rationale: Weight loss is strongly supported by evidence for improving joint function and reducing pain in osteoarthritis patients, as it reduces the mechanical load on joints. Tai Chi (B), while beneficial for balance and flexibility, does not directly reduce joint load. Ultrasound therapy (C) has limited evidence supporting its efficacy. Massage therapy (D) provides temporary relief but lacks long-term benefits in joint function improvement.

Question 35: Correct Answer: B) Hypocalcemia

Rationale: Hypocalcemia often presents with muscle weakness, lethargy, and ECG changes such as a prolonged QT interval due to delayed repolarization. Hypermagnesemia (A), while causing muscle weakness, typically shows a shortened QT interval. Hypercalcemia (C) would present with shortened QT intervals and other symptoms like polyuria and polydipsia. Hyponatremia (D), though causing lethargy, does not typically affect the QT interval in this manner.

Question 36: Correct Answer: C) The need for immediate medical attention if experiencing unusual bleeding or bruising.

Rationale: Emphasizing the need for immediate medical attention if experiencing unusual bleeding or bruising addresses the most critical safety concern associated with anticoagulant therapy, ensuring prompt intervention in case of adverse effects. While monitoring blood tests (A), dietary considerations (B), and consistent medication timing (D) are important aspects of anticoagulant management, recognizing and responding to signs of serious complications takes precedence in patient education for safety reasons.

Question 37: Correct Answer: C) Monitoring vital signs

Rationale: Monitoring vital signs is within the scope of practice for an LPN and can be appropriately delegated by an RN. Administering IV push medications (A) and conducting initial patient assessments (B) require the advanced skills and judgment of an RN. Developing a comprehensive discharge plan (D) involves critical thinking and coordination with multiple disciplines, which is beyond the typical scope of practice for an LPN.

Question 38: Correct Answer: A) Holistic assessment

Rationale: Holistic assessment is paramount as it considers all aspects of a patient's well-being, including physical, emotional, social, and spiritual needs. Evidence-based practice (B), while crucial for interventions, does not inherently address psychosocial needs. Multidisciplinary collaboration (C) involves teamwork but depends on initial holistic assessments to identify needs. Time management (D), although important for efficiency, does not ensure comprehensive care planning.

Question 39: Correct Answer: B) Administer calcium gluconate intravenously

Rationale: Calcium gluconate stabilizes the cardiac membrane, reducing the risk of life-threatening arrhythmias associated with hyperkalemia. Sodium bicarbonate (A) and insulin with glucose (C) also treat hyperkalemia but do not act as quickly to stabilize the heart. Furosemide (D) helps excrete potassium but is not an immediate intervention for acute hyperkalemia. Calcium gluconate's rapid action on cardiac cells makes it the priority intervention.

Question 40: Correct Answer: A) Fresh Frozen Plasma (FFP)

Rationale: Fresh Frozen Plasma (FFP) is rich in clotting factors, making it the most appropriate choice for patients with clotting factor deficiencies, often seen in liver disease. Platelets are used primarily for thrombocytopenia, cryoprecipitate is used for specific deficiencies like fibrinogen, and PRBCs are used to treat anemia. Therefore, FFP addresses the specific need for multiple clotting factors which are deficient in liver disease.

Question 41: Correct Answer: B) Acute Pain

Rationale: Acute pain is prioritized as it directly impacts the patient's vital signs and overall recovery. While "Risk for Infection" (A) is important, addressing acute pain (B) can reduce stress responses that may compromise immune function. "Impaired Physical Mobility" (C) and "Ineffective Airway Clearance" (D) are also significant but less immediate compared to managing acute pain, which can exacerbate other complications if not promptly addressed.

Question 42: Correct Answer: C) Providing supplemental

oxygen to maintain SpO2 between 88-92%
Rationale: The primary goal in managing an acute COPD exacerbation is to ensure adequate oxygenation while avoiding hypercapnia. Option C is correct as maintaining SpO2 between 88-92% optimizes oxygen delivery without causing CO2 retention. Option A, while important, should follow stabilization. Option B is beneficial but not the first priority. Option D helps reduce inflammation but is secondary to ensuring proper oxygenation.
Question 43: Correct Answer: B) Reduce the dosage of pregabalin gradually.
Rationale: Gradually reducing pregabalin dosage helps manage side effects while maintaining some level of pain control. Immediate discontinuation (A) could cause withdrawal symptoms and worsen pain. Switching to duloxetine (C), although an alternative, should be considered after attempting dose adjustment since abrupt changes can disrupt treatment efficacy. Advising tolerance (D) without addressing significant side effects like dizziness and somnolence is not advisable; managing side effects ensures patient safety and adherence to treatment plans.
Question 44: Correct Answer: A) Risk for Infection
Rationale: Prioritizing "Risk for Infection" is essential due to Sarah's non-healing foot ulcer and consistently high blood glucose levels, which increase her susceptibility to infections. While "Impaired Skin Integrity" (Option C) is significant, managing infection risk takes precedence to prevent further complications. "Imbalanced Nutrition" (Option B) and "Ineffective Health Maintenance" (Option D) are relevant but secondary concerns that can be addressed after stabilizing the infection risk.
Question 45: Correct Answer: A) Peer-reviewed journal articles
Rationale: Peer-reviewed journal articles are the most reliable source for obtaining evidence-based guidelines as they undergo rigorous review by experts in the field, ensuring the validity and reliability of the information. Nursing textbooks, while informative, may not always contain the latest research. Online medical forums can provide anecdotal experiences but lack scientific rigor. Continuing education workshops are beneficial but may vary in quality and depth of content. Therefore, peer-reviewed journal articles are preferred for up-to-date and scientifically validated guidelines.
Question 46: Correct Answer: A) Providing written instructions and a demonstration
Rationale: Providing written instructions and a demonstration is the most effective method because it combines visual, auditory, and kinesthetic learning styles, which enhances understanding and retention. Verbal explanations (Option B) are less effective without visual aids. Video tutorials (Option C) are useful but lack the personal touch of direct interaction. Follow-up calls (Option D) are supportive but do not ensure initial comprehension. Research supports multimodal teaching strategies for better patient education outcomes.
Question 47: Correct Answer: B) Peripheral neuropathy
Rationale: Peripheral neuropathy should be primarily considered due to the tingling and numbness in her feet, which are classic symptoms. This condition is common in patients with long-standing diabetes due to nerve damage from chronic hyperglycemia. While diabetic retinopathy (A) could explain blurred vision, it does not account for tingling and numbness in the feet. Autonomic neuropathy (C) might explain dizziness but is less likely to cause peripheral symptoms alone. Diabetic nephropathy (D) affects kidney function and typically presents with different symptoms such as proteinuria rather than sensory disturbances.
Question 48: Correct Answer: B) Case studies demonstrating successful implementation of evidence-based practice
Rationale: Case studies provide practical examples of how evidence-based practice is applied in real-world scenarios, making the concept more relatable and understandable. Textbooks are comprehensive but may be too theoretical. Online forums encourage discussion but lack structured learning. Lecture notes summarize key principles but do not offer practical application examples like case studies do, making them less effective for hands-on learning.
Question 49: Correct Answer: B) Arranging for home health services to monitor her blood pressure and glucose levels.
Rationale: The most crucial consideration for Mrs. Thompson's home care plan is arranging for home health services to monitor her blood pressure and glucose levels. This is essential due to her age and chronic conditions, which put her at high risk for complications. While options A, C, and D are important, they do not address the immediate need for ongoing monitoring of her hypertension and diabetes, which can significantly impact her recovery and overall health.
Question 50: Correct Answer: B) Provide education sessions highlighting evidence supporting the new protocol.
Rationale: Education sessions help staff understand and appreciate the rationale behind changes, fostering acceptance and adherence based on informed decision-making. Mandating compliance (A) can lead to resistance without understanding. Allowing choices (C) undermines consistency in care quality, while gradual changes without training (D) risk improper implementation. Education aligns with research emphasizing informed practice change strategies.
Question 51: Correct Answer: B) Evaluate the applicability of the guideline to the specific patient population.
Rationale: Evaluating the applicability of guidelines ensures they are relevant and suitable for specific patient populations, accounting for unique characteristics and needs. Direct application (A) ignores individual differences, while relying solely on personal experience (C) may lack current evidence. Seeking administrative approval (D) is procedural but does not assess clinical relevance. This approach aligns with contemporary research emphasizing tailored care.
Question 52: Correct Answer: A) Evaluate her adherence to the prescribed diuretic regimen.
Rationale: Evaluating adherence to diuretics helps determine if non-compliance or drug interaction is causing weight gain and edema, common issues in polypharmacy. Reducing salt intake (B) is beneficial but secondary. Increasing ACE inhibitor dosage (C) without assessment can be dangerous due to renal implications. Scheduling an echocardiogram (D), while important, does not directly address immediate medication adherence concerns related to polypharmacy issues.
Question 53: Correct Answer: A) Ensuring strict blood glucose control and regular wound assessments
Rationale: Strict blood glucose control prevents infection and promotes healing in diabetic patients. Regular wound assessments help monitor progress and detect complications early. Option B can worsen glucose control. Option C may lead to other complications like pressure ulcers. Option D neglects the importance of frequent dressing changes for infection prevention and wound healing monitoring.
Question 54: Correct Answer: B) Consistent belittling or humiliation by a partner
Rationale: Emotional abuse often manifests as consistent belittling or humiliation by a partner, which can severely impact the victim's mental health. While frequent unexplained injuries (A) and isolation from friends and family (D) can be signs of physical and social abuse respectively, they are not specific to emotional abuse. Unexplained financial difficulties (C) could indicate financial abuse but do not directly point to emotional abuse. Emotional abuse uniquely involves psychological manipulation and degradation.
Question 55: Correct Answer: C) Educating Mr. Lee on

managing his conditions at home.
Rationale: Educating patients (Option C) empowers them to manage their health post-discharge, which is crucial for long-term outcomes and aligns with contemporary nursing practice focusing on patient education and self-management. While Options A, B, and D are important aspects of discharge planning, they do not prioritize patient education which is essential for effective self-care and preventing readmissions.
Question 56: Correct Answer: B) Acute Pancreatitis
Rationale: Acute pancreatitis presents with severe abdominal pain radiating to the back, nausea/vomiting, epigastric tenderness, and Cullen's sign (periumbilical bruising). Acute Cholecystitis (A) involves right upper quadrant pain rather than epigastric pain. Peptic Ulcer Disease (C) may cause epigastric pain but lacks Cullen's sign or radiating back pain. Appendicitis (D) typically presents with right lower quadrant pain instead of epigastric pain. Maria's symptoms align best with acute pancreatitis.
Question 57: Correct Answer: A) Electrocardiogram (ECG)
Rationale: An ECG is essential for diagnosing myocardial infarction as it shows changes in heart activity indicative of ischemia or infarction. Although a chest X-ray (B) can reveal other conditions like pulmonary edema, it does not diagnose myocardial infarction. An echocardiogram (C) assesses heart structure and function but is less specific for acute MI diagnosis compared to an ECG. Cardiac catheterization (D) provides detailed coronary artery images but is more invasive and typically follows initial ECG confirmation. Thus, an ECG is the prioritized diagnostic test.
Question 58: Correct Answer: B) Arterial blood gas (ABG) analysis
Rationale: ABG analysis is crucial in assessing the severity of respiratory compromise in COPD patients as it provides information on oxygenation, ventilation, and acid-base balance. While a chest X-ray (A) can show structural changes and PFTs (C) can evaluate lung function, they do not provide immediate information on gas exchange. A sputum culture (D) identifies pathogens but does not assess respiratory compromise severity.
Question 59: Correct Answer: C) Tdap (Tetanus, diphtheria, and pertussis)
Rationale: The Tdap vaccine is recommended for pregnant women during each pregnancy to protect both the mother and infant from pertussis. This vaccination provides passive immunity to the infant until they can receive their own vaccinations. MMR (A), Varicella (B), and HPV (D) vaccines are not recommended during pregnancy due to potential risks; MMR and Varicella are live vaccines contraindicated in pregnancy. The HPV vaccine is not indicated for pregnant women but can be administered before or after pregnancy.
Question 60: Correct Answer: A) High-protein diet with controlled carbohydrate intake.
Rationale: A high-protein diet supports tissue repair and wound healing, essential for Mrs. Garcia's recovery post-amputation. Controlled carbohydrate intake is crucial for managing diabetes and preventing hyperglycemia, which can impair healing. A low-fat diet (Option B), high-carbohydrate diet (Option C), or low-sodium diet (Option D) do not directly address the dual need for wound healing and blood glucose control effectively.
Question 61: Correct Answer: B) To demonstrate understanding and empathy
Rationale: Reflective listening aims to show that the nurse understands and empathizes with the patient's experience, fostering trust and openness. Offering solutions (A), gathering history (C), or redirecting to medical facts (D), while important in other contexts, do not fulfill the primary purpose of reflective listening in therapeutic communication. Hence, demonstrating understanding and empathy is crucial.
Question 62: Correct Answer: B) Verifying the patient's blood type and crossmatch
Rationale: Verifying the patient's blood type and crossmatch is crucial to prevent hemolytic transfusion reactions, which can be life-threatening. While checking vital signs (A), obtaining informed consent (C), and monitoring urine output (D) are important, they do not directly address compatibility issues. Ensuring correct matching of blood types minimizes risks of adverse reactions, making it a priority over other assessments.
Question 63: Correct Answer: B) Neuropsychological testing
Rationale: Neuropsychological testing provides a detailed evaluation of various cognitive functions and helps differentiate between depression-related cognitive impairment and early dementia by assessing specific patterns of deficits. The GDS screens for depression but does not assess cognitive function comprehensively. An EEG evaluates electrical activity in the brain but is not specific for distinguishing between these conditions. A brain MRI can identify structural changes but does not provide functional assessment necessary for differential diagnosis between depression-related impairment and dementia.
Question 64: Correct Answer: D) Risk for ineffective cerebral tissue perfusion related to hypertension
Rationale: The priority nursing diagnosis is "Risk for ineffective cerebral tissue perfusion" due to her significantly elevated blood pressure, which poses an immediate threat of decreased brain perfusion leading to potential stroke or other complications. While "Risk for stroke" (Option A), "Acute pain" (Option B), and "Impaired vision" (Option C) are relevant concerns, addressing cerebral tissue perfusion takes precedence as it directly impacts her overall neurological status and urgent care needs.
Question 65: Correct Answer: B) Encourage each team member to present evidence-based practices supporting their opinion.
Rationale: Encouraging evidence-based discussions ensures that decisions are grounded in research and best practices, fostering informed collaboration. Voting (A) may not consider all perspectives equally, deferring to one member (C) undermines collaborative decision-making, and trial periods (D) could delay effective pain management. Therefore, option B is correct as it promotes comprehensive evaluation of all suggestions through interdisciplinary collaboration.
Question 66: Correct Answer: B) History of bipolar disorder
Rationale: Bipolar disorder is associated with a significantly higher risk of suicide compared to other psychiatric conditions. Patients with bipolar disorder experience extreme mood swings that can lead to impulsive behavior during depressive or manic episodes. While anxiety disorders, psychotic episodes, and personality disorders also increase suicide risk, the episodic nature and severity of mood changes in bipolar disorder present a more acute risk. Anxiety may contribute to chronic stress; psychotic episodes can involve harmful delusions; personality disorders often involve maladaptive coping strategies, but none match the acute fluctuation risks seen in bipolar disorder.
Question 67: Correct Answer: A) One-on-one education sessions
Rationale: One-on-one education sessions are most beneficial as they allow for personalized interaction, addressing specific patient concerns and tailoring information to individual needs. Group classes and interactive digital modules offer valuable information but lack the personalization of one-on-one sessions. Printed materials can be useful for reference but may not engage patients as effectively or address unique questions immediately. Personalized education ensures better understanding and adherence to management plans.
Question 68: Correct Answer: B) Hand hygiene compliance
Rationale: Hand hygiene compliance is the most critical skill to prevent surgical site infections. It significantly reduces the transmission of pathogens. While sterile dressing changes (A), proper wound irrigation technique (C), and timely administration of antibiotics (D) are important, they are

secondary to hand hygiene. Sterile dressing changes and wound irrigation are specific to wound care, and timely antibiotics are preventative measures, but none are as universally effective as hand hygiene in preventing infection.

Question 69: Correct Answer: C) Obtain an electrocardiogram (ECG)

Rationale: An ECG is crucial for identifying cardiac causes of chest discomfort and shortness of breath, such as myocardial infarction or arrhythmias. While auscultating lung sounds (Option A), measuring oxygen saturation (Option B), and assessing jugular vein distention (Option D) provide valuable information, they do not directly diagnose cardiac events, which require immediate attention.

Question 70: Correct Answer: A) Blood Pressure

Rationale: Mr. Johnson's blood pressure of 180/110 mmHg is critically high and indicates a hypertensive crisis, which can lead to stroke or other severe complications if not promptly managed. While his heart rate (HR), respiratory rate (RR), and oxygen saturation (SpO2) are important, they are within acceptable ranges given his clinical presentation. Immediate intervention to lower his blood pressure is crucial to prevent further neurological damage.

Question 71: Correct Answer: D) Spiral CT angiography

Rationale: Spiral CT angiography is the most appropriate diagnostic test for confirming a pulmonary embolism due to its high sensitivity and specificity. Chest X-ray cannot visualize emboli directly, D-dimer assay is sensitive but not specific, and V/Q scan can be useful but less definitive than CT angiography. Therefore, spiral CT angiography provides the most conclusive evidence of pulmonary embolism.

Question 72: Correct Answer: C) Recommend setting up reminders on her smartphone.

Rationale: Setting up reminders on Ms. Garcia's smartphone leverages technology she likely uses daily, providing consistent prompts that can significantly improve adherence through automation and convenience. While A is important, it may not address forgetfulness directly. B helps organize pills but doesn't actively remind her when to take them. D involves support but may not be sustainable long-term or respect Ms. Garcia's independence as effectively as C does in promoting self-management with minimal disruption to daily routines.

Question 73: Correct Answer: B) Colonoscopy every 10 years

Rationale: Colonoscopy every 10 years is the gold standard for colorectal cancer screening in average-risk adults aged 50-75 due to its comprehensive visualization and ability to remove polyps. FIT (A) is effective but requires annual testing. Flexible sigmoidoscopy (C) examines only the lower colon and should be combined with FIT every 10 years. Double-contrast barium enema (D) is less commonly used due to lower sensitivity compared to colonoscopy.

Question 74: Correct Answer: B) Enroll him in a diabetes self-management education (DSME) program.

Rationale: Enrolling Mr. Lee in a DSME program provides comprehensive education tailored to his needs, involving interactive sessions that cover diet, exercise, monitoring blood glucose levels, and problem-solving skills critical for effective diabetes management. Option A gives useful information but lacks interactive engagement necessary for behavior change. Option C offers valuable resources but may not be as effective without interactive learning components. Option D ensures continuous care but does not provide immediate educational support essential for initial self-management adherence.

Question 75: Correct Answer: C) The legal scope of practice for each team member

Rationale: Ensuring that tasks are delegated within each team member's legal scope of practice is paramount to maintaining patient safety and adhering to professional standards. While educational background (A), workload distribution (B), and interpersonal relationships (D) are important considerations, they do not supersede legal constraints governing what each healthcare provider is permitted to do by law.

Question 76: Correct Answer: B) Encouraging small, incremental changes tailored to the patient's preferences

Rationale: Small, incremental changes are more sustainable and tailored approaches respect individual preferences, leading to better adherence. Option A may be overwhelming and difficult to sustain. Option C involves external support but may not be feasible for all patients. Option D focuses on negative reinforcement, which is less effective than positive encouragement.

Question 77: Correct Answer: B) Impaired Gas Exchange

Rationale: Prioritizing "Impaired Gas Exchange" is critical due to John's low SpO2 (85%) and increased respiratory rate (28 breaths/min), indicating inadequate oxygenation. "Ineffective Airway Clearance" (Option A) is important but secondary as the primary concern is impaired oxygenation. "Activity Intolerance" (Option C) and "Anxiety" (Option D) are relevant but less immediate priorities compared to ensuring adequate gas exchange. Addressing impaired gas exchange first stabilizes the patient's oxygen levels, which is crucial for overall management.

Question 78: Correct Answer: B) Hepatitis B vaccine

Rationale: Healthcare workers are at higher risk of exposure to bloodborne pathogens; thus, ensuring immunity against Hepatitis B is crucial to protect both themselves and their patients from potential transmission. While Hepatitis A can be significant, it is less commonly transmitted in healthcare settings compared to Hepatitis B. The Rabies and Typhoid vaccines are more relevant for specific exposures rather than routine hospital work environments. Therefore, maintaining up-to-date Hepatitis B vaccination status is essential for Ms. Lee's occupational safety and public health responsibilities.

Question 79: Correct Answer: D) Recent physical activity

Rationale: Recent physical activity (D) can significantly alter respiratory rate by increasing it due to heightened metabolic demands. This makes it challenging to assess the patient's baseline respiratory status accurately. While level of consciousness (A), use of supplemental oxygen (B), and patient position (C) are important considerations, they do not typically cause such immediate and pronounced changes in respiratory rate as recent physical exertion does. For an accurate assessment, ensure the patient has rested adequately before measuring their respiratory rate.

Question 80: Correct Answer: B) Gabapentin

Rationale: Gabapentin is specifically indicated for neuropathic pain, including diabetic peripheral neuropathy, due to its mechanism of action on calcium channels in nerve cells. Ibuprofen (A) and acetaminophen (C) are primarily used for nociceptive pain and have limited efficacy in treating neuropathic pain. Oxycodone (D), while effective for severe nociceptive pain, is not first-line therapy for neuropathic pain due to potential for addiction and side effects. Contemporary research supports gabapentin's role in modulating neurotransmitter release, making it the most appropriate choice.

Question 81: Correct Answer: D) Central venous pressure (CVP)

Rationale: CVP is the most reliable measure of extracellular fluid volume status as it directly reflects the blood volume in the central veins. Skin turgor can be affected by age and skin elasticity, blood pressure can fluctuate due to various factors, and serum sodium levels indicate osmolarity rather than volume status. Accurate assessment of CVP helps guide fluid management strategies.

Question 82: Correct Answer: C) Assessing pain using a standardized pain scale

Rationale: Assessing pain using a standardized pain scale is crucial for effective pain management as it provides an objective measure of the patient's pain level, guiding appropriate interventions. Administering analgesics on schedule (Option A) is important but must be based on accurate assessment. Educating patients (Option B) and encouraging early reporting (Option D) are supportive measures but secondary to proper assessment. Without accurate assessment, other interventions may be ineffective or inappropriate.

Question 83: Correct Answer: C) Implement bed rest with bathroom privileges.

Rationale: For patients with CHF exacerbation, bed rest with bathroom privileges is often recommended to reduce cardiac workload and prevent fatigue. Encouraging ambulation (Option A) or scheduling frequent physical therapy sessions (Option B) can exacerbate symptoms due to increased cardiac demand. Unrestricted activity (Option D) may lead to overexertion and further decompensation. Bed rest helps manage symptoms while allowing minimal necessary movement.

Question 84: Correct Answer: B) Shingrix

Rationale: Shingrix is specifically recommended for adults aged 50 years and older to prevent shingles. It provides strong protection against shingles and its complications. Hepatitis A (A), Meningococcal ACWY (C), and Rabies (D) vaccines are not specifically targeted at preventing shingles; they are used for different indications such as hepatitis prevention, meningitis prevention, and rabies exposure prophylaxis respectively. Shingrix's efficacy in older adults makes it a critical component of preventive healthcare in this age group.

Question 85: Correct Answer: A) Dullness to percussion over affected area

Rationale: Dullness to percussion over the affected area is indicative of pleural effusion, where fluid accumulates in the pleural space, replacing air-filled lung tissue. Hyperresonance (B) suggests pneumothorax or emphysema, conditions where air is trapped in the pleural space or alveoli. Increased tactile fremitus (C) indicates lung consolidation, as seen in pneumonia. Wheezing (D) is typically associated with airway obstruction or bronchospasm rather than fluid accumulation in the pleural space. Thus, dullness to percussion is the most specific sign of pleural effusion.

Question 86: Correct Answer: B) John's HbA1c level will be maintained below 7% over the next six months.

Rationale: The correct answer is B). HbA1c levels provide a long-term measure of blood glucose control and reflect overall management effectiveness. Option A) is subjective and less specific. Option C) focuses on immediate blood glucose levels but doesn't provide long-term assessment. Option D) relates to intervention adherence rather than outcome measurement.

Question 87: Correct Answer: A) Cardiovascular system

Rationale: The cardiovascular system should be prioritized because dizziness and fainting (syncope) are often associated with cardiovascular issues such as arrhythmias, orthostatic hypotension, or heart failure. The respiratory system (B) could cause dizziness through hypoxia but is less likely to cause fainting. The gastrointestinal system (C) may lead to dizziness through dehydration or electrolyte imbalance but is not directly linked to syncope. The musculoskeletal system (D) is unrelated to these symptoms. A thorough cardiovascular assessment can help identify potential causes like arrhythmias or blood pressure abnormalities.

Question 88: Correct Answer: B) Assess the patient's underlying causes of aggression.

Rationale: The correct answer is B) Assess the patient's underlying causes of aggression. Before applying restraints, it is crucial to identify and address any underlying issues that may be causing the aggressive behavior, such as pain, fear, or medication side effects. This approach aligns with contemporary research emphasizing patient-centered care and minimizing restraint use. Option A is incorrect because immediate application without assessment may violate patient rights and safety protocols. Option C involves obtaining a physician's order but should follow assessment. Option D is part of documentation but does not directly address managing aggression or restraint use.

Question 89: Correct Answer: B) Interactive workshops

Rationale: Interactive workshops are most effective because they engage patients actively, allowing for personalized education and immediate feedback. Lecture-based sessions (A) may not cater to individual needs, while written materials (C) might not address literacy issues. Multimedia presentations (D), although engaging, lack the personal interaction that workshops provide. Research supports interactive methods as they enhance understanding and retention, especially in diverse populations where customization is key.

Question 90: Correct Answer: B) Family medical history

Rationale: Family medical history is essential for identifying hereditary conditions as it provides insight into diseases that may run in the patient's family, allowing for early detection and preventive measures. Social habits (A), past surgical history (C), and immunization records (D) are important for overall health assessment but do not specifically highlight hereditary risks. Understanding familial patterns of illness can guide genetic counseling and inform risk stratification, making it a crucial element in comprehensive health history collection.

Question 91: Correct Answer: C) Assess for signs of deep vein thrombosis (DVT).

Rationale: Redness, warmth, and swelling in the calf are classic signs of DVT, which can lead to serious complications like PE. The priority is to assess for DVT to initiate appropriate treatment promptly. Applying warm compresses (Option A) can worsen inflammation if DVT is present. Elevating the leg and applying compression stockings (Option B) may be part of DVT management but should follow proper assessment. Increased fluid intake (Option D) is beneficial but not a priority in this context.

Question 92: Correct Answer: C) Encourage pursed-lip breathing.

Rationale: The ABG results indicate respiratory acidosis due to CO_2 retention from COPD exacerbation. Encouraging pursed-lip breathing helps improve ventilation and reduce CO_2 levels naturally without invasive measures. Increasing oxygen flow rate (A) could worsen CO_2 retention in COPD patients by diminishing their hypoxic drive to breathe. Preparing for intubation (B) is unnecessary unless there is severe respiratory distress or failure unresponsive to other treatments. Administering sodium bicarbonate (D) does not address the underlying issue of CO_2 retention and is not the first-line treatment for respiratory acidosis in COPD patients.

Question 93: Correct Answer: D) Physical Therapy

Rationale: Contemporary research highlights physical therapy as the most effective non-pharmacologic treatment for chronic lower back pain due to its focus on strengthening, flexibility, and functional movement. While acupuncture (A) and yoga (B) offer benefits in pain reduction and flexibility, they lack the comprehensive approach of physical therapy. CBT (C), though beneficial for managing pain perception and psychological aspects, does not directly address the physical components of lower back pain.

Question 94: Correct Answer: D) Performing continuous patient assessments

Rationale: Continuous patient assessments provide real-time data on the patient's condition, allowing for timely adjustments to the care plan. While reviewing patient satisfaction surveys (A), monitoring changes in clinical indicators (B), and conducting interdisciplinary team meetings (C) are valuable, they do not offer the same immediacy and detail as ongoing assessments. Continuous evaluation ensures that interventions remain relevant and effective, reflecting best practices in dynamic patient care.

Question 95: Correct Answer: A) Hyperkalemia

Rationale: Hyperkalemia is a frequent and severe complication in patients with CKD, leading to cardiac arrhythmias due to the heart's sensitivity to potassium levels. While hypocalcemia can also affect cardiac function, it is less directly related to arrhythmias compared to hyperkalemia. Hypernatremia and hypomagnesemia can cause neuromuscular and cardiovascular disturbances but are less common and less directly impactful in CKD. The primary focus on hyperkalemia stems from its direct effect on cardiac cell membrane potential, making it the most critical electrolyte imbalance to monitor in CKD.

Question 96: Correct Answer: D) Randomized controlled trials (RCTs)

Rationale: RCTs provide the most reliable data as they eliminate bias and allow for direct comparison between intervention and control groups, thus offering high-quality evidence on the program's effectiveness. Patient self-reports (Option A) can be subjective and prone to bias. Pre- and post-test assessments (Option B) are useful but do not control for external variables. Patient satisfaction surveys (Option C), while important, do not objectively measure clinical outcomes or educational impact. Therefore, RCTs are considered the gold standard in evaluating educational interventions.

Question 97: Correct Answer: C) Reduction in episodes of aggressive behavior with minimal restraint use.

Rationale: The correct answer is C) Reduction in episodes of aggressive behavior with minimal restraint use. This indicator reflects effective management strategies that minimize reliance on restraints while addressing behavioral issues, aligning with contemporary principles advocating for minimal restraint use. Option A focuses on fall prevention but does not assess overall behavioral management success. Option B concerns physiological stability but does not evaluate behavioral outcomes. Option D pertains to documentation frequency rather than effectiveness in managing behavior or reducing restraint reliance.

Question 98: Correct Answer: A) To reduce the incidence of bloodstream infections

Rationale: Chlorhexidine-impregnated dressings are primarily used to reduce the incidence of bloodstream infections by providing continuous antimicrobial activity at the catheter insertion site. While preventing local skin irritation (B), minimizing allergic reactions (C), and promoting faster healing (D) are beneficial, they are secondary objectives. The primary goal is to prevent bloodstream infections by reducing microbial colonization at the insertion site, which chlorhexidine effectively achieves through its broad-spectrum antimicrobial properties.

Question 99: Correct Answer: A) Identity vs. Role Confusion

Rationale: Adolescents aged 12-18 are in Erikson's "Identity vs. Role Confusion" stage, where they seek to establish their personal identity while grappling with social roles and expectations from peers and family members.

Question 100: Correct Answer: C) Sarah's ejection fraction will improve by 10% within three months.

Rationale: The correct answer is C) because it provides a specific, measurable, achievable, relevant, and time-bound (SMART) outcome. Ejection fraction directly measures cardiac output improvement. Option A) is subjective and not easily measurable. Option B) is measurable but does not directly assess cardiac output improvement. Option D) is an action plan rather than an outcome measure.

Question 101: Correct Answer: A) Ensuring strict blood glucose control

Rationale: Strict blood glucose control is essential for wound healing in diabetic patients because hyperglycemia impairs leukocyte function and collagen synthesis. While applying a hydrocolloid dressing (Option B), administering prophylactic antibiotics (Option C), and elevating the foot (Option D) are all beneficial, they do not address the underlying issue of poor glycemic control, which is critical for effective wound healing.

Question 102: Correct Answer: C) Montreal Cognitive Assessment (MoCA)

Rationale: The MoCA includes tasks such as drawing a clock and copying a cube that specifically assess visuospatial abilities. The MMSE has limited evaluation of visuospatial skills, while SLUMS focuses more broadly on different cognitive domains without specific emphasis on visuospatial abilities. The GDS is used for assessing depression and does not evaluate cognitive functions directly. Thus, MoCA stands out for its inclusion of visuospatial assessment components.

Question 103: Correct Answer: A) Decrease in HbA1c levels

Rationale: Decrease in HbA1c levels directly reflects improved glycemic control, a critical outcome for diabetic education. B (Increase in knowledge test scores), C (Reduction in hospital readmissions), and D (Improvement in dietary habits) are secondary indicators. HbA1c is a validated clinical measure that aligns with research linking educational interventions to long-term diabetes management.

Question 104: Correct Answer: B) Provide range-of-motion exercises every 2 hours.

Rationale: Providing range-of-motion exercises every 2 hours (Option B) helps prevent complications such as contractures and pressure ulcers, ensuring patient safety while using restraints. Checking restraint tightness every 4 hours (Option A) is insufficient; it should be done more frequently. Monitoring vital signs once per shift (Option C) is inadequate; they should be monitored more frequently in restrained patients. Allowing family members to adjust restraints (Option D) is unsafe and not recommended due to lack of proper training.

Question 105: Correct Answer: B) Improving patient safety

Rationale: Bedside shift reports primarily improve patient safety by ensuring accurate information transfer between nurses with the patient's involvement. While enhancing nurse accountability (A), increasing staff satisfaction (C), and promoting family involvement (D) are secondary benefits, they stem from the accurate communication that directly impacts patient safety. The presence of patients during these reports allows for immediate clarification of discrepancies and reinforces transparency in care delivery. This practice reduces errors and enhances trust between patients, families, and healthcare providers.

Question 106: Correct Answer: B) Advocate for Mr. Johnson's autonomy and support his decision to pursue palliative care.

Rationale: The principle of autonomy emphasizes respecting a patient's right to make decisions about their own care. While involving the ethics committee (Option C) is important, it does not directly address advocacy for Mr. Johnson's autonomy. Respecting the family's wishes (Option A) and following physician's orders (Option D) without considering Mr. Johnson's preferences undermine his autonomy and ethical principles in nursing practice.

Question 107: Correct Answer: C) Assessing renal function and adjusting dosage accordingly

Rationale: In patients with CKD, renal function significantly affects drug clearance. Adjusting the dosage based on renal function helps prevent toxicity. While weight (A), liver function (B), and drug-drug interactions (D) are important, they are secondary to renal function in this context. Weight adjustments primarily apply to drugs with narrow therapeutic indices, liver function is crucial for hepatically metabolized drugs, and drug-drug interactions are essential but not as immediate as renal considerations in CKD patients.

Question 108: Correct Answer: B) Implement pursed-lip breathing techniques.

Rationale: Pursed-lip breathing helps to keep the airways open longer, reducing the work of breathing and improving ventilation. Deep breathing exercises (A) are beneficial but may not be as effective in maintaining airway patency during ADLs. Increasing fluid intake (C) can help thin secretions but does not directly enhance respiratory function. Continuous supplemental oxygen (D) is crucial for some patients but does not address the technique for improving ventilation during activities.

Question 109: Correct Answer: C) Shared goals and vision

Rationale: Shared goals and vision (C) align the team's efforts towards a common objective, fostering unity and purpose. Clear role definitions (A) are important but secondary to having a unified direction. Equal participation in decision-making (B), while ideal, may not always be practical or necessary for every situation. Frequent informal interactions (D), though beneficial for rapport-building, do not replace the necessity of a cohesive strategy centered on shared objectives. Research indicates that teams with a shared vision are more likely to achieve better patient outcomes due to their coordinated efforts.

Question 110: Correct Answer: B) Teaching him one-handed dressing techniques using adaptive clothing

Rationale: Teaching one-handed dressing techniques using adaptive clothing (Option B) empowers Mr. Lee to dress himself despite hemiparesis, promoting independence and self-efficacy. Encouraging use of only the unaffected side (Option A) might limit functionality and adaptability in real-life scenarios. Dressing him completely (Option C) undermines his autonomy and slows rehabilitation progress. Velcro fasteners (Option D), while helpful, do not address comprehensive dressing strategies as effectively as teaching adaptive techniques does. Thus, Option B provides the most holistic benefit for regaining independence in dressing.

Question 111: Correct Answer: B) Pressure-controlled ventilation

Rationale: Pressure-controlled ventilation is preferred for ARDS patients to prevent barotrauma and volutrauma by limiting peak airway pressures. Volume-controlled ventilation can risk high pressures, high-frequency oscillatory ventilation is less commonly used and more complex, and SIMV may not provide the consistent pressure control needed. Thus, pressure-controlled ventilation is optimal for lung protection in ARDS.

Question 112: Correct Answer: A) Mesenteric ischemia due to arterial embolism

Rationale: Postoperative patients with DVT history are at risk for arterial emboli, which can lead to mesenteric ischemia—a life-threatening condition characterized by severe abdominal pain and vomiting. Gastrointestinal perforation (B), acute pancreatitis (C), and small bowel obstruction (D) can present similarly but are less likely in this context given his DVT history and recent surgery. Mesenteric ischemia requires prompt diagnosis and intervention to prevent irreversible bowel damage.

Question 113: Correct Answer: D) Previous suicide attempt

Rationale: A previous suicide attempt is the strongest predictor of future suicide attempts and completion. While social isolation, family history of suicide, and substance abuse are significant risk factors, they do not carry as high a predictive value as a previous attempt. Social isolation can exacerbate feelings of hopelessness, family history can indicate genetic or learned behaviors, and substance abuse can impair judgment. However, a previous attempt directly indicates a higher level of intent and capability for self-harm.

Question 114: Correct Answer: A) Administer loop diuretics

Rationale: Loop diuretics (A) are effective in reducing potassium levels and managing fluid overload in heart failure patients. Potassium-sparing diuretics (B) would worsen hyperkalemia. Immediate dialysis (C) is generally reserved for severe, refractory cases or when other interventions fail. Encouraging high-potassium foods (D) would exacerbate hyperkalemia.

Question 115: Correct Answer: B) Restrict water intake

Rationale: The primary intervention for hyponatremia in a patient with chronic kidney disease is to restrict water intake to prevent further dilution of serum sodium. Administering hypertonic saline (A) can be risky and is typically reserved for severe cases. Isotonic saline (C) may not effectively correct hyponatremia in this context. Encouraging oral sodium intake (D) alone may not address the underlying issue of water retention.

Question 116: Correct Answer: B) Engaging in moderate-intensity aerobic physical activity for at least 150 minutes per week

Rationale: Engaging in moderate-intensity aerobic physical activity for at least 150 minutes per week is most effective in reducing cardiovascular risk. Physical activity helps lower blood pressure, improve lipid profiles, and enhance overall cardiovascular health. While reducing sodium intake (A), limiting alcohol consumption (C), and increasing dietary potassium (D) are beneficial, they do not provide as comprehensive a benefit as regular physical activity. Research supports that consistent exercise has the most profound impact on cardiovascular health compared to other single lifestyle modifications.

Question 117: Correct Answer: B) Hypokalemia

Rationale: Loop diuretics such as furosemide promote the excretion of potassium through the kidneys, leading to hypokalemia (low potassium levels). Hyperkalemia (high potassium levels), hypercalcemia (high calcium levels), and hyponatremia (low sodium levels) are less common with loop diuretics. Although hyponatremia can occur due to fluid loss, hypokalemia remains the most prevalent electrolyte disturbance associated with loop diuretic therapy.

Question 118: Correct Answer: D) Utilizing telehealth for continuous monitoring

Rationale: Telehealth allows for continuous and real-time monitoring of patients, which helps in early detection of complications and ensures timely interventions. While community-based exercise programs (A), individualized dietary plans (B), and health education seminars (C) are beneficial, they do not provide the same level of continuous oversight and immediate response as telehealth. Telehealth's ability to integrate various aspects of care, including remote consultations, monitoring, and follow-ups, makes it the most effective strategy for managing chronic diseases.

Question 119: Correct Answer: B) Utilizing a comprehensive medication review (CMR)

Rationale: A comprehensive medication review (CMR) is the most effective strategy as it involves an in-depth evaluation of all medications a patient is taking, including prescription, over-the-counter, and supplements. This process helps identify potential drug interactions, duplications, and unnecessary medications. Option A is less frequent and might miss interim changes. Option C can lead to errors due to lack of professional oversight. Option D might not address necessary medications and could lead to under-treatment.

Question 120: Correct Answer: B) Initiating intravenous heparin

Rationale: Intravenous heparin is the immediate treatment of choice for suspected PE to prevent further clot formation. Aspirin (A) is not sufficient for acute management. A chest X-ray (C) can help rule out other conditions but does not treat PE. Oral anticoagulants (D), such as warfarin, are typically started later after stabilization with heparin. Heparin provides rapid anticoagulation, reducing mortality in acute PE cases.

Question 121: Correct Answer: C) Mindfulness meditation

Rationale: Systematic reviews consistently highlight mindfulness meditation as an effective CAM therapy for managing chronic pain. It helps patients by promoting relaxation and altering pain perception through cognitive-behavioral mechanisms. Chiropractic care (A) can be effective but varies widely in outcomes. Herbal supplements (B), while beneficial, lack standardized dosing and comprehensive safety profiles. Homeopathy (D) has not demonstrated consistent efficacy in rigorous scientific studies. Thus, mindfulness meditation is the most reliable choice based on contemporary research.

Question 122: Correct Answer: A) "How often do you use your inhaler?"

Rationale: Understanding the frequency of inhaler use provides insight into how well Mr. Thompson manages his COPD symptoms and can indicate control levels or exacerbations. While B), C), and D) are relevant to environmental factors and medication adherence, they do not directly assess symptom management as effectively as A).

Question 123: Correct Answer: A) Barrel chest

Rationale: Barrel chest is a classic physical finding in COPD due to hyperinflation of the lungs. Clubbing of fingers (Option B) is more associated with chronic hypoxia from conditions like lung cancer or interstitial lung disease. Pitting edema (Option C) may occur in right heart failure secondary to COPD but is not specific to COPD itself. Splenomegaly (Option D) is unrelated to COPD and typically indicates hematologic or infectious processes.

Question 124: Correct Answer: B) Placing the arm above heart level

Rationale: Placing the arm above heart level can cause a falsely low blood pressure reading because gravity assists in pulling blood downwards, reducing the pressure in the arteries. Using a cuff that is too small (Option A) would actually result in a falsely high reading due to increased resistance. Deflating the cuff too slowly (Option C) can lead to venous congestion, falsely elevating readings. Measuring after exercise (Option D) typically results in higher readings due to increased cardiac output and vascular resistance.

Question 125: Correct Answer: C) ST-Elevation Myocardial Infarction (STEMI)

Rationale: The presence of ST-segment elevation in specific ECG leads (II, III, and aVF) along with symptoms like acute chest pain and diaphoresis strongly indicates STEMI. Stable angina (A) typically does not present with such severe symptoms or ECG changes. NSTEMI (B) would show elevated cardiac enzymes without ST elevation. Unstable angina (D) involves worsening chest pain but lacks the characteristic ECG findings of STEMI.

Made in the USA
Monee, IL
13 September 2026

63042954R00070